Video Atlas of Intraoperative Applications of Near Infrared Fluorescence Imaging

Essa M. Aleassa • Kevin M. El-Hayek
Editors

Video Atlas of Intraoperative Applications of Near Infrared Fluorescence Imaging

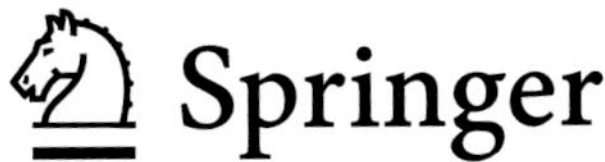

Springer

Editors
Essa M. Aleassa
Department of General Surgery,
Digestive Disease and Surgery Institute
Cleveland Clinic Foundation
Cleveland, OH
USA

Kevin M. El-Hayek
Division of General Surgery
Division of Surgical Oncology
MetroHealth System
Cleveland, OH
USA

ISBN 978-3-030-38094-6   ISBN 978-3-030-38092-2   (eBook)
https://doi.org/10.1007/978-3-030-38092-2

This Springer imprint is published by the registered company Springer Nature Switzerland AG
The registered company address is: Gewerbestrasse 11, 6330 Cham, Switzerland

Preface

In the not-too-distant past, the mark of an excellent physician was one who could diagnose and treat patients simply with a thorough history and physical exam. In many circles, the use of advanced imaging to aid in diagnosing diseases was considered a compromise to the art of medicine. Despite these early sentiments, the ability to visualize patient anatomy and pathology has continued to advance with improved imaging technology. In the majority of clinical scenarios, preoperative imaging helps surgeons plan the surgical approach and course of action.

While the concept of preoperative imaging is established, the trend to incorporate real-time intraoperative image guidance has also emerged. This concept originated with the desire to improve one's ability to accurately target pathology and to have objective information throughout the changing environment in the operating room. Two well-established examples of real-time imaging are fluoroscopy and ultrasonography. These modalities have been used to help orthopedic surgeons orient fractured bone and hepatobiliary surgeons locate lesions within the liver, respectively. Always seeking to further optimize surgical outcomes, additional modalities have been explored with varying levels of success. Near-infrared (NIR) imaging is one such tool that may further augment surgeons' skills in the operating room and thus outcomes.

In this dynamic textbook, we have compiled the first comprehensive video atlas of NIR imaging in the operating room. The work represents a head-to-toe guide for clinicians who are interested in applying real-time NIR imaging for their patients. Expert surgeons from around the globe were called upon to share their experience with NIR imaging, most commonly performed using indocyanine green (ICG) fluorescence. The chapters are structured to include a brief background and indications for use, followed by a technical description of the procedure. Each chapter is also accompanied by video examples and detailed information about necessary equipment, drug dosing, and alternative techniques. A pitfalls section serves as a "lessons learned" segment to bookend each chapter.

Authors represent a comprehensive list of surgical subspecialties ranging from neurosurgery to plastic surgery. While it is not meant to serve as an exhaustive summary of ICG use in surgery, the goal is to highlight the successful use of this technology in a number of settings. As the technology and applications continue to expand, we believe that this textbook will serve as a foundation upon which to build as clinicians gain more understanding of NIR imaging.

A work of this magnitude is not possible without the dedication of the authors to their patients and to expanding knowledge within the surgical community. We have relied on authors who have established themselves as pioneers in innovation, and we are grateful for their tireless work. In any large undertaking, there also needs to be a sturdy "glue" to hold things together. For this work, that glue is Development Editor for Springer Nature, Barbara Lopez-Lucio. Her ability to coordinate submissions and keep the project on task throughout the entire process cannot be understated. Thank you, Barbara.

Cleveland, OH, USA   Essa M. Aleassa, MD
Cleveland, OH, USA   Kevin M. El-Hayek, MD

Contents

Part VII   Applications in Urology

Part VIII   Applications in Breast Surgery

Part IX   Applications in Plastic Surgery

Part X   Other Applications

Contributors

Mahmoud Abu Gazala, MD Colorectal Department, Cleveland Clinic Florida, Weston, FL, USA

Essa M. Aleassa, MD Department of General Surgery, Digestive Disease and Surgery Institute, Cleveland Clinic Foundation, Cleveland, OH, USA
Department of Surgery, College of Medicine and Health Sciences, United Arab Emirates University, Al Ain, UAE

Rene Aleman, MD Bariatric and Metabolic Institute, Cleveland Clinic Florida, Weston, FL, USA

M. Al-Taher, MD Department of Surgery, Maastricht University Medical Center, Maastricht, The Netherlands

Michael J. Annunziata, BSc Case Western Reserve University School of Medicine, Cleveland, OH, USA

Takeshi Aoki, MD, PhD Division of Gastroenterological and General Surgery, Department of Surgery, Showa University, Tokyo, Japan

Annamaria Auricchio, MD Division of Surgical Oncology of the Gastrointestinal Tract, University of Campania "Luigi Vanvitelli", Naples, Italy

Nicoletta Basile, MD Division of Surgical Oncology of the Gastrointestinal Tract, University of Campania "Luigi Vanvitelli", Naples, Italy

Eren Berber, MD Department of General Surgery and Endocrine Surgery, Cleveland Clinic, Cleveland, OH, USA

Michael Bouvet, MD Department of Surgery, University of California San Diego, La Jolla, CA, USA

N. D. Bouvy, MD, PhD Department of Surgery, Maastricht University Medical Center, Maastricht, The Netherlands

Cagri Cakmakoglu, MD, FEBOPRAS Department of Plastic Surgery, Cleveland Clinic, Cleveland, OH, USA

Francesca Cardella, MD Division of Surgical Oncology of the Gastrointestinal Tract, University of Campania "Luigi Vanvitelli", Naples, Italy

Paolo Castellano, MD Division of Surgical Oncology of the Gastrointestinal Tract, University of Campania "Luigi Vanvitelli", Naples, Italy

Manish Chand, MBBS, BSc, FRCS, FASCRS, MBA, PhD Department of Surgery and Interventional Sciences, University College London Hospitals NHS Trust & GENIE Centre, University College London, London, UK

Jonathan C. DeLong, MD Department of Surgery, University of California San Diego, La Jolla, CA, USA

Juliana de Paula Machado Henrique, MD Department of General Surgery, The Bariatric and Metabolic Institute, Cleveland Clinic Florida, Weston, FL, USA

Giovanni Del Sorbo, MD Division of Surgical Oncology of the Gastrointestinal Tract, University of Campania "Luigi Vanvitelli", Naples, Italy

Fernando Dip, MD, FACS Hospital de Clinicas Jose de San Martin, Buenos Aires, Argentina

Risal S. Djohan, MD Department of Plastic Surgery, Dermatology and Plastic Surgery Institute, Cleveland Clinic, Cleveland, OH, USA
Department of Plastic Surgery, Cleveland Clinic, Cleveland, OH, USA

Kevin M. El-Hayek, MD Division of General Surgery, Division of Surgical Oncology, MetroHealth System, Cleveland, OH, USA
Case Western Reserve University School of Medicine, Cleveland, OH, USA

Silvia Erario, MD Division of Surgical Oncology of the Gastrointestinal Tract, University of Campania "Luigi Vanvitelli", Naples, Italy

Vahe Fahradyan, MD Department of Plastic Surgery, Dermatology and Plastic Surgery Institute, Cleveland Clinic, Cleveland, OH, USA

Gennaro Galizia, MD Department of Translational Medical Sciences, Division of Surgical Oncology of the Gastrointestinal Tract, University of Campania 'Luigi Vanvitelli' – School of Medicine, Naples, Italy

Maria Luisa Gasparri, MD, PhD Department of Gynecology and Obstetrics, "Sapienza" University of Rome, Rome, Italy

A. Daniel Guerron, MD Department of Surgery, Division of Metabolic and Weight Loss Surgery, Duke University, Durham, NC, USA

Kiyoshi Hasegawa, MD, PhD Hepato-Biliary-Pancreatic Surgery Division, Department of Surgery, Graduate School of Medicine, The University of Tokyo, Tokyo, Japan

David A. Iannitti, MD Department of Hepatopancreaticobiliary Surgery, Carolinas Medical Center, Atrium Health, Charlotte, NC, USA

Takeaki Ishizawa, MD, PhD Hepato-Biliary-Pancreatic Surgery Division, Department of Surgery, Graduate School of Medicine, The University of Tokyo, Tokyo, Japan

Daisuke Ito, MD Hepato-Biliary-Pancreatic Surgery Division, Department of Surgery, Graduate School of Medicine, The University of Tokyo, Tokyo, Japan

Shiksha Joshi, MD Department of General Surgery, The Bariatric and Metabolic Institute, Cleveland Clinic Florida, Weston, FL, USA

Bora Kahramangil, MD Department of General Surgery, Cleveland Clinic Florida, Weston, FL, USA

Yoshikuni Kawaguchi, MD, PhD Hepato-Biliary-Pancreatic Surgery Division, Department of Surgery, Graduate School of Medicine, The University of Tokyo, Tokyo, Japan

Rebecca Knackstedt, MD, PhD Department of Plastic Surgery, Cleveland Clinic, Cleveland, OH, USA

B. Knapen, MD Department of Surgery, Maastricht University Medical Center, Maastricht, The Netherlands

Kosuke Kobayashi, MD Hepato-Biliary-Pancreatic Surgery Division, Department of Surgery, Graduate School of Medicine, The University of Tokyo, Tokyo, Japan

Tomotake Koizumi, MD, PhD Division of Gastroenterological and General Surgery, Department of Surgery, Showa University, Tokyo, Japan

Norihiro Kokudo, MD, PhD National Center for Global Health and Medicine (NCGM), Tokyo, Japan

Jordan Lam, MBBS Department of Neurosurgery, Keck School of Medicine of USC, Los Angeles, CA, USA

Eva Lieto, MD Division of Surgical Oncology of the Gastrointestinal Tract, University of Campania "Luigi Vanvitelli", Naples, Italy

Emanuele Lo Menzo, MD, PhD, FACS, FASMBS Department of General Surgery, The Bariatric and Metabolic Institute, Cleveland Clinic Florida, Weston, FL, USA

Andrea Mabilia, MD Division of Surgical Oncology of the Gastrointestinal Tract, University of Campania "Luigi Vanvitelli", Naples, Italy

Doaa A. Mansour, MD, FRCS, FACS Division of Gastroenterological and General Surgery, Department of Surgery, Showa University, Tokyo, Japan

John B. Martinie, MD Department of Hepatopancreaticobiliary Surgery, Carolinas Medical Center, Atrium Health, Charlotte, NC, USA

Marcin Matuszewski, MD, PhD Department of Urology, Medical University of Gdansk, Gdansk, Pomorskie, Poland

Derek Muehrcke, MD Department of Cardiothoracic Surgery, Flagler Hospital, Saint Augustine, FL, USA

Michael D. Mueller, MD Department of Obstetrics and Gynecology, University Hospital of Bern and University of Bern, Bern, Switzerland

Masahiko Murakami, MD, PhD Division of Gastroenterological and General Surgery, Department of Surgery, Showa University, Tokyo, Japan

Shinich Ohba, MD, PhD Department of Otolaryngology, Head and Neck Surgery, Juntendo University, Tokyo, Japan

Heidi Paine, MBChB, BSc Department of General Surgery, London Deanery, London, UK

Andrea Papadia, MD, PhD Department of Obstetrics and Gynecology, Ospedale Regionale di Lugano, Ente Ospedialiero Cantonale, Svizzera Italiana, Lugano, Switzerland

Karol Polom, MD, PhD Department of Oncological Surgery, Medical University of Gdansk, Gdansk, Pomorskie, Poland

Wojciech Polom, MD, PhD Department of Urology, Medical University of Gdansk, Gdansk, Pomorskie, Poland

Anda Petronela Radan, MD Department of Obstetrics and Gynecology, University Hospital of Bern and University of Bern, Bern, Switzerland

Shivani Rangwala, MD Department of Neurosurgery, Keck School of Medicine of USC, Los Angeles, CA, USA

Raul J. Rosenthal, MD, FACS, FASMBS Department of General Surgery, The Bariatric and Metabolic Institute, Cleveland Clinic Florida, Weston, FL, USA

Jonathan Russin, MD Department of Neurosurgery, Keck School of Medicine of USC, Los Angeles, CA, USA

Kiyoshi Saito, MD, PhD Department of Neurosurgery, Fukushima Medical University, Fukushima, Japan

Jun Sakuma, MD, PhD Department of Neurosurgery, Fukushima Medical University, Fukushima, Japan

Takashi Sakurai, MD Department of Breast Surgery, JCHO Saitama Medical Center, Saitama, Japan

Patrick N. Salibi, MD Department of Hepatopancreaticobiliary Surgery, Carolinas Medical Center, Atrium Health, Charlotte, NC, USA

Taku Sato, MD, PhD Department of Neurosurgery, Fukushima Medical University, Fukushima, Japan

Graham S. Schwarz, MD, FACS Department of Plastic Surgery, Dermatology and Plastic Surgery Institute, Cleveland Clinic, Cleveland, OH, USA
Department of Plastic Surgery, Cleveland Clinic, Cleveland, OH, USA

Hirohito Seki, MD, PhD Department of Breast Surgery, JCHO Saitama Medical Center, Saitama, Japan

Yasuo Sekine, MD, PhD Department of Thoracic Surgery, Tokyo Women's Medical University Yachiyo Medical Center, Yachiyo, Chiba, Japan

Ken Shimizu, MD Department of Pathology, JCHO Saitama Medical Center, Saitama, Japan

Saman Sizdahkhani, MD Department of Neurosurgery, Keck School of Medicine of USC, Los Angeles, CA, USA

L. P. S. Stassen, MD, PhD Department of Surgery, Maastricht University Medical Center, Maastricht, The Netherlands

Jesse K. Sulzer, MD, PhD Department of Hepatopancreaticobiliary Surgery, Carolinas Medical Center, Atrium Health, Charlotte, NC, USA

Kyouichi Suzuki, MD, PhD Department of Neurosurgery, Japanese Red Cross Fukushima Hospital, Fukushima, Japan

Samuel Szomstein, MD, FACS, FASMBS Department of General Surgery, The Bariatric and Metabolic Institute, Cleveland Clinic Florida, Weston, FL, USA

Masahiro Takada, MD, PhD Department of Breast Surgery, Kyoto University Hospital, Kyoto, Japan

Nobuyuki Takemura, MD, PhD Hepat-Biliary Pancreatic Surgery Division, Department of Surgery, National Center for Global Health and Medicine, Tokyo, Japan

Masakazu Toi, MD, PhD Department of Breast Surgery, Kyoto University Hospital, Kyoto, Japan

Voranaddha Vacharathit, MD Department of General Surgery, Digestive Disease and Surgery Institute, Cleveland Clinic, Cleveland, OH, USA

J. van den Bos, MD Department of Surgery, Maastricht University Medical Center, Maastricht, The Netherlands

Junjie Wang, MBBS, MRCOG Department of Gynaecological Oncology, KK Women's & Children's Hospital, Singapore, Singapore

Leonard K. Welsh, MD Department of Surgery, Division of Metabolic and Weight Loss Surgery, Duke University, Durham, NC, USA

Steven D. Wexner, MD, PhD(Hon) Department of Colorectal Surgery, Digestive Disease Center, Cleveland Clinic Florida, Weston, FL, USA

Thomas Y. Xia, BS, BA School of Medicine, Case Western Reserve University, Cleveland, OH, USA

Junkichi Yokoyama, MD, PhD Department of Otolaryngology, Head and Neck Surgery, Kyorin University, Mitaka, Tokyo, Japan

Department of Otolaryngology, Head and Neck Surgery, Edogawa Hospital, Tokyo, Japan

Jin S. Yoo, MD Department of Surgery, Division of Metabolic and Weight Loss Surgery, Duke University, Durham, NC, USA

Jarmila Anna Zdanowicz, MD Department of Obstetrics and Gynecology, University Hospital of Bern and University of Bern, Bern, Switzerland

Introduction to Near-Infrared Fluoroscopy in the Operating Room

1

Voranaddha Vacharathit, Essa M. Aleassa, and Kevin M. El-Hayek

First characterized in 1800 by William Herschel, infrared radiation (IR) is an electromagnetic radiation with wavelengths beyond visible red light, in the 700 nm–1 mm range. Fluorescence imaging in the near-infrared (NIR) window utilizes photoexcitation of a molecule (fluorophore) with subsequent measurement of the emitted photon at a lower wavelength, in this case in the 650–900 nm NIR range. The first application of NIR in surgery was much later, in 1948, when fluorescein was used to aid in brain tumor resection [1]. Since then, the field has continued to evolve at a steady pace. Advantages and limitations of this imaging modality in the operating room are summarized in Table 1.1. In brief—for a specialty that places great emphasis on visualizing structures of interest, be they pathological or innate— NIR provides real-time surgical guidance with nonionizing radiation, high signal-to-background ratio, and the advantage of subsurface imaging to a certain extent [2]. However, applying this technology in the operating room requires some understanding of its limitations. Most of these limitations and difficulties are linked to non-standardized protocols, which may lead to suboptimal visualization of the desired structure. For instance, the optimal concentration of the fluorophore may be different for visualization of structures in the obese patient or for viewing different kinds of structures (i.e., vascular vs biliary). Correction for these may not be intuitive, or as simple as increasing the fluorophore concentration, for example, as this may paradoxically result in self-quenching and decreased fluorescence signal [3]. Overall, it is clear that working toward a standardized protocol in the OR will aid in a uniform and reproducible application of NIR technology.

NIR imaging requires three factors: (1) a source of photoexcitation (i.e., laser diode excitation), that stimulates a (2) fluorophore. The fluorophore emits NIR wavelength light that is captured by a (3) camera with a collection of optics and filtration sensitive to NIR in that particular wavelength to distinguish it from the background signal or the fluorescence of other fluorophores that may be used simultaneously. We

V. Vacharathit
Department of General Surgery, Digestive Disease and Surgery Institute, Cleveland Clinic, Cleveland, OH, USA

E. M. Aleassa (✉)
Department of General Surgery, Digestive Disease and Surgery Institute, Cleveland Clinic Foundation, Cleveland, OH, USA

Department of Surgery, College of Medicine and Health Sciences, United Arab Emirates University, Al Ain, UAE

K. M. El-Hayek
Division of General Surgery, Division of Surgical Oncology, MetroHealth System, Cleveland, OH, USA

Case Western Reserve University School of Medicine, Cleveland, OH, USA

© Springer Nature Switzerland AG 2020
E. M. Aleassa, K. M. El-Hayek (eds.), *Video Atlas of Intraoperative Applications of Near Infrared Fluorescence Imaging*, https://doi.org/10.1007/978-3-030-38092-2_1

Table 1.1 Advantages of near-infrared fluorescence imaging in the operating room

Advantages	Limitations
Low background autofluorescence, scattering, low absorption leading to high SBR	5–10 mm depth (attenuated by absorption and scatter in surrounding tissue)
Can be used with many surgical modalities (open, laparoscopic, robotic, microscopic)	Most systems use qualitative rather than quantitative information unless with specific measurements of tissue absorption, scatter, and anisotropy
Many targets (nerves, lymph, blood vessels, cancer cells, ureter, bile ducts) with potential for targeting down to molecular level	Imaging optimized differently for different fluorophores and targets (distance to target, timing, dose, fluorophore, patient BMI—many variables to consider)
Can visualized some depth below surface	Can have false-positive appearance from overcorrection of attenuation
Nonionizing radiation	Lack of many FDA-approved targeting agents
No staining of surgical field	Quenching
Real-time guidance system	Non-standardized imaging platform

SBR signal-to-background ratio, *BMI* body mass index, *FDA* US Food and Drug Administration

will limit our discussion of these three elements to the fluorophore itself, as this is the only element directly handled by the clinician.

Fluorophores

There is currently only one fluorophore approved by the US Food and Drug Administration (FDA): indocyanine green (ICG). It is a tricarbocyanine, water-soluble compound that contains both hydrophilic and hydrophobic elements with an excitation wavelength of 778 nm and emission wavelength of 830 nm, although the exact wavelengths may change based on the concentration and solvent properties [4, 5]. In vivo, ICG forms a complex with human lipoprotein and albumin with a short half-life of 150–180 seconds and is subsequently cleared by the liver [6]. Importantly, ICG is a nonspecific contrast dye. Therefore, although ICG tends to accumulate in solid tumors—thought to be due to vascular permeability and other molecular factors related to the tumor microenvironment called the enhanced permeability and retention (EPR) effect first described in 1986—there is no actual molecular targeting of this dye to tumor-specific ligands [7]. Risk of adverse events is low and seems to be related to non-immunogenic anaphylactoid reactions. The maximum recommended dosage of ICG in adults is 2 mg/kg [8]. Patients with iodine allergies should be excluded or pretreated.

Methylene blue (MB) is a photoactive phenothiazine dye initially used as an antimalarial drug at the end of the nineteenth century. The FDA approved MB for other indications, as it has been found to have fluorescent properties with emission in the 700 nm range when diluted [9]. This is at a much lower concentration that would otherwise be used for a conventional sentinel lymph node biopsy, where the blue stain can be visualized with the naked eye. Because it is excreted via the kidneys, MB is an optimal dye for the visualization of ureters. Potential adverse effects of high-dose MB, though rare, include local skin toxicities, cardiac arrhythmias, decreased cardiac output, increased pulmonary vascular resistance, and neurotoxicity with concomitant use of serotonin reuptake inhibitors, serotonin and norepinephrine reuptake inhibitors, and monoamine oxidase inhibitors. MB should be avoided in patients with glucose-6-phosphate dehydrogenase (G6PD) deficiency, as it may cause hemolytic anemia.

A notable "pro-dye" is 5-aminolevulinic acid (5-ALA), a naturally occurring precursor molecule in the protoporphyrin IX (PpIX) biosynthesis pathway, the latter of which then forms heme B when bound to ferrous iron. 5-ALA was approved by the FDA in 2017 for image-guided neurosurgery in patients with suspected high-grade gliomas. However, it is not uniquely a fluorophore. Rather, its derivative, PpIX emits NIR fluorescence at 635 nm when activated by light in the 375–440 nm range. Exogenous delivery of 5-ALA allows for increased PpIX concentration, which in turn allows for NIR visualization of certain cancer types based on 5-ALA accumulation [10]. Although it is a non-specific pro-dye with no specific targeting component, at the tissue level, 5-ALA is actively transported into cells rather than through passive diffusion. Interestingly, 5-ALA can be orally administered and can cross the blood-brain barrier.

Other fluorophores are actively under study. Rather than dye accumulation in the target tissue by the passive effect of EPR, the newer generations of fluorophores are tethered to a specific targeting ligand that allows homing to the tissue of interest. Some examples of these homing molecules are trastuzumab antibody (targets HER2 receptor in breast cancers), XQ-2d DNA aptamer (targets pancreatic ductal adenocarcinoma cells), vascular endothelial growth factor antibody, folate receptor targeting, carbonic anhydrase IX antibody, and epidermal growth factor (EGF) (targets cancers that overexpress EGF receptors) [11, 12]. Another exciting development is the creation of "activatable" NIR probes where the dye, delivered in an "off" state, is evenly distributed in all tissues but only fluoresces when activated by specific conditions (for instance, probe-ligand internalization by tumor cells, which then results in activation of the fluorophore by pH-induced linker molecule cleavage) [13].

Applications

Representative current applications of NIR using MB, ICB, and 5-ALA are summarized in Table 1.2 with corresponding papers cited [8, 14–35]. Although studies quote different concentrations and dosages of fluorophores, mode of delivery, and timing to visualization, we present the most common protocols quoted in the literature and, if possible, protocols that have undergone optimization or are a product of an aggregate review. The details of these applications and video chapters are presented in the textbook for more detailed descriptions.

Table 1.2 Current intraoperative applications of near-infrared fluoroscopy using fluorophore [8, 14–35]

Structure	Fluorophore	Timing	Delivery	Applications
Arterial system	ICG 5 mg	1 min PI	Angiography after flap harvest	Free flap viability [14, 15]
Venous system	ICG 2.5 mg	1-10 min PI	Portal vein or intravenous	Hepatic perfusion for formal segmentectomy [16]
Lymphatic system	ICG 2-6 mg depending on BMI	3-15 min PI	Subareolar injection, peritumor injection	Breast cancer SLNB [17, 18]
	ICG 5 mg	15 min-3 hour PI	Subcutaneous peritumor	Skin cancer SLN mapping [19]
	ICG 0.5–1.5 mg	Immediately PI-12 hour	First web space foot or second webspace hand or interstitial injection	Lymphography, lymphaticovenular anastomosis (chronic lymphadema), reverse mapping [8, 20]
	ICG 2.5 mg	15-30 min PI	4 quadrant injections in target area of interest	Esophageal, bladder, prostate, colorectal, gastric, endometrial SLN mapping [21]
Digestive system	ICG 1.25 mg	Visible for 1–7 days	Peritumor injection	Endoscopic tumor marking [22]
	ICG 2 mg/kg	Immediately PI	Intravenous	Neoplasia within Barrett's esophagus [23]
	ICG 0.2 mg/kg-7.5 mg	Immediately after division of mesentery or anastomosis creation	Intravenous	Anastomotic perfusion for leak risk assessment [24]

(continued)

Table 1.2 (continued)

Structure	Fluorophore	Timing	Delivery	Applications
Endocrine system	MB 0.4 mg/kg	41 seconds PI	Intravenous	Parathyroid glands parathyroid adenomas, thyroid gland [25, 26]
Nervous system	5-ALA 20 kg/kg	3 hour post ingestion	Oral	Malignant glioma [27, 28]
Urinary system	MB 0.25 mg/kg	10–60 min PI	Intravenous	Ureters [29]
Hepatobiliary system	ICG 0.5 mg/kg	24 hour PI	Intravenous	HCC, colorectal liver metastases [30]
	ICG 0.5 mg/kg	72 hour PI	Intravenous	Peritoneal mets from HCC [31]
	ICG 2.5 mg	15-45 min PI	Intravenous or intrabiliary	Biliary anatomy [32]
	ICG 2.5 mg	3–5 min PI	Intravenous	Pancreatic neuroendocrine tumors, cystic neoplasms (defect in fluorescence) [33]
	MB 1 mg/kg	5-15 min PI	Intravenous	Solitary fibrous tumor [34]
	MB 1 mg/kg	Immediately PI-1 hour	Intravenous	Insulinoma[a] [35]

ICG indocyanine green, *MB* methylene blue, *5-ALA* 5-aminolevulinic acid, *HCC* hepatocellular carcinoma, *PI* post-injection
[a]animal study

Augmented Reality

A discussion of such a versatile imaging platform as NIR fluorescence imaging with its many potential surgical applications would not be complete without mentioning augmented or computer-assisted reality. As it is, image-guided NIR fluoroscopy can be used in open, laparoscopic, endoscopic, microscopic, and robotic operations, making it an extremely versatile real-time guidance system. The overlay of fluorescence on the white light surgical field by screen integration allows for "enhanced reality." However, this is only the first step. Along with other imaging modalities such as preoperative imaging (CT scans, MRI, ultrasound, PET scans), the goal is to create one cohesive and integrated patient-specific road map for surgery. In its best embodiment, this would allow a three-dimensional "virtual reality" system capable of overlapping multiple sources of information such as prior scans into the physical surgical field with integration of real-time data such as NIR fluoroscopy so as to provide intraoperative navigation. While the field is still in its infancy, promising steps have been taken by different institutions to explore this novel operative aid, mainly in the field of urologic surgery [36]. Further work and research are needed in this field to push surgical constraints beyond the limitations of the naked eye.

This textbook is the first resource to highlight clinical uses of NIR with accompanying video descriptions. This textbook serves as a general reference for physicians and health-care providers who are interested in the clinical use of this technology. It will certainly be an evolving field in medicine.

References

1. Moore GE, et al. The clinical use of fluorescein in neurosurgery; the localization of brain tumors. J Neurosurg. 1948;5(4):392–8.
2. Vahrmeijer AL, et al. Image-guided cancer surgery using near-infrared fluorescence. Nat Rev Clin Oncol. 2013;10(9):507–18.
3. Matsui A, et al. Real-time intraoperative near-infrared fluorescence identification of the extrahepatic bile ducts using clinically-available contrast agents. Surgery. 2010;148(1):87–95.

4. Yuan B, et al. Emission and absorption properties of indocyanine green in Intralipid solution. J Biomed Opt. 2004;9(3):497–503.
5. Gurfinkel M, et al. Pharmacokinetics of ICG and HPPH-car for the detection of normal and tumor tissue using fluorescence, near-infrared reflectance imaging: a case study. Photochem Photobiol. 2000;72:94–102.
6. Shimizu S, et al. New method for measuring ICG Rmax with a clearance meter. World J Surg. 1995;19:113–8.
7. Matsumura Y, Maeda H. A new concept for macromolecular therapeutics in cancer chemotherapy: mechanism of tumoritropic accumulation of proteins and the antitumor agent smancs. Cancer Res. 1986;46:6387–92.
8. Marshall MV, et al. Near-infrared fluorescence imaging in humans with indocyanine green: a review and update. Open Surg Oncol J. 2010;2(2):12–25.
9. Matsui A, et al. Real-time, near-infrared, fluorescence-guided identification of the ureters using methylene blue. Surgery. 2010;148(1):78–86.
10. Xiao Q, et al. Fluorescent contrast agents for tumor surgery. Exp Ther Med. 2018;16(3):1577–85.
11. Owens EA, et al. Tissue-specific near-infrared fluorescence imaging. Acc Chem Res. 2016;49(9):1731–40.
12. Pogue BW, et al. Perspective review of what is needed for molecular-specific fluorescence-guided surgery. J Biomed Opt. 2018;23(10):1–9.
13. Lee H, et al. A folate receptor-specific activatable probe for near-infrared fluorescence imaging of ovarian cancer. Chem Commun (Camb). 2014;50(56):7507–10.
14. Losken A, et al. Assessment of zonal perfusion using intraoperative angiography during abdominal flap breast reconstruction Plast Reconstr Surg. 2012;129(4):618e–24e.
15. Burnier P, et al. Indocyanine green applications in plastic surgery: a review of the literature. J Plast Reconstr Aesthet Surg. 2017;70(6):814–27.
16. Aoki T, et al. Image-guided liver mapping using fluorescence navigation system with indocyanine green for anatomical hepatic resection. World J Surg. 2008;32(8):1763–7.
17. Hirano, et al. A comparison of indocyanine green fluorescence imaging plus blue dye and blue dye alone for sentinel node navigation surgery in breast cancer patients. Ann Surg Oncol. 2012;19(13):4112–6.
18. Samorani D, et al. The use of indocyanine green to detect sentinel nodes in breast cancer: a prospective study. Eur J Surg Oncol. 2015;41(1):64–70.
19. Tsujino A, et al. Fluorescence navigation with indocyanine green for detecting sentinel nodes in extramammary Paget's disease and squamous cell carcinoma. J Dermatol. 2009;36(2):90–4.
20. Yamamoto T, et al. Indocyanine green-enhanced lymphography for upper extremity lymphedema: a novel severity staging system using dermal backflow patterns. Plast Reconstr Surg. 2011;128(4):941–7.
21. Manen V, et al. A practical guide for the use of indocyanine green and methylene blue in fluorescence-guided abdominal surgery. J Surg Oncol. 2018;118:283–300.
22. Watanabe M, et al. Intraoperative identification of colonic tumor sites using a near-infrared fluorescence endoscopic imaging system and indocyanine green. Dig Surg. 2017;34(6):495–501.
23. Ortiz-Fernandez-Sordo J et al. Evaluation of a novel infra-red endoscopy system in the assessment of early neoplasia in Barretts esophagus: pilot study from a single center. Dis Esophagus. 2018;31(3).
24. Van den Bos J, et al. Near-infrared fluorescence imaging for real-time intraoperative guidance in anastomotic colorectal surgery: a systematic review of literature. J Laparoendosc Adv Surg Tech A. 2018;28(2):157–67.
25. Van der Vorst JR, et al. Intraoperative near-infrared fluorescence imaging of parathyroid adenomas using low-dose methylene blue. Head Neck. 2014;36(6):853–8.
26. Hillary SL, et al. Use of methylene blue and near-infrared fluorescence in thyroid and parathyroid surgery. Langenbeck's Arch Surg. 2018;403(1):111–8.
27. Stummer W, et al. Fluorescence-guided surgery with 5-aminolevulinic acid for resection of malignant glioma: a randomised controlled multicentre phase III trial. Lancet Oncol. 2006;7(5):392–401.
28. Hadjipanayis CG, et al. What is the surgical benefit of utilizing 5-Aminolevulinic acid for fluorescence-guided surgery of malignant gliomas? Neurosurgery. 2015;77(5):663–73.
29. Verbeek FPR, et al. Intraoperative near-infrared fluorescence-guided identification of the ureters using low-dose methylene blue: a first-in-human experience. J Urol. 2013;190(2):574–9.
30. Nanaseko Y, et al. Fluorescence-guided surgery for liver tumors. J Surg Oncol. 2018;118:324–31.
31. Miyazaki, et al. Indocyanine green fluorescence-navigated laparoscopic metastasectomy for peritoneal metastasis of hepatocellular carcinoma: a case report. Surg Case Rep. 2018;4(1):130.
32. Vlek SL, et al. Biliary tract visualization using near-infrared imaging with indocyanine green during laparoscopic cholecystectomy: results of a systematic review. Surg Endosc. 2017;31(7):2731–42.
33. Shirata, et al. Usefulness of indocyanine green-fluorescence imaging for real-time visualization of pancreas neuroendocrine tumor and cystic neoplasm. J Surg Oncol. 2018;118(6):1012–20.
34. Van der Vorst JR, et al. Near-infrared fluorescence imaging of a solitary fibrous tumor of the pancreas using methylene blue. World J Gastrointest Surg. 2012;4(7):180–4.
35. Winer J, et al. Intraoperative localization of insulinoma and normal pancreas using invisible near-infrared fluorescent light. Ann Surg Oncol. 2010;17(4):1094–100.
36. van Oosterom MN, et al. Computer-assisted surgery: virtual- and augmented-reality displays for navigation during urological interventions. Curr Opin Urol. 2018;28(2):205–13.

Applications in Endocrine Surgery

Jonathan C. DeLong and Michael Bouvet

Background

Surgical excision is the only definitive treatment for primary hyperparathyroidism (PHPT), which is marked by benign adenomatous proliferation of one or more glands leading to excessive parathyroid hormone secretion and hypercalcemia. There are four parathyroid glands that are located in an upper and lower position adjacent to the thyroid gland. Successful surgical treatment is dependent on the localization and removal of all aberrant parathyroid glands which can be a challenge due to their variable location, particularly in the lower glands. In PHPT, the disease is typically limited to a single adenoma, but multiglandular lesions can be identified in 10–15% of patients [1, 2]. Preoperative ultrasound and nuclear scintigraphy (sestamibi) can assist with preoperative localization to help guide the surgeon, but the sensitivity for detection of parathyroid glands is variable and user dependent. Computed tomog-

raphy (CT), single-photon emission computed tomography (SPECT), and magnetic resonance imaging (MRI) protocols are also available for high-resolution axial imaging [3]. These preoperative localization techniques allow for efficient, focused dissections that may avoid the need for routine four-gland exploration, reducing the risk of bilateral recurrent laryngeal nerve injury.

Preoperative localization techniques are widely available and routinely performed. By contrast, intraoperative techniques for the detection of parathyroid glands are more limited. Intraoperative sestamibi scanning using a gamma probe has been attempted, but it is cumbersome and not widely accepted. Rather, the surgeon is dependent on classic techniques such as intraoperative parathyroid hormone (PTH) assays, and pathological frozen section to confirm all abnormal parathyroid glands are resected.

Indocyanine green (ICG) fluorescence angiography is a type of augmented reality technology that can be used intraoperatively to identify and confirm the location of parathyroid glands. The technique involves intravenous injection of the organic dye that emits a fluorescent signal when excited by near-infrared light. Due to the increased vascularity of endocrine glands relative to surrounding tissues, the parathyroid glands emit a strong fluorescent signal that can be identified by a specialized camera system and displayed visually on a monitor (see Fig. 2.1). Because near-infrared

Electronic Supplementary Material The online version of this chapter (https://doi.org/10.1007/978-3-030-38092-2_2) contains supplementary material, which is available to authorized users.

J. C. DeLong · M. Bouvet (✉)
Department of Surgery, University of California San Diego, La Jolla, CA, USA
e-mail: mbouvet@ucsd.edu

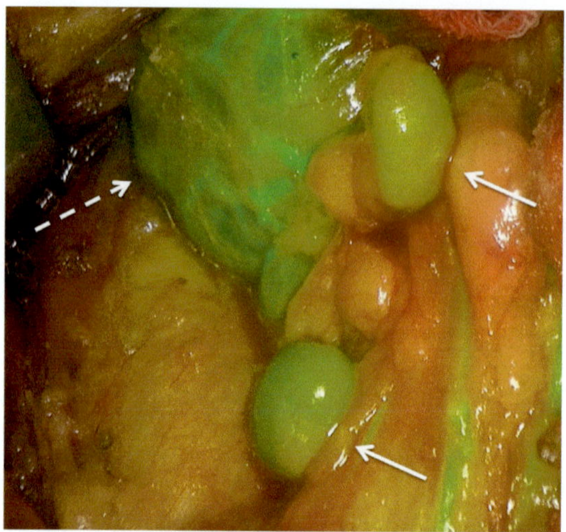

Fig. 2.1 ICG fluorescence angiography enhancing two parathyroid glands (solid arrows) and the thyroid gland (dashed arrow). The fluorescence signal detected from the imaging system is represented by a computer-generated green overlay. Enhancement is proportional to blood flow

fluorescence cannot be seen with the naked eye, a computer-generated bright green overlay is displayed on top of the standard image, creating a green glow where the strength and saturation of the green color correlate to the strength of the fluorescent signal detected by the imaging system [4]. The technique was first shown to be successful in the identification of parathyroid glands in a series of three dogs undergoing thyroid surgery in 2015 [5]. The use of ICG in humans, however, dates back much further as it was originally used as an agent to help assess hepatic function and cardiac output begining in the 1960s [6]. ICG has been established as a safe and inexpensive fluorophore for use in human surgery.

Indications

ICG fluorescence angiography can be used to assess perfusion of the parathyroid glands during parathyroid surgery. Because the technique is reliant upon blood supply, it will detect both normal and aberrant parathyroid glands so long as the blood supply is preserved. In the case where preoperative imaging indicates the location of the diseased gland, ICG fluorescence can confirm the location of an adenoma by its enhanced perfusion. If multiglandular disease is suspected, the technique can be used to help identify the four parathyroid glands during the neck exploration. This confirmatory technique may limit the amount of dissection necessary for the surgeon to confidently identify parathyroid tissue, which would preserve the vascularity for the normal parathyroid glands left in place. It may also reduce operative times.

Reoperation is an area where ICG fluorescence may be especially useful. Patients who undergo redo neck explorations for recurrent hyperparathyroidism have an increased risk of complication including recurrent laryngeal nerve injury, decreased cure rates, and permanent hypocalcemia due to devascularization of the parathyroid glands from excessive dissection [7]. Increased risk is inherent to redo surgery due to scar tissue from prior dissections and distortion or obliteration of surgical planes. Further, glands may be harder to find due to an increased risk of an ectopic location of the parathyroid glands in redo surgery. Using ICG fluorescence as an adjunct to preoperative imaging may improve the safety and success of repeat surgery [8].

Since ICG fluorescence angiography requires that the parathyroid glands be well perfused, successful identification of the gland with this technique also facilitates assessment of the perfusion of parathyroid glands during head and neck surgery. This may allow for the prediction and possible prevention of postoperative hypoparathyroidism and subsequent hypocalcemia. Assessment of parathyroid perfusion is also useful for decision-making during subtotal parathyroidectomy where three and a half glands are removed. ICG fluorescence angiography can be used to assess the perfusion of the gland and allow the surgeon to leave the half of the gland with the best perfusion behind. After splitting the gland in half, the surgeon can confirm adequate perfusion of the remnant parathyroid tissue. In a series of six patients where this technique was employed, all were found to have adequate remnant parathyroid perfusion, and none were found to have postoperative hypoparathyroidism [9]. In the event that a parathyroid gland is identified but the blood supply has been disrupted, ICG fluorescence angiography can also be used as criteria for autotransplantation, which has been used by some authors with favorable results [10].

Technical Description of the Procedure

Indocyanine Green Fluorescence

Indocyanine green (ICG) is an inert, non-toxic tricarbocyanine dye with a variety of uses in fluorescence-guided surgery (FGS) and an excellent safety profile. It has had applications for human use since the 1960s when researchers at the Mayo Clinic used the intravenous agent to assess cardiac output and hepatic function [11]. The dye preparation is stored in a powdered form and suspended in sterile water at a concentration of 2.5 mg ICG per ml by convention as the dye is typically packaged in 25 mg vials. During FGS, the anesthesiologist administers ICG dose intravenously when the surgeon is ready to evaluate the target. Upon injection, the negatively charged dye becomes tightly bound to plasma proteins, keeping it confined to the vascular compartment until it reaches the hepatocytes. ICG is excreted through first-pass metabolism as the hepatocytes clear the concentrated dye through the bile, which makes the technique useful for hepatobiliary surgery. The mean half-life of the circulating dye is 3.4 min (SD 0.7 min) and is dependent on normal functioning hepatocytes [12]. Dosage ranges from 2.5 mg to 10 mg per dosing with most authors reporting peak fluorescence 30 seconds to 3 min after administration.

Fluorescent particles emit fluorescent light when excited by light within a specific wavelength range. For particles that emit fluorescence in the visible range, like fluorescein, this is seen as a glow. ICG emits fluorescence in the near-infrared range, which is not visible to the naked eye, so we must use a specialized camera and computer-generated imaging to visualize the fluorescent signal. The excitation of ICG occurs at 780–805 nm and emits a fluorescent signal that can be captured by cameras that are specialized to capture light at

825 nm. Tissues are more translucent in the near-infrared range than in visible wavelengths, so ICG circulating within deep structures can be seen at a depth of up to several millimeters depending on hemaglobin concentration [13]. Fluorescent signal is converted to an augmented reality bright green overlay where the strength of the signal correlates to the saturation of the green color.

Equipment

There are numerous commercially available fluorescence laparoscopes on the market that are used for minimally invasive laparoscopic surgery. These cameras have a standard, or "bright light," mode as well as a fluorescent mode that is capable of detecting ICG fluorescence. Our institution has experience with Novadaq PINPOINT Endoscopic Fluorescence Imaging System (Bonita Springs, FL) and Stryker AIM (San Jose, CA). An additional system is available through Karl Storz (El Segundo, CA). The laparoscope is directed into the surgical field of interest and the parathyroid glands can be evaluated. More recently, a handheld imaging device has been developed for use in this application. The device is covered with a sterile drape and used for intraoperative evaluation of the parathyroid glands and can be used for other open FGS applications (see Fig. 2.2). In recent years, minimally invasive techniques for thyroid and parathyroid have emerged using robotic surgical platforms. Similar to the aforementioned laparoscopes, the da Vinci robotic surgical platform has Firefly, which is their version of fluorescence mode.

Adjustments and Configurations

The laparoscopic and handheld imaging systems allow for adjustments to a number of settings. Adjusting the brightness or backlight (Novadaq and Stryker terminologies, respectively) will adjust the amount of light in the standard image, while adjusting the contrast or gain will adjust the sensitivity or amplification of the fluorescent signal. Adjustments to these settings will allow

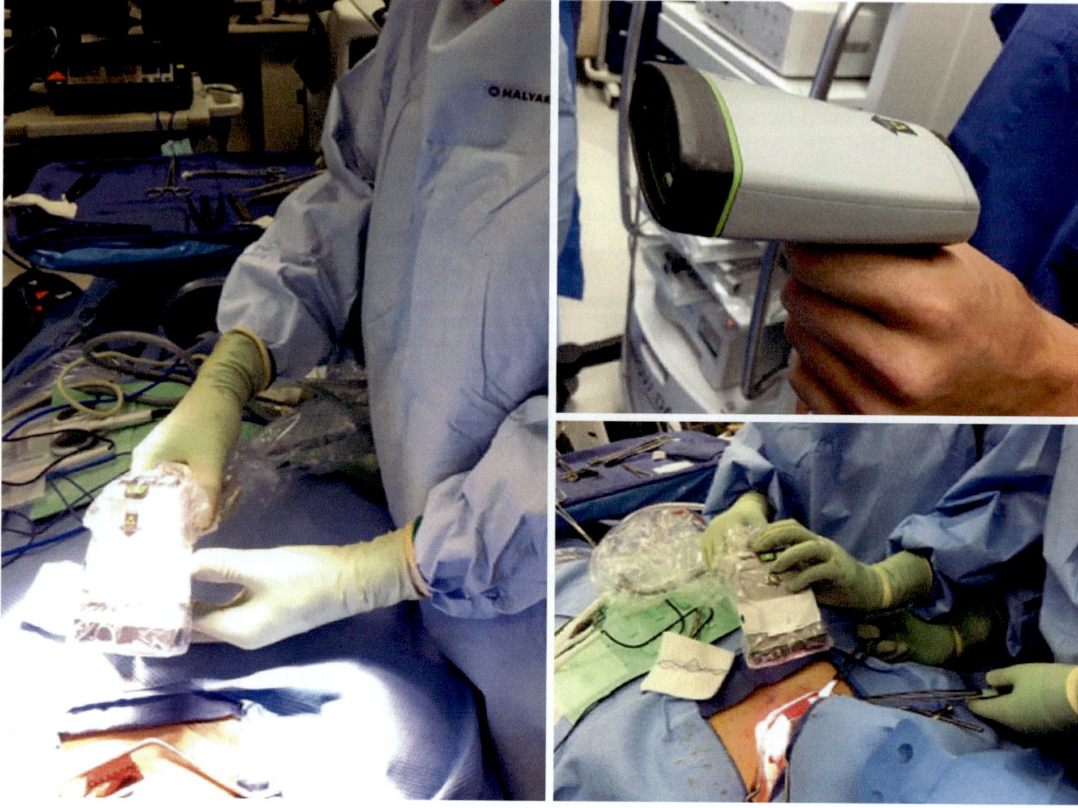

Fig. 2.2 Use of handheld ICG fluorescence imaging system directed at cervical neck incision for parathyroid surgery

the surgeon to optimize the target-to-background ratio which is a measure of the maximal fluorescence in the target tissue with the least amount of background noise. Adjustments to the dosing of ICG and the focal length (distance the camera is held from the target tissue) will also impact fluorescence intensity. We hold the camera approximately 20 cm from the target tissue. Depending on the device and filters that are used, some manufacturers recommend dimming the overhead and room lights which we recommend doing routinely for optimal results.

Surgical Procedure

Parathyroid glands are accessed through a standard, transverse surgical incision. We perform a focused unilateral neck dissection if preoperative imaging indicates laterality and post-excision PTH assay results are reassuring. If preoperative imaging does not indicate laterality or if PTH does not decrease as expected, a four-gland exploration is performed. We retract the strap muscles laterally and mobilize the thyroid gland for exposure. Care is taken to identify and preserve the recurrently laryngeal nerve. We continue the dissection until a candidate parathyroid gland is identified noting any abnormalities in size, shape, and texture. When a suspected parathyroid gland is identified and exposed, 3 mL of ICG (concentration 2.5 mg/mL) is administered as an intravenous push by the anesthesiologist, and the fluorescence imaging systems is directed into the operative field. In our experience, exposed parathyroid adenomas exhibit fluorescence within 1 minute of injection. If a parathyroid is not localized, further dissection is performed and ICG fluorescence imaging is repeated. Once a gland has been successfully localized with the technique, the vascular pedicle of the parathyroid is ligated, and a sample is sent to pathology for frozen section confirmation. A PTH assay is also routinely sent. See Video 2.1 for a video demonstration of the technique.

Other Techniques

There are a number of other techniques that have been used to localize parathyroid glands using fluorescence. The most popular involves autofluorescence of the parathyroid gland itself. Researchers at Vanderbilt hypothesized that parathyroid glands contain an unknown intrinsic fluorescent-emitting substance that can be detected with a fluorescence spectrometer [14]. A specific fluorophore has not yet been identified, but autofluorescence of the parathyroid glands has consistently been found in 90–98% of parathyroid glands, independent of perfusion [15, 16]. Parathyroid autofluorescence can be detected using a spectrometer or with a modified near-infrared camera system. Some authors have used the Fluobeam® 800 imaging system (Fluoptics, Grenoble, France), a commercially available system with reported success. The handheld device consists of a laptop with "Fluoptics©" software installed and a handheld camera with a near-infrared emitter (750 nm) and an integrated fluorescence detector (850–900 nm). Because this technique is not reliant upon an intravenous agent, it can successfully locate parathyroid glands even after the blood supply has been disrupted. This is because the technique relies on the intrinsic autofluorescent properties of the parathyroid gland itself rather than an exogenously delivered fluorophore. Since the parathyroid glands retain autofluorescence after devascularization, this technique cannot be used to assess viability of the glands or be used as a surrogate marker to predict postoperative hypocalcemia. However, unlike ICG angiography, the autofluorescence of the parathyroid glands is considerably brighter than the adjacent thyroid gland, improving the target-to-background ratio when this technique is used [17]. When compared to ICG fluorescence for the detection of parathyroid glands, there were simi-

lar parathyroid gland detection rates, but the autofluorescence technique was found to detect glands faster than the naked eye in up to half of the cases [15]. This indicates there may be a role for autofluorescence for navigation and localization of parathyroid glands rather than confirmation. But like ICG, the depth of penetration of the fluorescence signal is limited.

Robotic surgery is another technique where fluorescence angiography may be useful. Because the robotic platform lacks haptic feedback, adjunctive strategies for identifying targeted anatomy may be useful. Minimally invasive head and neck endocrine surgeries have emerged in recent years for the removal of thyroid glands [18]. When performed there the bilateral transaxillary approach, typically only the lower parathyroid glands are visualized with this technique. When ICG fluorescence was used during robotic thyroidectomy, some authors report improved rate of parathyroid identification and a reduced number of incidental parathyroidectomy [19]. Routine use of ICG fluorescence during robotic thyroid surgery may ameliorate the increased risk of transient hypocalcemia that has been reported with this approach [20].

Other techniques have been used for intraoperative localization of parathyroid glands including intravenous use of methylene blue. Like ICG, methylene blue emits fluorescence in the near-infrared range, but it is dosed only once at the beginning of the case. Success of the technique improved with increased dosing with identification of parathyroid glands in up to 97% of cases [21]. However, this technique was associated with cases of toxic metabolic encephalopathy because methylene blue acts as a monoamine oxidase inhibitor. Further, it has not shown to improve outcomes and was associated with cutaneous complications [22]. The use of aminolevulinic acid, an oral photosensitizer, has also been used for the intraoperative localization of parathyroid glands. However, this technique was only successful in identifying the parathyroid glands half of the time [23]. For the other half of patients, this technique inadequately enhanced the parenchyma of the parathyroid gland, limiting its clinical utility. Further, this technique requires oral administration of the photosensitizer prior to surgery and avoidance of light for up to 48 hours after surgery, making its routine use impractical.

Future Applications

In the future, ICG fluorescence techniques could be integrated with other available FGS technologies. A key application that would be of particular value is with fluorescent identification of the recurrent laryngeal nerve. Translational research is quickly evolving in the field of fluorescent nerve enhancement, and this technology may be available for use in the near future [24]. Additionally, integration with augmented reality platforms such as the Microsoft HoloLens may allow for the development of further applications in digital surgery.

Interpretation

All current commercially available FGS imaging systems provide qualitative data on fluorescence intensity in the form of color saturation of the computer-displayed image. As discussed previously, saturation can be manipulated by the surgeon through imaging system user controls, changes to the focal length between the camera and the target tissue, and by adjusting the dose of the ICG dye. Given these numerous components that make up the signal intensity that is captured by the device, there is no standard unit of fluorescence intensity that has been reproducibly described. Instead, surgeons rely on qualitative interpretation of the images obtained during surgery.

Some authors use a numerical scoring system to describe the strength of fluorescent enhancement that was first described by Fortuny et al. [25]. The numerical scale is used to describe the fluorescence perceived by the surgeon and can be used intraoperatively or postoperatively during analysis. On the scale, 0 denotes that little to no fluorescent intensity has been appreciated, 1 indicates that moderate fluorescence was seen, and a score of 2 denotes strong fluorescent intensity (see Fig. 2.3). If a candidate structure does not fluoresce when evaluated with ICG fluorescence angiography (score = 0), there are two likely explanations. First, it is possible that the structure may not be a parathyroid gland, but rather a lymph node or scar from prior surgery. The other

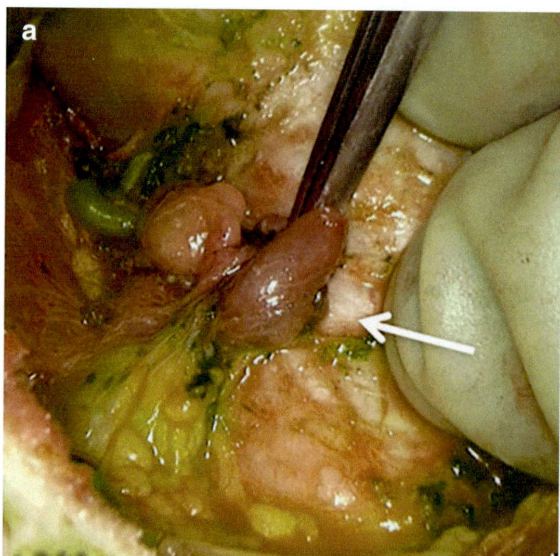
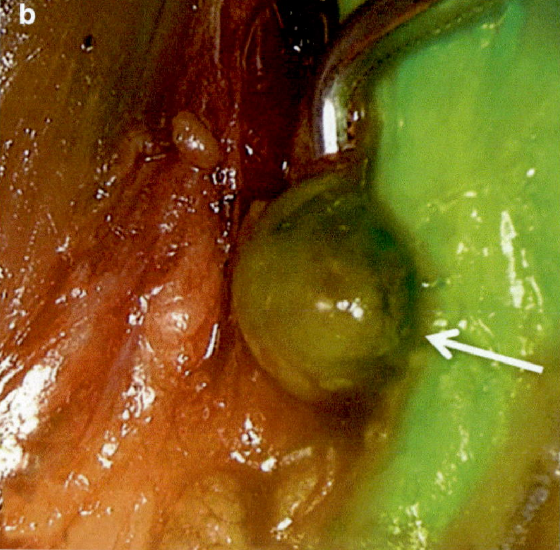

Fig. 2.3 A numerical scoring system was developed to describe the amount of fluorescent enhancement of the parathyroid glands where (**a**) 0 = no fluorescent enhancement, (**b**) 1 = moderate or partial gland enhancement, and (**c**) 2 = strong fluorescent enhancement

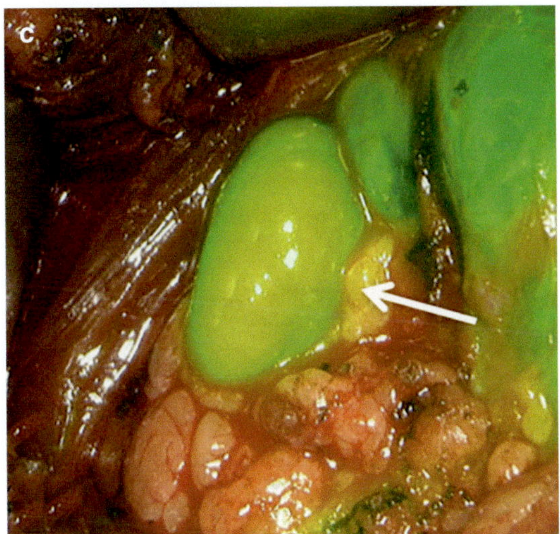

Fig. 2.3 (continued)

of the target tissue compared to the fluorescent enhancement of the surrounding tissues, or the "noise." Since ICG is administered intravenously and is not targeted to the parathyroid glands specifically, the utility of this technique for localizing parathyroid glands within or on the thyroid gland is limited because both structures will be illuminated. The target-to-background ratio limitation is less pronounced when using the parathyroid autofluorescence technique. While the thyroid gland does have some autofluorescent properties, authors report that parathyroid glands are up to three times brighter [15].

Another limitation of ICG fluorescence angiography is that it is reliant upon an intact vascular supply to the parathyroid tissue; however, as discussed, this also serves as one of the technique's strengths. If the surgeon dissects the parathyroid gland to the point that its major blood supply has been disrupted, the technique will not work. Conversely, the surgeon can evaluate and confirm adequate perfusion of an identified parathyroid gland at the end of a case. Further, the uptake of ICG is independent of gland histology, so this technique cannot be used to differentiate a parathyroid adenoma from normal parathyroid tissue. For this reason, ICG fluorescence angiography will not replace intraoperative rapid PTH assays or frozen sections to guide parathyroid resections for primary hyperparathyroidism.

The depth of penetration of the fluorescent signal has also been identified as a limitation. ICG can be detected through 2–3 millimeters of tissue, which makes it useful for guiding surgical navigation for indications like laparoscopic cholecystectomy [26]. However, during parathyroid surgery, we do not consistently identify parathyroid glands with ICG fluorescence until they are dissected and exposed. Increasing the depth of penetration or optimizing the display of the fluorescent signal would increase the utility of this technique by helping surgeons locate difficult to identify or aberrantly located glands.

ICG fluorescence is currently a qualitative technique and relies on the surgeon to interpret and assess the perfusion of the tissue. There are no consistent numbers or measures that can be used to quantify fluorescent intensity. The surgeon's

possibility is that the parathyroid gland may be completely dissected off the vascular pedicle, preventing the delivery of ICG necessary to enhance the parathyroid tissue. If this is suspected, frozen section can be used to confirm, and autotransplant can be considered. Similarly, if a parathyroid gland is found to have moderate or partial fluorescent intensity (score = 1), it may be partially devascularized. When a subtotal parathyroid resection is to be completed, the surgeon should attempt to remove the part of the parathyroid gland with the least amount of enhancement, leaving the well-vascularized tissue in place. The dosing of ICG can be safely repeated several times during a case, but since the ICG does not wash out completely between administrations, care should be taken to note the fluorescent intensity of target tissues before each additional dosing to help guide interpretations.

Limitations

There are a number of limitations to ICG fluorescence angiography for use in parathyroid surgery. The most glaring is the target-to-background ratio challenges given the close proximity of the thyroid gland. As discussed previously, the target-to-background ratio is the fluorescent enhancement assessment therefore is subjective and reliant upon past experience. And finally, ICG preparations contain sodium iodide, which prevents use in patients with iodine allergies. Despite this, ICG has an excellent safety profile as there have only been 17 adverse reactions reported in 34 years [27]. In those cases, all patients had an allergy to iodine and all patients had known renal insufficiency. Renal insufficiency alone, however, was not associated with adverse events. We recommend excluding all patients with iodine allergies from this technique.

ICG fluorescence angiography has the potential to assist surgeons in identifying parathyroid glands rapidly with minimal risk. It does not significantly add to case time, and the imaging systems are becoming widely available. With the high safety profile of the dye and wide availability of near-infrared fluorescence imaging systems, ICG should be considered as an adjunctive method for parathyroid gland localization during parathyroid surgery.

References

1. Ruda JM, Hollenbeak CS, Stack BC Jr. A systematic review of the diagnosis and treatment of primary hyperparathyroidism from 1995 to 2003. Otolaryngol Head Neck Surg. 2005;132(3):359–72.
2. Madkhali T, Alhefdhi A, Chen H, Elfenbein D. Primary hyperparathyroidism. Ulus Cerrahi Derg. 2016;32(1):58–66.
3. Warren Frunzac R, Richards M. Computed tomography and magnetic resonance imaging of the thyroid and parathyroid glands. Front Horm Res. 2016;45:16–23.
4. DeLong JC, Ward EP, Lwin TM, Brumund KT, Kelly KJ, Horgan S, et al. Indocyanine green fluorescence-guided parathyroidectomy for primary hyperparathyroidism. Surgery. 2018;163(2):388–92.
5. Suh YJ, Choi JY, Chai YJ, Kwon H, Woo JW, Kim SJ, et al. Indocyanine green as a near-infrared fluorescent agent for identifying parathyroid glands during thyroid surgery in dogs. Surg Endosc. 2015;29(9):2811–7.
6. van den Biesen PR, Jongsma FH, Tangelder GJ, Slaaf DW. Yield of fluorescence from indocyanine green in plasma and flowing blood. Ann Biomed Eng. 1995;23(4):475–81.
7. Simental A, Ferris RL. Reoperative parathyroidectomy. Otolaryngol Clin N Am. 2008;41(6):1269–74, xii.
8. Chakedis JM, Maser C, Brumund KT, Bouvet M. Indocyanine green fluorescence-guided redo parathyroidectomy. BMJ Case Rep. 2015;2015
9. Zaidi N, Bucak E, Okoh A, Yazici P, Yigitbas H, Berber E. The utility of indocyanine green near infrared fluorescent imaging in the identification of parathyroid glands during surgery for primary hyperparathyroidism. J Surg Oncol. 2016;113(7):771–4.
10. Jin H, Dong Q, He Z, Fan J, Liao K, Cui M. Application of a fluorescence imaging system with indocyanine green to protect the parathyroid gland Intraoperatively and to predict postoperative parathyroidism. Adv Ther. 2018;35(12):2167–75.
11. Fox IJ, Wood EH. Indocyanine green: physical and physiologic properties. Proc Staff Meet Mayo Clin. 1960;35:732–44.
12. Desmettre T, Devoisselle JM, Mordon S. Fluorescence properties and metabolic features of indocyanine green (ICG) as related to angiography. Surv Ophthalmol. 2000;45(1):15–27.
13. Gao Y, Li M, Song ZF, Cui L, Wang BR, Lou XD, et al. Mechanism of dynamic near-infrared fluorescence cholangiography of extrahepatic bile ducts and applications in detecting bile duct injuries using indocyanine green in animal models. J Huazhong Univ Sci Technolog Med Sci. 2017;37(1):44–50.
14. Paras C, Keller M, White L, Phay J, Mahadevan-Jansen A. Near-infrared autofluorescence for the detection of parathyroid glands. J Biomed Opt. 2011;16(6):067012.
15. DiMarco A, Chotalia R, Bloxham R, McIntyre C, Tolley N, Palazzo FF. Autofluorescence in parathyroidectomy: signal intensity correlates with serum calcium and parathyroid hormone but routine clinical use is not justified. World J Surg. 2019;43(6):1532–7.
16. Kahramangil B, Berber E. Comparison of indocyanine green fluorescence and parathyroid autofluorescence imaging in the identification of parathyroid glands during thyroidectomy. Gland Surg. 2017;6(6):644–8.
17. Ladurner R, Al Arabi N, Guendogar U, Hallfeldt K, Stepp H, Gallwas J. Near-infrared autofluorescence imaging to detect parathyroid glands in thyroid surgery. Ann R Coll Surg Engl. 2018;100(1):33–6.
18. Miyano G, Lobe TE, Wright SK. Bilateral transaxillary endoscopic total thyroidectomy. J Pediatr Surg. 2008;43(2):299–303.
19. Yu HW, Chung JW, Yi JW, Song RY, Lee JH, Kwon H, et al. Intraoperative localization of the parathyroid glands with indocyanine green and firefly(R) technology during BABA robotic thyroidectomy. Surg Endosc. 2017;31(7):3020–7.
20. Lee KE, Kim E, Koo do H, Choi JY, Kim KH, Youn YK. Robotic thyroidectomy by bilateral axillo-breast approach: review of 1,026 cases and surgical completeness. Surg Endosc. 2013;27(8):2955–62.
21. Tummers QR, Schepers A, Hamming JF, Kievit J, Frangioni JV, van de Velde CJ, et al. Intraoperative guidance in parathyroid surgery using near-infrared fluorescence imaging and low-dose methylene blue. Surgery. 2015;158(5):1323–30.

22. Lieberman ED, Thambi R, Pytynia KB. Methylene blue and parathyroid adenoma localization: three new cases of a rare cutaneous complication. Ear Nose Throat J. 2016;95(2):70–2.
23. Prosst RL, Weiss J, Hupp L, Willeke F, Post S. Fluorescence-guided minimally invasive parathyroidectomy: clinical experience with a novel intraoperative detection technique for parathyroid glands. World J Surg. 2010;34(9):2217–22.
24. Walsh EM, Cole D, Tipirneni KE, Bland KI, Udayakumar N, Kasten BB, et al. Fluorescence imaging of nerves during surgery. Ann Surg. 2019;270(1):69–76.
25. Vidal Fortuny J, Karenovics W, Triponez F, Sadowski SM. Intra-operative indocyanine green angiography of the parathyroid gland. World J Surg. 2016;40(10):2378–81.
26. DeLong JC, Hoffman RM, Bouvet M. Current status and future perspectives of fluorescence-guided surgery for cancer. Expert Rev Anticancer Ther. 2016;16(1):71–81.
27. Perry D, Bharara M, Armstrong DG, Mills J. Intraoperative fluorescence vascular angiography: during tibial bypass. J Diabetes Sci Technol. 2012;6(1):204–8.

3

Bora Kahramangil and Eren Berber

Indications

Adrenalectomy is the preferred treatment for adrenal tumors with hormonal activity, pressure symptoms, and/or concern for adrenocortical carcinoma, as well as adrenal metastases from certain malignant tumors. Historically, adrenalectomy was performed by making a laparotomy. Since the initial description of laparoscopic adrenalectomy [1], minimally invasive adrenalectomy has gained popularity and become the standard of care. Minimally invasive adrenalectomy is performed at different centers using laparoscopic [2] or robotic [3] techniques depending on central expertise.

Adrenal glands are located superior to the kidneys in the retroperitoneum, and their exposure can be challenging. A successful adrenalectomy depends on the correct identification of the gland itself, its vasculature, and the correct dissection plane. Laparoscopic ultrasound is an intraoperative adjunct, which can help locate the adrenal glands. Its use relies on achieving a good contact between the tissue and the probe and may require periodic interruptions of dissection to reemphasize tissue planes during the procedure [4].

Indocyanine green (ICG) near-infrared fluorescence imaging has recently become available for use in adrenalectomy [5]. Its main advantages are the ability to switch back and forth between fluoresced and non-fluoresced views without interrupting the procedure. Furthermore, ICG has long been used for other procedures and is safe with few adverse reactions [6]. Recent literature has suggested that ICG is more useful in tumors of adrenocortical tissue origin and when cortical-sparing adrenalectomy is attempted for a pheochromocytoma [7]. ICG fluorescence imaging systems are available for laparoscopic [8] as well as robotic platforms [9]. The following is the description of the use of ICG in robotic adrenalectomy.

Electronic Supplementary Material The online version of this chapter (https://doi.org/10.1007/978-3-030-38092-2_3) contains supplementary material, which is available to authorized users.

B. Kahramangil
Department of General Surgery, Cleveland Clinic Florida, Weston, FL, USA

E. Berber (✉)
Department of General Surgery and Endocrine Surgery, Cleveland Clinic, Cleveland, OH, USA
e-mail: berbere@ccf.org

Technical Description of the Procedure

We prefer a hybrid laparoscopic/robotic technique for our adrenalectomies, which we have previously described in detail (Video 3.1) [10]. We utilize both posterior retroperitoneal and lateral transabdominal approaches with similar technical principals depending on the suitability for the patient. Briefly, the initial access is gained laparoscopically, surgical field insufflated, and laparoscopic ultrasound performed to help locate the adrenal gland. Next, the da Vinci Si or Xi (Intuitive Surgical Inc., Sunnyvale, CA) robotic platform is docked and the adrenal dissection carried robotically. After the adrenal gland is freed from the surrounding retroperitoneal structures, the robot is undocked and the specimen is retrieved laparoscopically.

The use of ICG is not recommended during pregnancy and in patients with iodine allergy, history of anaphylactic reaction to another dye, chronic kidney disease, chronic liver disease [7]. In all other patients, ICG has become a routine part of our surgical technique. An ICG solution with a concentration of 2.5 mg/ml is prepared in the operating room by dissolving 25 mg of ICG (Akorn Inc., Lake Forrest, IL) in 10 ml of normal saline. Five milligrams (2 ml) of ICG is administered intravenously by the anesthesiologist after the exposure of the retroperitoneum. Although a single injection is typically adequate, additional doses of ICG may be administered in longer cases if found necessary by the surgeon. In our clinical practice, we use the robotic Firefly technology (Intuitive Surgical Inc., Sunnyvale, CA) to visualize ICG fluorescence. The PINPOINT system (Stryker Inc., Kalamazoo, MI) is available for laparoscopic adrenalectomy.

Interpretation

Knowledge of the ICG pharmacokinetics is essential to optimally benefit from ICG fluorescence [11]. Fluorescence can first be detected 20–30 seconds after the intravenous administration of ICG. Initially, a bright fluorescence is detected both in the adrenal gland and the surrounding retroperitoneum. Optimal contrast is achieved at 5 minutes post-injection, when the ICG clears from the retroperitoneum. From this point on the adrenal gland appears bright green on a background of dark, non-fluorescing retroperitoneum (Fig. 3.1). ICG fluorescence in the adrenal gland typically persists for about 20 minutes [9]. When the retroperitoneal fat is not abundant and the adrenal tumor is large, the adrenal fluorescence may become apparent even with the overlying retroperitoneum intact (Fig. 3.2). In most cases, however, the retroperitoneal has to be peeled off, and the intensity of the fluorescence increases as one gets closer to the adrenal gland. ICG becomes the most useful once dissecting the lateral borders of the adrenal gland from the surrounding retroperitoneum, where the surgeon can switch back and forth between the fluoresced and non-fluoresced views to stay in the correct dissection plane. With consistent use and increasing expertise, ICG can become a valuable intraoperative adjunct.

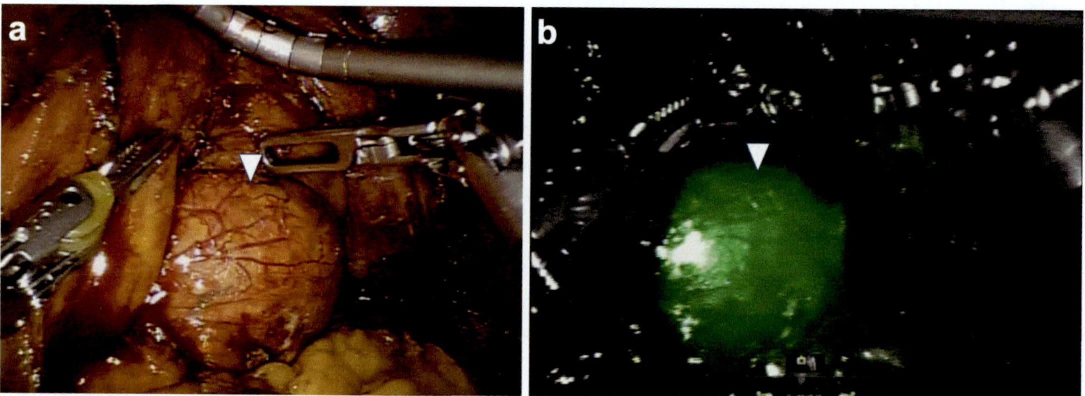

Fig. 3.1 An adrenocortical tumor (arrowhead) demonstrating bright indocyanine green (ICG) fluorescence. Non-fluoresced robotic (**a**) and ICG-fluoresced (**b**) views

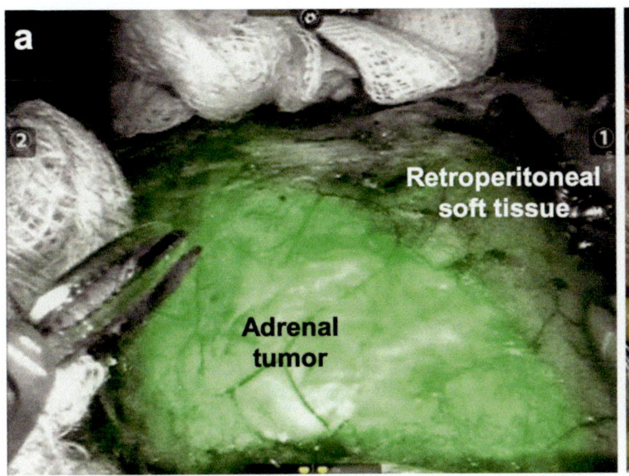

Fig. 3.2 A case where the indocyanine green (ICG) fluorescence delineated the border between the adrenal tumor and the normal retroperitoneal soft tissue even before the dissection of the overlying retroperitoneum. (**a**) ICG-fluoresced view and (**b**) non-fluoresced robotic view

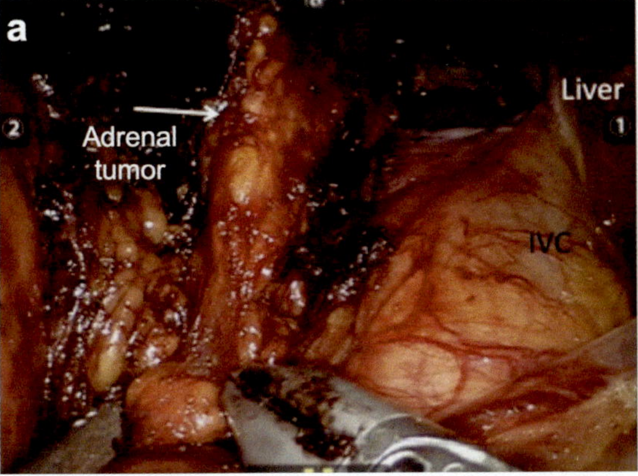

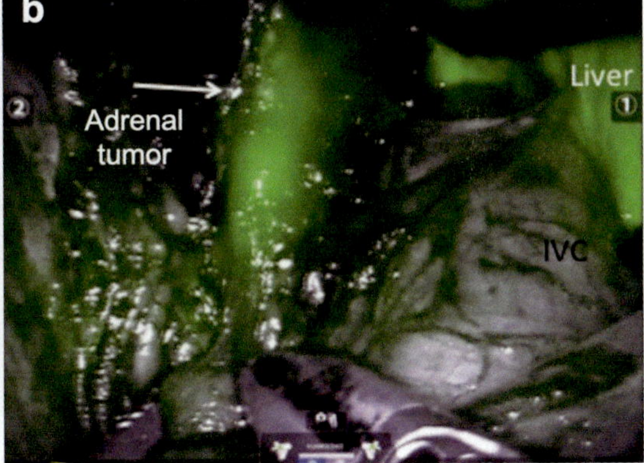

Fig. 3.3 Indocyanine green (ICG) fluorescence during the removal of a right-sided adrenal tumor. Non-fluoresced robotic (**a**) and ICG-fluoresced (**b**) views. A bright fluorescence with similar intensity to that of the adrenal can be detected from the liver. (IVC inferior vena cava)

Pitfalls

Despite its clinical utility, ICG fluorescence imaging has some shortcomings in adrenal surgery. Once ICG is administered intravenously, it binds to plasma proteins, trapping it in the intravascular space and allowing it to serve in an identical manner to a real-time angiography in organs with abundant blood supply. ICG is ultimately excreted by the liver [11, 12]. As a result, the liver is another organ with bright ICG fluorescence, which persists throughout the surgery (Fig. 3.3). This may limit the utility of the ICG in right-sided adrenal tumors where the background liver fluorescence may make the interpretation of the fluorescence patterns and the identification of correct dissection margins difficult. This limitation becomes even more pronounced in the posterior retroperitoneal approach to right-sided adrenal tumors due to the small surgical field and limited room for retraction.

It has been reported in the literature that the detection of fluorescence is more consistent from the adrenal cortex than from the medulla [7]. This is true for both the healthy adrenal cortex and the tumors originating from the adrenal cortex. The practical implication of this is that when attempting a unilateral adrenalectomy for a pheochromocytoma, ICG may not be very helpful due to an inability to detect a strong fluorescence from the tumor (Fig. 3.4). In the rare circumstance when a cortical-sparing adrenalectomy is attempted, however, the lack of fluorescence from the tumorous medulla may actually be useful in delineating it from the healthy cortex (Fig. 3.5). When dealing with bilateral pheochromocytomas or a new pheochromocytoma in a contralateral adrenalectomized patient, ICG may be a valuable addition to the surgical arma-ment. Similar to pheochromocytomas, when attempting an adrenalectomy for an adrenal metastasis, ICG may be of limited utility due to the lack of fluorescence.

Finally, the mapping of the adrenal vascular anatomy with ICG merits mentioning. The imaging modality does not allow for the visualization of the adrenal vein with ICG fluorescence, as the whole adrenal gland takes up the dye. Although the ICG uptake in the small adrenal arteries before the onset of dissection was more consistent, we do not see clinical utility in the identification of the adrenal vein.

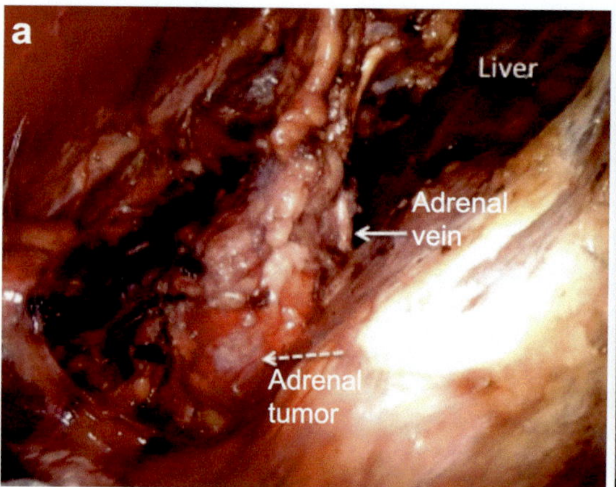

Fig. 3.4 A pheochromocytoma not demonstrating indocyanine green (ICG) fluorescence. Non-fluoresced robotic (**a**) and ICG-fluoresced (**b**) views. Even after the tumor was dissected off the surrounding retroperitoneal tissues, it did not demonstrate fluorescence, limiting its utility. In this case, strong fluorescence was noted in the liver and in the adrenal vein

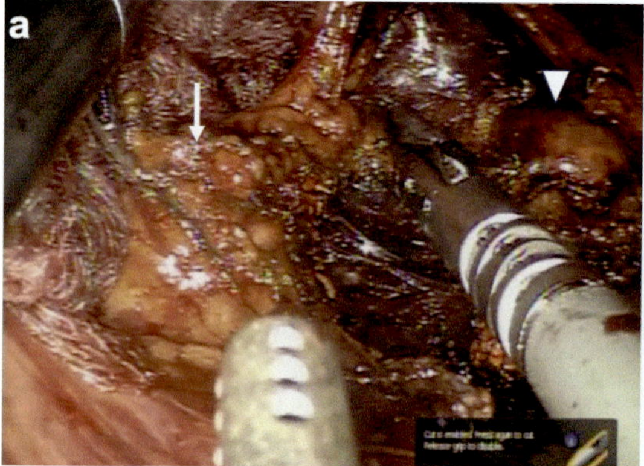
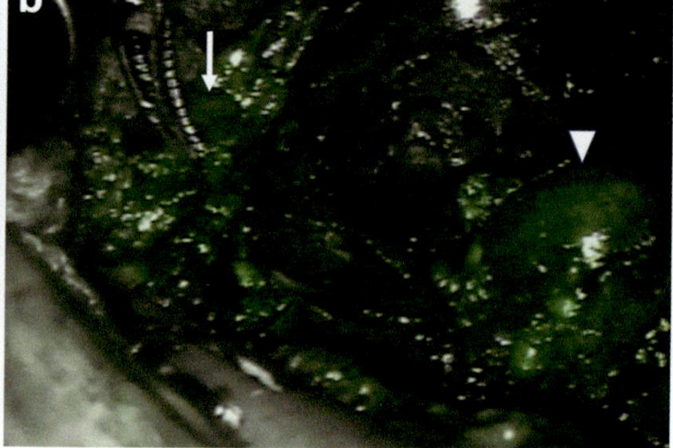

Fig. 3.5 The use of indocyanine green (ICG) fluorescence to confirm perfusion of the remnant cortex during cortical-sparing adrenalectomy. Non-fluoresced robotic (**a**) and ICG-fluoresced (**b**) views. Arrows point at the healthy adrenal cortical remnant and the arrowheads at the resected pheochromocytoma. In the fluoresced view, the adrenal cortex appears green indicating good perfusion

Literature Review

Since the initial description of laparoscopic adrenalectomy [1] and the subsequent description of robotic adrenalectomy [13, 14], minimally invasive surgery has become the standard of care in treating adrenal gland tumors. Regardless of the technique and platform used, a successful adrenalectomy depends on the correct identification of the adrenal gland within the retroperitoneal fat and division of the adrenal vein. There has been an increasing number of studies in the literature, which describe the use of ICG to identify vital structures. The following is a review of the literature on the use of ICG in human studies.

Manny et al. described the first clinical use of ICG for adrenalectomy in 2013 [5]. Using a 5-mg injection of intravenous ICG, authors could successfully conduct robotic partial adrenalectomy in three patients. Robotic Firefly technology was used for ICG fluorescence imaging. The conclusion from this study was that the use of ICG was safe and could facilitate partial adrenalectomy.

First robotic total adrenalectomy series using ICG to guide resection was reported by our group in 2015 [9]. In this pilot study of ten patients, ICG doses ranging from 7.5 to 18.8 mg were used. The time to achieve optimal fluorescence was 5 minutes, and the fluorescence persisted for up to 20 minutes. ICG fluorescence allowed superior border distinction in eight of the ten patients.

Also in 2015, DeLong et al. reported the use of ICG in four patients undergoing laparoscopic adrenalectomy [8]. Authors were able to successfully visualize the adrenal arteries and veins using ICG, as well as the border between the adrenal gland and the surrounding periglandular fat.

In a prospective study of 40 patients and 43 adrenalectomies, Colvin et al. studied the utility of ICG fluorescence imaging during robotic adrenalectomy [4]. In 46.5% of the patients, ICG resulted in superior border distinction than non-fluoresced view. Overall, ICG was found more useful in tumors of adrenocortical origin.

The optimal dose of ICG was 5 mg per injection. The injections could be repeated up to two to three times when deemed necessary by the operating surgeon.

Arora et al. evaluated the role of ICG in laparoscopic adrenalectomy in a retrospective review of 55 patients [15]. One case had to be converted to open due to an inability to achieve hemostasis. An average ICG dose of 14.4 mg was administered. ICG fluorescence was noted to persist for 15 minutes. There was no ICG-related complication.

Most recently in 2018, our group analyzed the utility of ICG in 100 patients undergoing robotic adrenalectomy and attempted to determine the patient population who would benefit most from the use of ICG [7]. Of the 100 adrenal tumors, 74 fluoresced upon ICG administration, whereas 26 did not. Overall, ICG fluorescence helped achieve a superior border distinction than the non-fluoresced robotic view in 41% of the cases. The biggest utility for ICG was found in patients with tumors of adrenocortical origin operated through a lateral transabdominal approach. The utility in pheochromocytomas was limited as the ICG uptake was inconsistent in these tumors. One specific use was in cortical-sparing adrenalectomy where the normal, fluorescing adrenal cortex could be distinguished from non-fluorescing pheochromocytoma. Of note, the utility of ICG was limited in right-sided adrenal tumors approached posterior retroperitoneally due to the bright ICG fluorescence of the liver.

Conclusion

ICG fluorescence imaging is a useful intraoperative adjunct for laparoscopic and robotic adrenalectomy. It has the highest utility in adrenocortical tumors and cortical-sparing adrenalectomy for pheochromocytoma. One should be cognizant of the possible hindrance from the background liver fluorescence in right-sided adrenal tumors, which may become more problematic in the posterior retroperitoneal approach due to the small working space.

References

1. Gagner M, Lacroix A, Bolte E. Laparoscopic adrenalectomy in Cushing's syndrome and pheochromocytoma. N Engl J Med. 1992;327(14):1033.
2. Chen Y, Scholten A, Chomsky-Higgins K, Nwaogu I, Gosnell JE, Seib C, et al. Risk factors associated with perioperative complications and prolonged length of stay after laparoscopic adrenalectomy. JAMA Surg. 2018;153(11):1036–41.
3. Kahramangil B, Berber E. Comparison of posterior retroperitoneal and transabdominal lateral approaches in robotic adrenalectomy: an analysis of 200 cases. Surg Endosc. 2018;32(4):1984–9.
4. Colvin J, Zaidi N, Berber E. The utility of indocyanine green fluorescence imaging during robotic adrenalectomy. J Surg Oncol. 2016;114(2):153–6.
5. Manny TB, Pompeo AS, Hemal AK. Robotic partial adrenalectomy using indocyanine green dye with near-infrared imaging: the initial clinical experience. Urology. 2013;82(3):738–42.
6. Hope-Ross M, Yannuzzi LA, Gragoudas ES, Guyer DR, Slakter JS, Sorenson JA, et al. Adverse reactions due to indocyanine green. Ophthalmology. 1994;101(3):529–33.
7. Kahramangil B, Kose E, Berber E. Characterization of fluorescence patterns exhibited by different adrenal tumors: determining the indications for indocyanine green use in adrenalectomy. Surgery. 2018;164(5):972–7.
8. DeLong JC, Chakedis JM, Hosseini A, Kelly KJ, Horgan S, Bouvet M. Indocyanine green (ICG) fluorescence-guided laparoscopic adrenalectomy. J Surg Oncol. 2015;112(6):650–3.
9. Sound S, Okoh AK, Bucak E, Yigitbas H, Dural C, Berber E. Intraoperative tumor localization and tissue distinction during robotic adrenalectomy using indocyanine green fluorescence imaging: a feasibility study. Surg Endosc. 2016;30(2):657–62.
10. Taskin HE, Berber E. Robotic adrenalectomy. Cancer J. 2013;19(2):162–6.
11. Kahramangil B, Berber E. The use of near-infrared fluorescence imaging in endocrine surgical procedures. J Surg Oncol. 2017;115(7):848–55.
12. Aoki T, Murakami M, Yasuda D, Shimizu Y, Kusano T, Matsuda K, et al. Intraoperative fluorescent imaging using indocyanine green for liver mapping and cholangiography. J Hepatobiliary Pancreat Sci. 2010;17(5):590–4.
13. Piazza L, Caragliano P, Scardilli M, Sgroi AV, Marino G, Giannone G. Laparoscopic robot-assisted right adrenalectomy and left ovariectomy (case reports). Chir Ital. 1999;51(6):465–6.
14. Hubens G, Ysebaert D, Vaneerdeweg W, Chapelle T, Eyskens E. Laparoscopic adrenalectomy with the aid of the AESOP 2000 robot. Acta Chir Belg. 1999;99(3):125–7; discussion 7-9.
15. Arora E, Bhandarwar A, Wagh A, Gandhi S, Patel C, Gupta S, et al. Role of indo-cyanine green (ICG) fluorescence in laparoscopic adrenalectomy: a retrospective review of 55 cases. Surg Endosc. 2018;32(11):4649–57.

Part II

Applications in Neurosurgery

Clipping Cerebral Aneurysm

Taku Sato, Kyouichi Suzuki, Jun Sakuma,
and Kiyoshi Saito

Introduction

The goal of cerebral aneurysm (CA) surgery is to achieve complete exclusion of the aneurysm from the circulation while preserving the patency of the parent, branching, and perforating arteries, which can be prevented by intraoperative adjuncts. In particular, indocyanine green (ICG) angiography-based near-infrared (NIR) fluorescence imaging has become more popular in the recent years due to its convenience and accuracy. However, its application has various pitfalls that should be considered.

This chapter will focus on the intraoperative ICG angiography in CA surgeries. In addition, it will describe a novel useful intraoperative laser light imaging to simultaneously visualize light and near-infrared fluorescence for ICG angiography.

Electronic Supplementary Material The online version of this chapter (https://doi.org/10.1007/978-3-030-38092-2_4) contains supplementary material, which is available to authorized users.

T. Sato (✉) · J. Sakuma · K. Saito
Department of Neurosurgery, Fukushima Medical University, Fukushima, Japan
e-mail: tak-s@fmu.ac.jp

K. Suzuki
Department of Neurosurgery, Japanese Red Cross Fukushima Hospital, Fukushima, Japan

Background

CAs occur in 3–5% of the general population and are characterized by localized structural deterioration of the arterial wall, with loss of internal elastic lamina and disruption of the media [1].

Ruptured CAs cause subarachnoid hemorrhage with up to 40–50% mortality [2]. They should be treated immediately to prevent recurrent rupture. Their current therapeutic options are limited to invasive therapies, namely, microsurgical clipping and endovascular intervention, both with non-negligible risk of procedural morbidity. Furthermore, ruptured CAs can cause various complications, such as cerebral vasospasm and hydrocephalus [3–5].

Unruptured CAs are incidentally discovered with an increasing frequency because of the widespread use of high-resolution magnetic resonance imaging. All unruptured CAs do not rupture during a lifelong follow-up [6]. The treatment is associated with 5% risks of morbidity and 1.7% mortality [7].

Several factors, including patient age and aneurysm location, size, and shape, should be considered when selecting microsurgical clipping or endovascular treatment.

Microsurgical Clipping for CAs

Microsurgical clipping is performed to obliterate CA through a craniotomy under general anesthesia. The surgeon must not only focus on preventing intraoperative aneurysm rupture but also identify carefully all relevant perforating arteries. During the microsurgical clipping, microscopic visual observation alone is not reliable enough to routinely prevent ischemic complications. Therefore, intraoperative adjuncts should be performed during microsurgical clipping.

Intraoperative Adjuncts

Intraoperative adjuncts are advanced to maximize the safety of microsurgical clipping.

Digital subtraction angiography (DSA) has become more widespread and revealed unexpected findings in approximately 7–12% of cases [8–10]. It can also confirm the complete obliteration of the aneurysm after clipping and the patency of parent or branching vessels. However, it is an expensive and invasive procedure, and its limited resolution does not allow complete confirmation of the patency of small perforating arteries. Other less invasive tools are available, which can help in confirming the blood vessels patency.

Doppler Ultrasonography

Doppler ultrasonography can noninvasively detect blood flow [11], based on two methods: the continuous-wave and the pulse-wave. Surgeons should exercise caution when using the continuous method because this may actually detect flow derived from vessels other than the target artery [12].

Neurophysiological Monitoring

Intraoperative neurophysiological monitoring of motor evoked potential (MEP), somatosensory evoked potential, and visual evoked potential (VEP) is useful for CA surgeries. MEP monitoring is the most reliable technique in detecting blood flow disturbance in the internal carotid and middle cerebral arteries that supply the corticospinal tract [13, 14], and VEP monitoring can prevent postoperative visual dysfunction [15]. However, neurophysiological monitoring cannot confirm the brain function at all. No reliable neu-

rophysiological monitoring can detect the blood flow disturbances of blood vessels, such as the hypothalamic artery branching from the anterior communicating artery complex.

Fluorescence Angiography

The application of ICG or fluorescein angiography in CA surgeries is widely performed [16, 17]. They are a real-time intraoperative imaging adjunct to identify the vascular structure, flow direction, and semiquantitative blood flow.

The usefulness of ICG angiography in microscopic surgeries was reported in 2005 [16]. The ICG fluorescence's excitation wavelength is between 700–850 nm, and its emission occurs between 780–950 nm. Therefore, the attenuation of fluorescence of ICG is less than that of fluorescein due to the longer wavelength. ICG angiography is better in confirming the patency of the thick parent artery than fluorescein angiography. The perforating artery in deep surgical field is less visualized by ICG angiography than fluorescein angiography due to the high fluorescence intensity [18].

Indications for ICG Angiography
- Microsurgery for all CAs
- No history of allergic reactions to ICG

Technical Description of the Procedures
1. Administration of ICG intravenously (the recommended dose is 0.2–0.5 mg/kg).
2. Illumination using a microscope-integrated light source with a wavelength covering the ICG absorption band.
3. Observation of ICG fluorescence's excitation in the clipped CA and parent and perforating arteries.
4. Upon noticing a remnant CA or an obliteration of the parent and perforating arteries, repositioning of the aneurysmal clip or addition of aneurysmal clips should be performed.

Interpretation
ICG angiography can visualize the observed obstructive CA and perforating arteries around the CA.

Pitfalls

- ICG angiography can visualize vessels within the operative microscopic field only and can hardly visualize vascular structures in deep locations or covered by blood clots [19].
- The absence of ICG filling is not a definitive indicator of complete occlusion at all.
- In normal physiological conditions, ICG takes about 10 minutes to be cleared from the body. If another dose was administered before the previous dose been cleared, the fluorescence emission of both doses could overlap and might affect the neurosurgeon assessment [20, 21].
- ICG angiography can detect blood flow but cannot show any quantitative information. Therefore, it is not possible to determine if the blood flow volume is sufficient to prevent infarction. Therefore, other intraoperative adjuncts such as neurophysiological monitoring should be performed with ICG angiography simultaneously.
- ICG angiography is also recommended before clip placement. If it was performed only after the clip placement, the patency of other blood vessels by the clip cannot be concluded.
- The rate of mistaken clip placements eluded by microscopic visual detection and was identified by ICG angiography is 6.1%, and the rate of mistaken clip placements eluded by ICG angiography and were identified by DSA is 4.5%. DSA remains the best tool for the detection for CA remnants [22].

Analysis of Blood Flow Dynamics

The fluorescence intensity inside the vessels and CA can be measured and its variation over time can be translated to intensity curves with specific software integrated in the surgical microscope [21]. This technique enables objective and semiquantitative analyses demonstrated through color map and ICG intensity-time curve.

Endoscope-Assisted ICG Angiography

ICG angiography can hardly visualize deep structures or those covered by brain parenchyma or other structures. An integration of ICG angiography with a neurosurgical endoscope could visualize these blind spots [23, 24].

Dual-Image Videoangiography (DIVA)

Remnant CA or obliteration of the parent and perforating arteries in ICG angiography is noticeably shown in white with a black background. ICG flow alone, but not other structures, can be observed using ICG angiography.

DIVA, which is a novel high-resolution intraoperative imaging system, was developed to simultaneously visualize both visible light and NIR fluorescence images of ICG angiography. Images from the color video and NIR fluorescence emission windows were merged for visualization on a monitor screen simultaneously (Figs. 4.1, 4.2, and 4.3) [25]. In the control system, NIR images can be changed to a designated color from a pal-

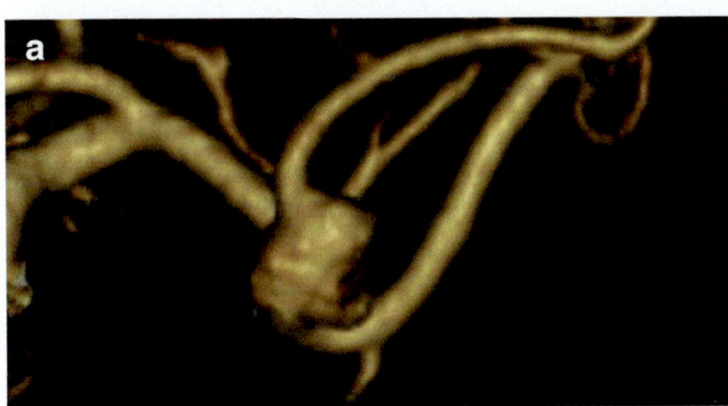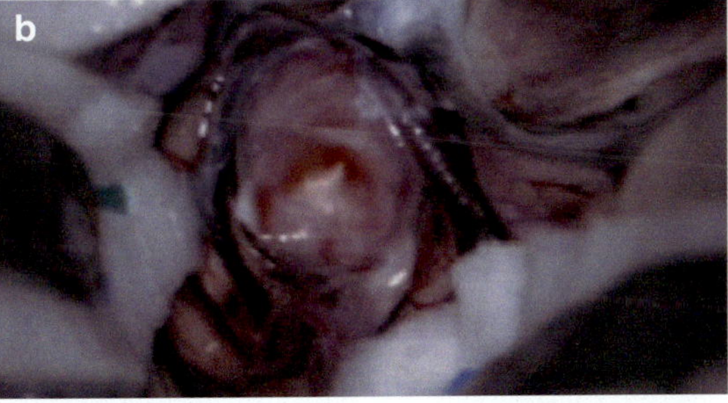

Fig. 4.1 Case 1. Preoperative three-dimensional CT angiography (anteroposterior view) showing a left middle cerebral artery aneurysm (**a**). Microscopic view of the cerebral aneurysm before clipping (**b**). Indocyanine green (ICG) videoangiography shows the parent and branching arteries (**c**). Dual-image videoangiography simultaneously visualizes both light and near-infrared fluorescence images from ICG videoangiography (**d**). (Reprinted with permission from Sato et al. [25])

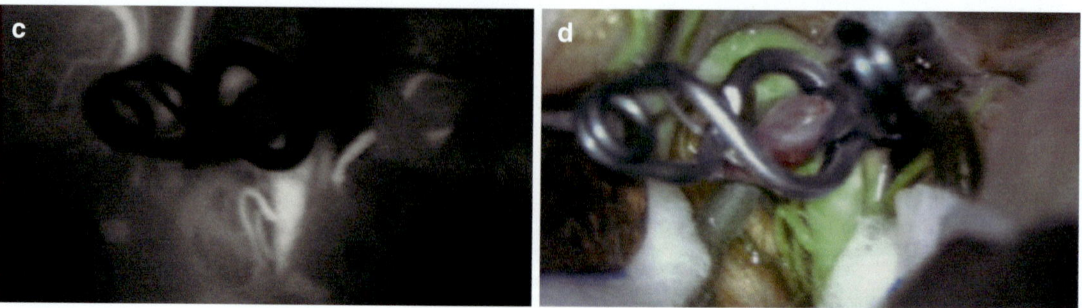

Fig. 4.1 (continued)

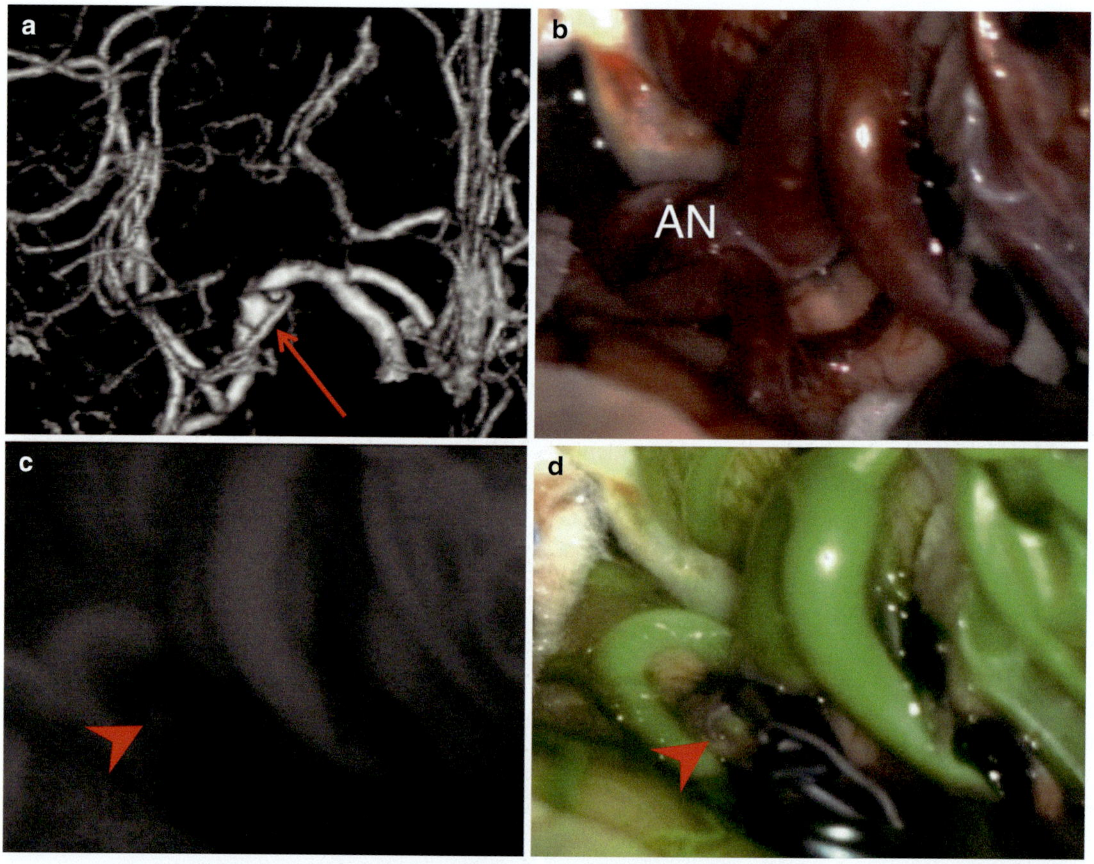

Fig. 4.2 Case 2. Preoperative three-dimensional angiography (3D-CTA) (anteroposterior (A-P) view) showing aneurysm of the right M1 segment of the middle cerebral artery (arrow) (**a**). Microscopic view of the aneurysm before clipping (**b**). AN, aneurysm. ICG videoangiography after clipping shows faint fluorescence in the aneurysmal dome (arrowhead) (**c**). Using dual-image videoangiography, the anatomical relationship between the clip and remnant flow and the cerebral aneurysm is clearly visualized (arrowhead) (**d**). Postoperative 3D-CTA (A-P view) demonstrating complete clipping of the cerebral aneurysm (arrow) (**e**). (Reprinted with permission from Sato et al. [25])

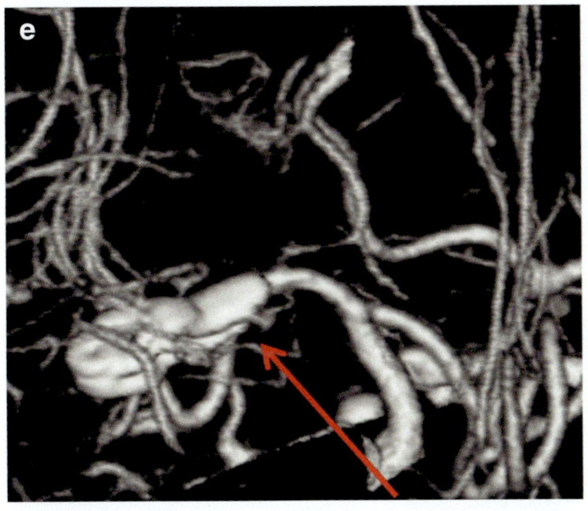

Fig. 4.2 (continued)

ette of more than 256 visible colors. Green was selected as a nonbiological color.

Surgeons can also switch between a white-light binocular view to a simultaneous right monocular DIVA image and a left monocular white-light image. Thus, performing surgery while simultaneously observing both the light and DIVA-processed images was possible [26]. DIVA may be a standard system in microscopic CA surgeries due to its usefulness.

We also developed a laser light source that can be integrated to the DIVA system (see Chap. 6) [27]. The novel laser light source composes of four bands at 464 (blue), 532 (green), 640 (red), and 785 nm (near-infrared region). Laser light

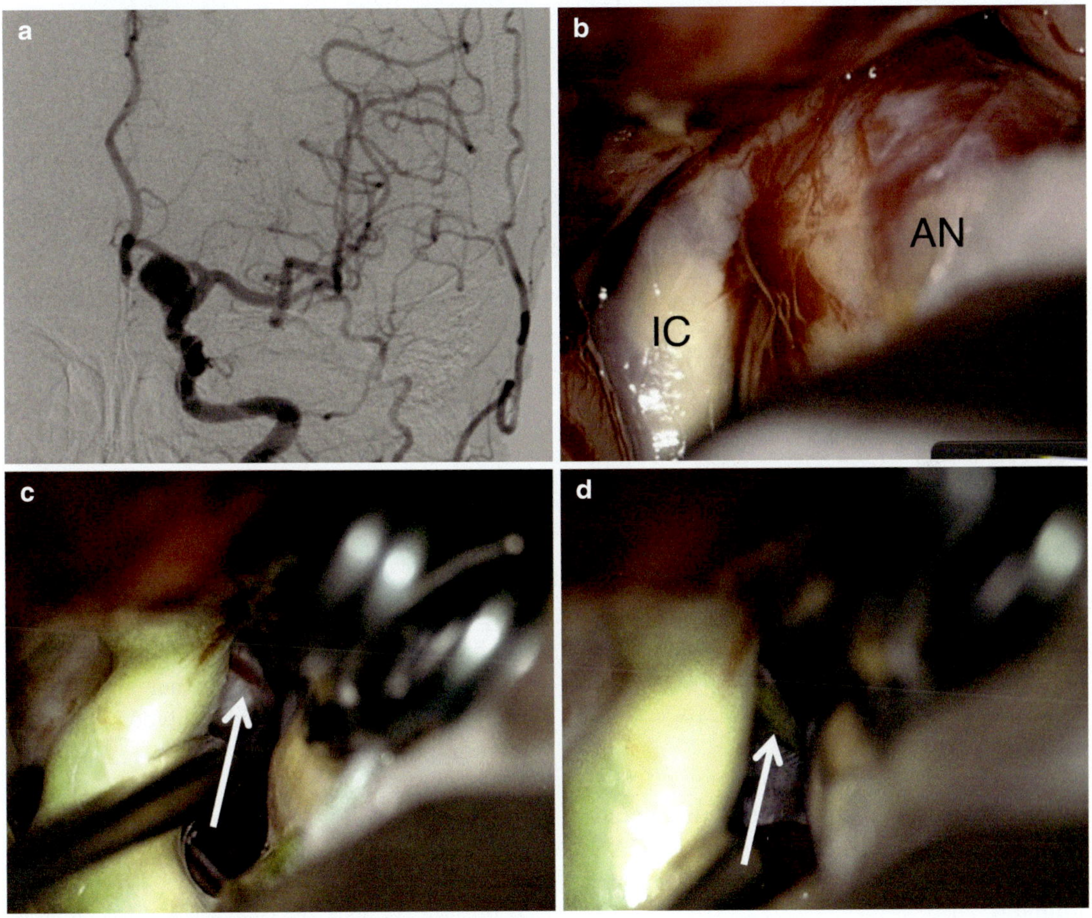

Fig. 4.3 Case 3. Preoperative angiography (anteroposterior view) showing left internal carotid paraclinoid aneurysm (**a**). Microscopic view of the aneurysm before clipping (**b**). Dual-image videoangiography (DIVA) after clipping showing no fluorescence in the superior hypophysial artery (SHA) (arrow) (**c**). A repeated attempt of DIVA clearly showing fluorescence flow in the SHA (arrow) (**d**). (Reprinted with permission from Sato et al. [28])

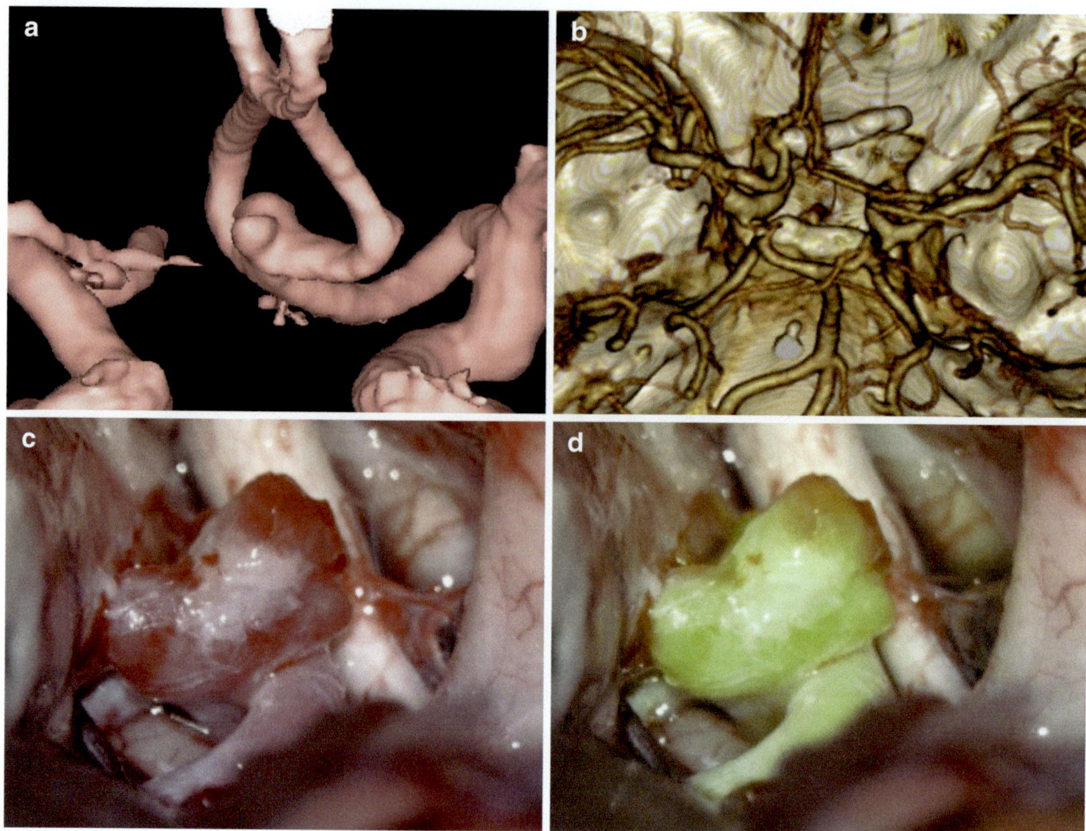

Fig. 4.4 Case 4. Preoperative magnetic resonance angiography (A-P view) showing an anterior communicating artery aneurysm (**a**). Postoperative three-dimensional computed tomography angiography (superior view) showing no aneurysm remnant after clipping (**b**). Microscopic view of the aneurysm (**c**). Dual-image videoangiography integrated with a laser light source showing the anatomical relationship between the aneurysm, hypothalamic artery, anterior cerebral artery, and surrounding brain tissues (**d**). (Reprinted with permission from Sato et al. [29])

has some advantages over xenon light. DIVA with the laser light source can clearly visualized the natural color of the operative field with enhanced blood flow (Fig. 4.4 and Video 4.1).

Conclusion

ICG angiography is an essential intraoperative adjunct to observe the occlusion of CA by microsurgical clipping and perforating arteries around it.

DIVA, a high-resolution intraoperative imaging system used to simultaneously visualize both visible light and NIR fluorescence images of ICG angiography, would be a standard microscopic adjunct in microscopic CA surgeries for its usefulness. Conversely, the combination of all available intraoperative adjuncts complements each other since some problems remain to be solved in ICG angiography.

References

1. Brisman JL, Song JK, Newell DW. Cerebral aneurysms. N Engl J Med. 2006;355:928–39.
2. Nieuwkamp DJ, Setz LE, Algra A, Linn FH, de Rooij NK, Rinkel GJ. Changes in case fatality of aneurysmal subarachnoid haemorrhage over time, accord-

ing to age, sex, and region: a meta-analysis. Lancet Neurol. 2009;8:635–42.

3. Kodama N, Sasaki T, Kawakami M, Sato M, Asari J. Cisternal irrigation therapy with urokinase and ascorbic acid for prevention of vasospasm after aneurysmal subarachnoid hemorrhage. Outcome in 217 patients. Surg Neurol. 2000;53:110–7; discussion 117–8.

4. Sato T, Sasaki T, Sakuma J, Watanabe T, Ichikawa M, Ito E, et al. Quantification of subarachnoid hemorrhage by three-dimensional computed tomography: correlation between hematoma volume and symptomatic vasospasm. Neurol Med Chir (Tokyo). 2011;51:187–94.

5. Jabbarli R, Bohrer AM, Pierscianek D, Muller D, Wrede KH, Dammann P, et al. The chess score: a simple tool for early prediction of shunt dependency after aneurysmal subarachnoid hemorrhage. Eur J Neurol. 2016;23:912–8.

6. Korja M, Lehto H, Juvela S. Lifelong rupture risk of intracranial aneurysms depends on risk factors: a prospective finnish cohort study. Stroke. 2014;45:1958–63.

7. Kotowski M, Naggara O, Darsaut TE, Nolet S, Gevry G, Kouznetsov E, et al. Safety and occlusion rates of surgical treatment of unruptured intracranial aneurysms: a systematic review and meta-analysis of the literature from 1990 to 2011. J Neurol Neurosurg Psychiatry. 2013;84:42–8.

8. Klopfenstein JD, Spetzler RF, Kim LJ, Feiz-Erfan I, Han PP, Zabramski JM, et al. Comparison of routine and selective use of intraoperative angiography during aneurysm surgery: a prospective assessment. J Neurosurg. 2004;100:230–5.

9. Tang G, Cawley CM, Dion JE, Barrow DL. Intraoperative angiography during aneurysm surgery: a prospective evaluation of efficacy. J Neurosurg. 2002;96:993–9.

10. Chiang VL, Gailloud P, Murphy KJ, Rigamonti D, Tamargo RJ. Routine intraoperative angiography during aneurysm surgery. J Neurosurg. 2002;96:988–92.

11. Stendel R, Pietila T, Al Hassan AA, Schilling A, Brock M. Intraoperative microvascular doppler ultrasonography in cerebral aneurysm surgery. J Neurol Neurosurg Psychiatry. 2000;68:29–35.

12. Kodama N, Endo Y, Oinuma M, Sakuma J, Suzuki K, Matsumoto M, et al. The principles and pitfalls on using doppler ultrasonography during surgery. No Shinkei Geka. 2005;33:109–17 (in Japanese).

13. Suzuki K, Kodama N, Sasaki T, Matsumoto M, Konno Y, Sakuma J, et al. Intraoperative monitoring of blood flow insufficiency in the anterior choroidal artery during aneurysm surgery. J Neurosurg. 2003;98:507–14.

14. Horiuchi K, Suzuki K, Sasaki T, Matsumoto M, Sakuma J, Konno Y, et al. Intraoperative monitoring of blood flow insufficiency during surgery of middle cerebral artery aneurysms. J Neurosurg. 2005;103:275–83.

15. Sasaki T, Itakura T, Suzuki K, Kasuya H, Munakata R, Muramatsu H, et al. Intraoperative monitoring of visual evoked potential: introduction of a clinically useful method. J Neurosurg. 2010;112:273–84.

16. Raabe A, Nakaji P, Beck J, Kim LJ, Hsu FP, Kamerman JD, et al. Prospective evaluation of surgical microscope-integrated intraoperative near-infrared indocyanine green videoangiography during aneurysm surgery. J Neurosurg. 2005;103:982–9.

17. Suzuki K, Kodama N, Sasaki T, Matsumoto M, Ichikawa T, Munakata R, et al. Confirmation of blood flow in perforating arteries using fluorescein cerebral angiography during aneurysm surgery. J Neurosurg. 2007;107:68–73.

18. Matano F, Mizunari T, Murai Y, Kubota A, Fujiki Y, Kobayashi S, et al. Quantitative comparison of the intraoperative utility of indocyanine green and fluorescein videoangiographies in cerebrovascular surgery. Oper Neurosurg (Hagerstown). 2017;13:361–6.

19. Khurana VG, Seow K, Duke D. Intuitiveness, quality and utility of intraoperative fluorescence videoangiography: Australian neurosurgical experience. Br J Neurosurg. 2010;24:163–72.

20. Killory BD, Nakaji P, Gonzales LF, Ponce FA, Wait SD, Spetzler RF. Prospective evaluation of surgical microscope-integrated intraoperative near-infrared indocyanine green angiography during cerebral arteriovenous malformation surgery. Neurosurgery. 2009;65:456–62; discussion 462.

21. Kamp MA, Slotty P, Turowski B, Etminan N, Steiger HJ, Hanggi D, et al. Microscope-integrated quantitative analysis of intraoperative indocyanine green fluorescence angiography for blood flow assessment: First experience in 30 patients. Neurosurgery. 2012;70:65–73; discussion 73–4.

22. Riva M, Amin-Hanjani S, Giussani C, De Witte O, Bruneau M. Indocyanine green videoangiography in aneurysm surgery: systematic review and meta-analysis. Neurosurgery. 2018;83:166–80.

23. Bruneau M, Appelboom G, Rynkowski M, Van Cutsem N, Mine B, De Witte O. Endoscope-integrated icg technology: first application during intracranial aneurysm surgery. Neurosurg Rev. 2013;36:77–84; discussion 84–5.

24. Nishiyama Y, Kinouchi H, Senbokuya N, Kato T, Kanemaru K, Yoshioka H, et al. Endoscopic indocyanine green video angiography in aneurysm surgery: an innovative method for intraoperative assessment of blood flow in vasculature hidden from microscopic view. J Neurosurg. 2012;117:302–8.

25. Sato T, Suzuki K, Sakuma J, Takatsu N, Kojima Y, Sugano T, et al. Development of a new high-resolution intraoperative imaging system (dual-image videoangiography, DIVA) to simultaneously visualize light and near-infrared fluorescence images of indocyanine green angiography. Acta Neurochir. 2015;157:1295–301.

26. Sato T, Bakhit MS, Suzuki K, Sakuma J, Fujii M, Murakami Y, Ito Y, Sure U, Saito K. A novel intraoperative laser light imaging system to simultaneously visualize visible light and near-infrared fluorescence

for indocyanine green videoangiography. Cerebrovasc Dis Extra. 2018;8:96–100.

27. Sato T, Bakhit MS, Suzuki K, Sakuma J, Fujii M, Murakami Y, et al. Utility and safety of a novel surgical microscope laser light source. PLoS One. 2018;13:e0192112.

28. Sato T, Sakuma J, Suzuki K, Oda K, Kuromi Y, Yamada M, et al. Usefulness of a new high-resolution intraoperative imaging system to simultaneously visualize visible light and near-infrared fluorescence for indocyanine green angiography. Surg Cereb Stroke. 2016;44:362–6. (in Japanese).

29. Sato T, Itakura T, Suzuki K, Sakuma J, Fujii M, Bakhit M, et al. Motor evoked potential monitoring and novel laser light imaging system to simultaneously visualize light and near-infrared fluorescence images in aneurysmal surgery. Surg Cereb Stroke, in press. (in Japanese).

Saman Sizdahkhani, Jordan Lam,
Shivani Rangwala, and Jonathan Russin

Overview of Cerebral Bypass

Cerebral bypass surgery was first conceived by Yasargil in the 1960s far before fluorescence imaging was available [1]. Although its initial application was for the treatment of ischemic stroke, the indication for cerebral revascularization has broadened to include complex aneurysms such as moyamoya disease and is increasingly being used to exclude blood flow from complex skull base tumors [2]. In this chapter, we will briefly review the types of cerebral bypass prior to discussing their specific indications.

Bypass techniques may be regarded as extracranial to intracranial (EC-IC) or intracranial-intracranial (IC-IC). The EC-IC group can further be separated into pedicle-based and non-pedicle-based bypass grafts. Pedicle-based grafts utilize an extracranial donor vessel to redistribute flow intracranially, and non-pedicle grafts may include arterial or venous donor vessels which serve as interposition grafts in high-flow settings. IC-IC bypass, on the other hand, redistributes intracranial blood flow utilizing neighboring vessels and their natural arborization patterns.

Flow dynamics are essential in determining the type of bypass indicated – as vascular flow patterns will dictate the success of a graft. EC-IC bypass grafts can be classified into standard, intermediate, and high flow. Standard flow supplies roughly 20–60 ml/min and is generally a pedicled graft, a common example of which is a superficial temporal artery to middle cerebral artery end-to-side anastomosis [3]. Intermediate flow grafts provide roughly 60–100 ml/min and encompass radial artery interposition grafts usually originating at the proximal external carotid artery (ECA) and terminating at the middle cerebral artery (MCA), anterior cerebral artery (ACA), or (posterior cerebral artery) PCA at their M2, A2, or P2 levels [4]. High-flow bypasses supply 100–200 ml/min and therefore employ interposition saphenous vein grafts [5, 6]. In comparison to radial artery grafts, saphenous vein grafts may traverse greater distances and therefore originate proximal to the ECA such as at the subclavian artery. As a result of being higher flow, as expected, the recipient vessels intracranially are larger proximal branches of the MCA, ACA, or PCA.

IC-IC bypass will be considered within an independent flow category since flow dynamics in this situation are dependent on local territories

Electronic Supplementary Material The online version of this chapter (https://doi.org/10.1007/978-3-030-38092-2_5) contains supplementary material, which is available to authorized users.

S. Sizdahkhani (✉) · J. Lam · S. Rangwala
J. Russin
Department of Neurosurgery, Keck School of Medicine of USC, Los Angeles, CA, USA
e-mail: saman.sizdahkhani@med.usc.edu

© Springer Nature Switzerland AG 2020
E. M. Aleassa, K. M. El-Hayek (eds.), *Video Atlas of Intraoperative Applications of Near Infrared Fluorescence Imaging*, https://doi.org/10.1007/978-3-030-38092-2_5

being revascularized, especially for in situ bypasses. These bypasses should involve vessels with matching diameter. A common example of an IC-IC bypass with utilization of a neighboring vascular territory includes bypassing proximal posterior inferior cerebellar artery (PICA) aneurysms with a PICA-PICA side-to-side anastomosis. A similar application is for the treatment of complex MCA aneurysms, which can be done with an interposition graft or with an in situ M2 to M2 side-to-side anastomosis of neighboring parallel M2 vessels. These are generally performed to treat an ipsilateral fusiform or distal aneurysm and result in occlusion of the diseased vessel [4, 7]. Of note, IC-IC grafts carry higher risk of perioperative ischemia due to the requirement of temporary vessel occlusion. Therefore, technical expertise is required of the surgeon which is often acquired via numerous bypass graft exercises using animal models ex vivo.

Fluorescence in Cerebral Bypass

Fluorescence used in cerebrovascular neurosurgery includes the two fluorophores sodium fluorescein (FL) and indocyanine green (ICG). These bind tightly to plasma proteins and assist in the real-time assessment of vascular flow during open neurosurgical procedures. Their use in video angiography (VA) is made possible by operative microscopes with integrated fluorescence filters and software.

An important complication of cerebral bypass is failure of graft patency. Use of fluorescence allows for real-time verification and subsequent correction of vascular flow and patency during open neurosurgical procedures. This provides a significant advantage to the current gold standard of imaging digital subtraction angiography (DSA), where unexpected findings are identified postoperatively, prompting reoperation. Furthermore, fluorescence has multiple advantages even over other intraoperative monitoring methods. Intraoperative catheter angiography provides an accurate method of confirming vessel patency or blood flow but is more time-consuming, costly, and associated with various disadvantages such as radiation exposure, contrast allergy, puncture site complications, and risk of permanent neurological deficit secondary to ischemic stroke [8, 9]. Intraoperative magnetic resonance imaging (iMRI) is noninvasive and can reconstruct three-dimensional (3D) images and detect ischemic changes through diffusion-weighting. However, iMRI is even more expensive, time-consuming, and logistically challenging, limited to centers with such operating room facilities [10]. A quick, cost-effective, and safe option that allows for visualization and quantification of vessel blood flow is Doppler ultrasound. However, the wide field of view limits spatial resolution, visualization is limited to the section of imaged vessel, and deeper access can be problematic due to the size of the probe. A newer technology called laser speckle imaging has been reported to offer real-time noninvasive imaging with good spatial resolution but has not been integrated with the microscope and has not shown to be superior to video fluorescence angiography [11].

Indocyanine Green

The excitation and emission spectra of ICG are 600–900 nm and 750–950 nm, respectively, and its first safe use for intracranial vascular lesions was described in 2003 by Raabe et al. [12]. Its intraoperative use and integration with the microscope with the INFRARED 800 module (Zeiss Meditec, Oberkochen, Germany) have been validated and published in numerous studies, all of which demonstrate ICG-VA's high spatial resolution, ability to directly visualize blood flow and patency, and correlation with postoperative digital subtraction angiography [13–17]. ICG-VA is particularly useful in high-flow bypass grafts where its utility assists surgeons reach 100% patency rates due to the ability to directly visualize the site of anastomosis. Furthermore, software has recently been developed which can utilize real-time ICG-VA data to assist in both visualization of surrounding structures and dynamics of cerebral blood flow (CBF) [18, 19]. Dual-image video angiography, called DIVA for short, combines fluorescent ICG-VA images with visible light to allow the surgeon to instantaneously visualize the anatomical relationship of vessels with nearby cortex, tissue, or vessels that are not fluorescent due to poor flow.

As ICG-VA alone allows for only a visual, qualitative understanding of blood flow, the FLOW 800 module (Zeiss Meditec, Oberkochen, Germany) is capable of analyzing ICG-VA data to calculate semi-quantitative measures of blood flow. These include maximal fluorescence, time to half maximal fluorescence ($t_{1/2\ max}$), and slope of fluorescence increase (blood flow index, BFI). Based on relative fluorescence dynamics, FLOW 800 develops a color delay map, providing information on the relative direction and sequence of blood flow [20]. FLOW 800 has been used to examine blood flow in cerebral bypass grafts and cerebral perfusion distal to the bypass, confirming its utility as a tool to navigate intraoperative decision making [19, 21–23]. A number of small, recent studies have used FLOW 800 ICG-VA to examine cerebral perfusion and postoperative hyperperfusion syndrome (HPS). Investigators found that FLOW 800 parameters could identify delayed cerebral perfusion and predict HPS [21, 24–26]. One study was able to predict vasospasm and delayed cerebral perfusion in patients with subarachnoid hemorrhage secondary to a ruptured aneurysm, providing an added benefit for this subset of patients undergoing bypass [27]. Despite concordance of FLOW 800 data with intraoperative and postoperative angiography [19], other methods have shown discordance including LSI and Doppler [28]. Prinz et al. [28] note the shortfalls of FLOW 800: the $t_{1/2\ max}$ parameter relates to a single point in time compared with real-time measurements such as Doppler and LSI; blood velocity cannot be calculated due to the lack of consideration of vessel size. FLOW 800 nevertheless provides a useful tool for comparing changes in blood flow intraoperatively.

In addition to FLOW 800, ICG-VA holds a number of other advantages to FL. ICG is cleared rapidly and can be repeated within 10 minutes with adequate visualization allowing for more frequent examination of flow during bypass surgery; FL-VA in contrast is retained by vessel

Table 5.1 Key comparisons of sodium fluorescein and indocyanine green

	Sodium fluorescein	Indocyanine green
Excitation	460–500 nm	600–900 nm
Emission	540–690 nm	750–950 nm
Clearance	20–30 minutes	<10 minutes
Microscope module	INFRARED 800	YELLOW 560
Real-time microscope visualization	Yes	No
Quality at high magnifications	Stable	Degrades
Deep visualization	Better	Poorer
Perforator visualization	Better	Poorer
Quantitative flow measurement	No	FLOW 800

walls and cannot be reinjected before another 20–30 minutes [29, 30]. ICG has also been shown to be superior for visualization of large arteries such as the parent vessel in bypass [30].

Reported drawbacks of ICG-VA include worse visualization of perforators and deeper fields and degradation of image quality at higher magnifications, although the former two have been disputed in the literature [12, 30, 31]. Table 5.1 summarizes key comparisons of ICG and FL.

Sodium Fluorescein

The excitation and emission spectra of FL are in the range 460–500 nm and 540–690 nm, respectively [30]. Although fluorescein is a highly useful tool for vascular lesions, it was first utilized for detection and resection of intracranial tumors [32]. Its use in tumor surgery derived from its infiltration of the tumor bed at locations where the blood-brain barrier is broken – a nonspecific and unreliable mechanism for true assessment of tumor borders. With respect to vascular lesions, however, fluorescein is useful as its direct visibility allows for inspection and manipulation of vessels [33].

Since its recent integration with microscopy, several qualities of FL-VA have made its use in cerebral bypass popular. The YELLOW 560 module (Zeiss Meditec, Oberkochen, Germany) allows real-time visualization through the microscopy oculars, unlike ICG-VA. This means that manipulation is possible during angiography which Narducci et al. note is important for deeper bypasses such as external carotid-middle cerebral artery (ECA-MCA), but less so for superficial anastomoses such as the superficial temporal artery (STA) where manipulation is less likely to be required [34]. Other advantages of FL-VA at deeper fields include better visualization of vasculature, maintenance of image quality throughout higher magnifications compared to ICG-VA, and reported use of a light-emitting pencil-type probe to enhance visualization [29, 34, 35]. Furthermore, FL-VA has been reported to be better for visualizing perforating vessels than ICG-VA [30, 34, 35].

Pitfalls

Disadvantages of ICG and FL in VA are as each previously discussed. However, there are a few important limitations common to both fluorophores which are intrinsic to VA and indeed any optically based methods of imaging in general.

One major limitation of VA is the narrow field of view, limited by the field of the microscope and angle of surgical approach. Whereas DSA gives a complete picture of cerebral blood flow, VA has more restricted views and can only visualize one section of vessel at a time. This has the disadvantage of not being able to compare flow further downstream or in different vascular territories.

Again, common to optically based imaging, VA has the disadvantage of only being able to visualize the direct line of sight. As a consequence, VA cannot visualize vessels covered by endogenous materials, such as brain tissue, clotted blood, or aneurysms, or exogenous materials, such as cottonoids, sealants, or clips [14, 16, 36, 37]. This may necessitate retraction and clearance of the surgical field. Other vessel characteristics such as wall thickness, thrombosis, atherosclerosis, or calcification may also

alter signal providing difficulties in determining patency [36].

Cerebral Bypass for Flow Augmentation

Cerebral bypass is conducted when there is a necessity either for (1) flow augmentation or (2) for flow replacement. Flow augmentation is useful in cases where CBF has been reduced due to chronic ischemic changes, such as progressive stenosis of the cerebral arteries. Examples of such conditions would be atherosclerosis and moyamoya disease, each of which result in progressive stenosis. Patients are considered candidates for bypass when they have reduced cerebrovascular reserve capacity (CVRC) – confirmed by perfusion imaging such as single-photon emission computed tomography (SPECT) or positron emission tomography (PET) which can quantify the decline in blood flow [38, 39]. Individual stroke risk is then applied based on these imaging findings [38]. Once it is deemed that a patient has reduced CVRC, then the typical flow augmenting bypass is considered, such as an STA-MCA bypass graft. Studies have shown that bypass grafting will lead to rescue of hemodynamics and improve neurological outcome if conduced at highly specialized centers with careful consideration of indications [40–42].

STA-MCA Bypass for Ischemia

A 41-year-old female presented as a transfer from an outside hospital after recently giving birth with acute onset of neurologic deficits. Preoperative imaging demonstrated a left vertebral dissection with severe stenosis and trace anterograde flow to the basilar artery (Video 5.1; 0:09). The contralateral vertebral artery terminated in PICA. The endovascular team did not feel it was safe to balloon angioplasty and stent the vertebral artery. Given that the patient had perfusion and neurological deficits, she was recommended for revascularization using a superficial temporal artery to superior cerebellar artery bypass (STA-SCA). The procedure began with dissection of the parietal branch of the STA. Once the artery was circumferentially dissected out, it was extended distally for approximately 8 cm from the root of the zygoma and cut, with back bleeding coagulated (Video 5.1; 0:23). The artery was heparinized with a heparin and milrinone solution, and a 5-mm arteriovenous malformation (AVM) clip was placed proximally. The graft was mobilized such that the craniotomy could be carried out without its disruption. A temporal craniotomy was performed, ensuring the floor of the middle fossa could be reached, drilling down the temporal squama as needed. The dura was opened and the temporal lobe was elevated in a subtemporal approach. The ambient cistern was opened sharply with brisk egress of cerebrospinal fluid and relaxation of the temporal lobe (Video 5.1; 0:30). Upon dissecting out the ambient cistern, the SCA was identified and it was traced anteriorly to confirm (Video 5.1; 0:48). The SCA was clearly dissected with a thrombosed false lumen (Video 5.1; 1:05). Intraoperative indocyanine green was performed, and there was some slow anterior grade flow through the dissection (Video 5.1; 1:11). Once this flow was confirmed, we proceeded with the bypass. The distal portion of the SCA, beyond the dissection, was circumferentially dissected, and a microgrid background was placed. The STA was mobilized intracranially, fish mouthed, and placed next to the recipient artery (Video 5.1; 1:26). Proximal and distal 3-mm AVM clips were placed on the recipient vessel. An arteriotomy was performed, and a running 10-0 nylon was used to perform an end-to-side anastomosis of the STA graft to the SCA vessel. The temporary clip was removed from the recipient artery, and there was no anastomotic leak appreciated. The background was removed, the proximal clip was removed from the donor graft, and good pulsatility was noted in the graft. Intraoperative indocyanine green confirmed patency of the bypass (Video 5.1; 2:16). A postoperative angiogram also demonstrated a patent bypass graft. Postoperative perfusion studies also demonstrated a decrease in mismatch volume from 50 to 26 cc.

STA-MCA Bypass for Moyamoya

Esposito et al. highlighted the importance of ICG-VA in (1) thorough mapping of the donor STA artery and (2) safe identification of the recipient artery to prevent revascularization to the wrong vascular territory [7]. "Transdural ICG videography may have advantages when used for a combined direct and indirect bypass procedure for moyamoya disease to clarify the relationship of the overlying middle meningeal artery with the underlying cortical arteries." [43]

A 60-year-old male presented with symptoms referable to a right frontal watershed ischemic infarct. His angiogram was significant for bilateral ICA stenosis as well as right MCA occlusion with moyamoya type vasculature (Video 5.2; 0:08). A right-sided STA to MCA bypass for revascularization was planned. The right STA was mapped out using Doppler, and the incision for the pterional craniotomy was made such that the base of the STA would originate at the base of the incision. The STA was dissected, and the distal 2 cm of the frontal branch of the STA was circumferentially dissected free from the adventitia. At this point, a temporary aneurysm clip was placed proximally on the STA, and the artery was divided distally (Video 5.2; 0:25). Two vascular clips were placed on the distal portion to prevent backbleeding. The graft was then flushed with a heparin milrinone solution and elevated such that it could be removed from the field during the craniotomy. The incision was extended and the musculocutaneous flap was reflected in preparation for a craniotomy. The patient's preoperative angiogram showed contributions from the middle meningeal to the intracranial vasculature; therefore, the dural opening was carefully planned to preserve the middle meningeal branches (Video 5.2; 0:38).

A recipient vessel was dissected out circumferentially, and a microsurgical background was placed. The donor STA was mobilized intracranially and fish mouthed in preparation for an end-to-side anastomosis (Video 5.2; 1:00). At this point, temporary AVM clips were placed proximally and distally on the recipient artery. An arteriotomy was performed, and a standard end-to-side anastomosis in a running fashion with a 10-0 nylon suture was completed (Video 5.2; 2:12). The temporary clips were then removed, and indocyanine green angiography was performed to verify the patency of the bypass. Postoperative imaging showed improvement in perfusion mismatch volume.

Cerebral Bypass for Flow Replacement

Flow replacement with bypass grafting is indicated for (1) treatment of giant or complex aneurysms not amenable to clip ligation or endovascular treatment and (2) skull base tumors large enough to necessitate vessel sacrifice [4, 44–46]. Prior to bypass for flow replacement, it is important to estimate the amount of flow that will be required. Such estimations can be made preoperatively with a balloon test occlusion (BTO). This test allows for understanding the degree of CBF in the region of interest on thermal diffusion and the CVRC after administration of acetazolamide [47]. During a BTO, the patient is kept awake such that a change in neurological status could be detected. This information is combined with perfusion response and change in CVRC to establish the flow required for the bypass graft [5].

Bypass for Giant and Complex Aneurysm

A 33-year-old male with a giant right-sided A1 aneurysm was treated with a complex extracranial to intracranial bypass for aneurysm trapping (Video 5.3). The aneurysm measured approximately 3 cm and was deemed not amenable to endovascular intervention due to its morphology. Shown here is the CT angiogram, with a 3D reconstruction, as well as the diagnostic angiogram. A brief overview of the final anastomosis is shown. In detail, the bypass was done utilizing a radial artery graft that originated at the superior temporal artery (STA) and terminated at the A2 segment of the anterior cerebral artery (ACA).

Not shown is the proximal STA dissection, the pterional craniotomy with orbitozygomatic extension, sylvian dissection, and interhemispheric dissection. The dissection was taken to the level of the ipsilateral ICA, where the A1 proximal to the aneurysm was directly visible. Similarly, the interhemispheric dissection was carried superiorly to reveal bilateral optic nerves and A2 segments, including visualization of the aneurysmal outflow. The ipsilateral A2 was then circumferentially dissected out, and a microgrid background was placed behind the intended anastomosis site. A radial artery graft which had been harvested from the patient's forearm was flushed and stripped of adventitia distally. It was placed intracranially adjacent to the ACA, and temporary aneurysm clips were placed proximally and distally on the A2 segment. An end-to-side microvascular anastomosis was performed with a 10-0 nylon in an interrupted manner connecting the radial artery graft to the A2 segment. The temporary clips were removed, and no bleeding was noted from the anastomosis. The graft was then heparinized and occluded distally with a temporary clip in preparation for anastomosis to the STA. A temporary clip was placed proximally on the STA, and an end-to-end anastomosis with the radial artery graft was then performed using an interrupted 10-0 nylon suture. Once the extracranial anastomosis was completed, the clips were removed, confirming no anastomotic leak and good pulsatility in the graft. Next, intracranial clip trapping of the aneurysm was performed. First, a temporary clip was placed on the ICA (Video 5.3; 0:57). Then, the proximal ACA at the bifurcation from the ICA was occluded with a fenestrated clip around the ICA (Video 5.3; 1:05). The temporary clip was then removed, and ICG was used to confirm the ICA-MCA junction was patent. At this point, dissection was taken medially over the optic nerve and the outflow of the aneurysm was. A fenestrated clip placed around the recurrent artery of Heubner was used to trap the aneurysm (Video 5.3; 1:19). At this point, indocyanine green was again used to confirm patency of the bypass and the bilateral A2s (Video 5.3; 1:25). Once patency was confirmed, attention was turned to the aneurysm. There did seem to be some delayed filling in the aneurysm with indocyanine green; however, this was delayed. Given the delay, we felt the aneurysm was likely to thrombose. The aneurysm was not cut open, and the decision was made to close allow for thrombosis over time.

A postoperative day one angiogram showed persistent, robust filling of the aneurysm through its neck (Video 5.3; 1:38); however, the decision was made to return to the operating room. A redo craniotomy and dissection were performed, with exposure of the ICA, and a temporary clip was placed. The previous permanent aneurysm clip on the origin of the ACA was removed (Video 5.3; 2:20). A slightly longer clip was then placed across the inflow to the aneurysm (Video 5.3; 2:38). The temporary clip was removed. At this point, ICG angiography was performed using the OR microscope (not shown). There was no filling appreciated in the aneurysm. Microscissors were then used to cut into the aneurysm, and there was still a small amount of bleeding coming from the aneurysm itself (Video 5.3; 3:15). After cutting more of the aneurysm wall and freeing it up to allow it to collapse, a second fenestrated clip was placed around the origin of the ACA (Video 5.3; 4:05). Once this was placed, there was a significant decrease in bleeding from the aneurysm; however, still a small amount of bleeding persisted. The posterior communicating and anterior choroidal artery were dissected out, and adhesions to the aneurysm wall were sharply dissected. A third fenestrated clip was placed between the posterior communicating and anterior choroidal arteries (Video 5.3; 5:24). At this point, there was no further bleeding from the aneurysm. A postoperative angiogram revealed no filling of the trapped giant anterior cerebral artery aneurysm (Video 5.3; 5:50).

Conclusion

Since the integration of fluorescent technology with microscopes, fluorescent angiography has become a routine tool in cerebral bypass surgery, providing real-time, intraoperative evaluation of bypass patency and offering a number of advantages including low cost, speed, and safety compared to alternatives. ICG and FL each offer their relative strengths and weaknesses, providing complementary options depending on the type and location of the bypass. Despite being limited by microscope optics, VA will continue to be a key tool in the neurovascular surgeon's armamentarium, and its use will continue to expand as technology advances.

References

1. Yasargil MG, Yonekawa Y. Results of microsurgical extra-intracranial arterial bypass in the treatment of cerebral ischemia. Neurosurgery. 1977;1:22–4.
2. Wessels L, Hecht N, Vajkoczy P. Bypass in neurosurgery-indications and techniques. Neurosurg Rev. 2018;42:389. https://doi.org/10.1007/s10143-018-0966-9.
3. Charbel FT, Meglio G, Amin-Hanjani S. Superficial temporal artery-to-middle cerebral artery bypass. Neurosurgery. 2005;56:186–90; discussion 186-190.
4. Tayebi Meybodi A, Huang W, Benet A, Kola O, Lawton MT. Bypass surgery for complex middle cerebral artery aneurysms: an algorithmic approach to revascularization. J Neurosurg. 2017;127:463–79. https://doi.org/10.3171/2016.7.JNS16772.
5. Matsukawa H, Miyata S, Tsuboi T, Noda K, Ota N, Takahashi O, Takeda R, Tokuda S, Kamiyama H, Tanikawa R. Rationale for graft selection in patients with complex internal carotid artery aneurysms treated with extracranial to intracranial high-flow bypass and therapeutic internal carotid artery occlusion. J Neurosurg. 2018;128:1753–61. https://doi.org/10.3171/2016.11.JNS161986.
6. Matsukawa H, Tanikawa R, Kamiyama H, Tsuboi T, Noda K, Ota N, Miyata S, Tokuda S. The valveless saphenous vein graft technique for EC-IC high-flow bypass: technical note. World Neurosurg. 2016;87:35–8. https://doi.org/10.1016/j.wneu.2015.12.009.
7. Esposito G, Fierstra J, Regli L. Distal outflow occlusion with bypass revascularization: last resort measure in managing complex MCA and PICA aneurysms. Acta Neurochir. 2016;158:1523–31. https://doi.org/10.1007/s00701-016-2868-3.
8. Alakbarzade V, Pereira AC. Cerebral catheter angiography and its complications. Pract Neurol. 2018;18:393–8. https://doi.org/10.1136/practneurol-2018-001986.
9. Hardesty DA, Thind H, Zabramski JM, Spetzler RF, Nakaji P. Safety, efficacy, and cost of intraoperative indocyanine green angiography compared to intraoperative catheter angiography in cerebral aneurysm surgery. J Clin Neurosci. 2014;21:1377–82. https://doi.org/10.1016/j.jocn.2014.02.006.

10. Pesce A, Frati A, D'Andrea G, Palmieri M, Familiari P, Cimatti M, Valente D, Raco A. The real impact of an intraoperative magnetic resonance imaging-equipped operative theatre in neurovascular surgery: the Sapienza University experience. World Neurosurg. 2018;120:190–9. https://doi.org/10.1016/j.wneu.2018.08.124.

11. Hecht N, Woitzik J, König S, Horn P, Vajkoczy P. Laser speckle imaging allows real-time intraoperative blood flow assessment during neurosurgical procedures. J Cereb Blood Flow Metab. 2013;33:1000–7. https://doi.org/10.1038/jcbfm.2013.42.

12. Raabe A, Beck J, Gerlach R, Zimmermann M, Seifert V. Near-infrared indocyanine green video angiography: a new method for intraoperative assessment of vascular flow. Neurosurgery. 2003;52:132–9; discussion 139.

13. Balamurugan S, Agrawal A, Kato Y, Sano H. Intra operative indocyanine green video-angiography in cerebrovascular surgery: an overview with review of literature. Asian J Neurosurg. 2011;6:88–93. https://doi.org/10.4103/1793-5482.92168.

14. Li J, Lan Z, He M, You C. Assessment of microscope-integrated indocyanine green angiography during intracranial aneurysm surgery: a retrospective study of 120 patients. Neurol India. 2009;57:453–9. https://doi.org/10.4103/0028-3886.55607.

15. Ma C-Y, Shi J-X, Wang H-D, Hang C-H, Cheng H-L, Wu W. Intraoperative indocyanine green angiography in intracranial aneurysm surgery: microsurgical clipping and revascularization. Clin Neurol Neurosurg. 2009;111:840–6. https://doi.org/10.1016/j.clineuro.2009.08.017.

16. Raabe A, Nakaji P, Beck J, Kim LJ, Hsu FPK, Kamerman JD, Seifert V, Spetzler RF. Prospective evaluation of surgical microscope-integrated intraoperative near-infrared indocyanine green videoangiography during aneurysm surgery. J Neurosurg. 2005;103:982–9. https://doi.org/10.3171/jns.2005.103.6.0982.

17. Woitzik J, Horn P, Vajkoczy P, Schmiedek P. Intraoperative control of extracranial-intracranial bypass patency by near-infrared indocyanine green videoangiography. J Neurosurg. 2005;102:692–8. https://doi.org/10.3171/jns.2005.102.4.0692.

18. Feletti A, Wang X, Tanaka R, Yamada Y, Suyama D, Kawase T, Sano H, Kato Y. Dual-image video-angiography during intracranial microvascular surgery. World Neurosurg. 2017;99:572–9. https://doi.org/10.1016/j.wneu.2016.12.070.

19. Shah KJ, Cohen-Gadol AA. The application of FLOW 800 ICG videoangiography color maps for neurovascular surgery and intraoperative decision making. World Neurosurg. 2019;122:e186–97. https://doi.org/10.1016/j.wneu.2018.09.195.

20. Jhawar SS, Kato Y, Oda J, Oguri D, Sano H, Hirose Y. FLOW 800-assisted surgery for arteriovenous malformation. J Clin Neurosci. 2011;18:1556–7. https://doi.org/10.1016/j.jocn.2011.01.041.

21. Rennert RC, Strickland BA, Ravina K, Bakhsheshian J, Russin JJ. Assessment of hemodynamic changes and hyperperfusion risk after extracranial-to-intracranial bypass surgery using intraoperative indocyanine green-based flow analysis. World Neurosurg. 2018;114:352–60. https://doi.org/10.1016/j.wneu.2018.03.189.

22. Rennert RC, Strickland BA, Ravina K, Bakhsheshian J, Fredrickson V, Carey J, Russin JJ. Intraoperative assessment of cortical perfusion after intracranial-to-intracranial and extracranial-to-intracranial bypass for complex cerebral aneurysms using flow 800. Oper Neurosurg (Hagerstown). 2018;16:583. https://doi.org/10.1093/ons/opy154.

23. Ye X, Liu X-J, Ma L, Liu L-T, Wang W-L, Wang S, Cao Y, Zhang D, Wang R, Zhao J-Z, Zhao Y-L. Clinical values of intraoperative indocyanine green fluorescence video angiography with Flow 800 software in cerebrovascular surgery. Chin Med J. 2013;126:4232–7.

24. Kobayashi S, Ishikawa T, Tanabe J, Moroi J, Suzuki A. Quantitative cerebral perfusion assessment using microscope-integrated analysis of intraoperative indocyanine green fluorescence angiography versus positron emission tomography in superficial temporal artery to middle cerebral artery anastomosis. Surg Neurol Int. 2014;5:135. https://doi.org/10.4103/2152-7806.140705.

25. Uchino H, Kazumata K, Ito M, Nakayama N, Kuroda S, Houkin K. Intraoperative assessment of cortical perfusion by indocyanine green videoangiography in surgical revascularization for moyamoya disease. Acta Neurochir. 2014;156:1753–60. https://doi.org/10.1007/s00701-014-2161-2.

26. Uchino H, Nakamura T, Houkin K, Murata J, Saito H, Kuroda S. Semiquantitative analysis of indocyanine green videoangiography for cortical perfusion assessment in superficial temporal artery to middle cerebral artery anastomosis. Acta Neurochir. 2013;155:599–605. https://doi.org/10.1007/s00701-012-1575-y.

27. Munakomi S, Poudel D. A pilot study on assessing the role of intra-operative Flow 800 vascular map model in predicting onset of vasospasm following micro vascular clipping of ruptured intracranial aneurysms. F1000Res. 2018;7:1188. https://doi.org/10.12688/f1000research.15627.1.

28. Prinz V, Hecht N, Kato N, Vajkoczy P. FLOW 800 allows visualization of hemodynamic changes after extracranial-to-intracranial bypass surgery but not assessment of quantitative perfusion or flow. Oper Neurosurg (Hagerstown). 2014;10:231–9. https://doi.org/10.1227/NEU.0000000000000277.

29. Lane B, Bohnstedt BN, Cohen-Gadol AA. A prospective comparative study of microscope-integrated intraoperative fluorescein and indocyanine videoangiography for clip ligation of complex cerebral aneurysms. J Neurosurg. 2015;122:618–26. https://doi.org/10.3171/2014.10.JNS132766.

30. Matano F, Mizunari T, Murai Y, Kubota A, Fujiki Y, Kobayashi S, Morita A. Quantitative comparison of the intraoperative utility of indocyanine green and fluorescein videoangiographies in cerebrovascular surgery. Oper Neurosurg (Hagerstown). 2017;13:361–6. https://doi.org/10.1093/ons/opw020.
31. Raabe A, Spetzler RF. Fluorescence angiography. J Neurosurg. 2008;108:429–30. https://doi.org/10.3171/JNS/2008/108/2/0429.
32. Moore GE, Peyton WT. The clinical use of fluorescein in neurosurgery; the localization of brain tumors. J Neurosurg. 1948;5:392–8. https://doi.org/10.3171/jns.1948.5.4.0392.
33. Ewelt C, Nemes A, Senner V, Wölfer J, Brokinkel B, Stummer W, Holling M. Fluorescence in neurosurgery: its diagnostic and therapeutic use. Review of the literature. J Photochem Photobiol B Biol. 2015;148:302–9. https://doi.org/10.1016/j.jphotobiol.2015.05.002.
34. Narducci A, Onken J, Czabanka M, Hecht N, Vajkoczy P. Fluorescein videoangiography during extracranial-to-intracranial bypass surgery: preliminary results. Acta Neurochir. 2018;160:767–74. https://doi.org/10.1007/s00701-017-3453-0.
35. Suzuki K, Kodama N, Sasaki T, Matsumoto M, Ichikawa T, Munakata R, Muramatsu H, Kasuya H. Confirmation of blood flow in perforating arteries using fluorescein cerebral angiography during aneurysm surgery. J Neurosurg. 2007;107:68–73. https://doi.org/10.3171/JNS-07/07/0068.
36. Chen SF, Kato Y, Oda J, Kumar A, Watabe T, Imizu S, Oguri D, Sano H, Hirose Y. The application of intraoperative near-infrared indocyanine green videoangiography and analysis of fluorescence intensity in cerebrovascular surgery. Surg Neurol Int. 2011;2:42. https://doi.org/10.4103/2152-7806.78517.
37. Januszewski J, Beecher JS, Chalif DJ, Dehdashti AR. Flow-based evaluation of cerebral revascularization using near-infrared indocyanine green videoangiography. Neurosurg Focus. 2014;36:E14. https://doi.org/10.3171/2013.12.FOCUS13473.
38. Grubb RL, Derdeyn CP, Fritsch SM, Carpenter DA, Yundt KD, Videen TO, Spitznagel EL, Powers WJ. Importance of hemodynamic factors in the prognosis of symptomatic carotid occlusion. JAMA. 1998;280:1055–60.
39. Klijn CJ, Kappelle LJ, Tulleken CA, van Gijn J. Symptomatic carotid artery occlusion. A reappraisal of hemodynamic factors. Stroke. 1997;28:2084–93.
40. Amin-Hanjani S, Barker FG, Charbel FT, Connolly ES, Morcos JJ, Thompson BG, Cerebrovascular Section of the American Association of Neurological Surgeons, Congress of Neurological Surgeons. Extracranial-intracranial bypass for stroke-is this the end of the line or a bump in the road? Neurosurgery. 2012;71:557–61. https://doi.org/10.1227/NEU.0b013e3182621488.
41. Hänggi D, Steiger H-J, Vajkoczy P, Cerebrovascular Section of the European Association of Neurological Surgeons (EANS). EC-IC bypass for stroke: is there a future perspective? Acta Neurochir. 2012;154:1943–4. https://doi.org/10.1007/s00701-012-1480-4.
42. Jussen D, Zdunczyk A, Schmidt S, Rösler J, Buchert R, Julkunen P, Karhu J, Brandt S, Picht T, Vajkoczy P. Motor plasticity after extra-intracranial bypass surgery in occlusive cerebrovascular disease. Neurology. 2016;87:27–35. https://doi.org/10.1212/WNL.0000000000002802.
43. Yokota H, Yonezawa T, Yamada T, Miyamae S, Kim T, Takamura Y, Masui K, Aketa S. Transdural indocyanine green videography for superficial temporal artery-to-middle cerebral artery bypass-technical note. World Neurosurg. 2017;106:446–9. https://doi.org/10.1016/j.wneu.2017.07.004.
44. Dengler J, Kato N, Vajkoczy P. The Y-shaped double-barrel bypass in the treatment of large and giant anterior communicating artery aneurysms. J Neurosurg. 2013;118:444–50. https://doi.org/10.3171/2012.11.JNS121061.
45. Kato N, Prinz V, Finger T, Schomacher M, Onken J, Dengler J, Jakob W, Vajkoczy P. Multiple reimplantation technique for treatment of complex giant aneurysms of the middle cerebral artery: technical note. Acta Neurochir. 2013;155:261–9. https://doi.org/10.1007/s00701-012-1538-3.
46. Yang T, Tariq F, Chabot J, Madhok R, Sekhar LN. Cerebral revascularization for difficult skull base tumors: a contemporary series of 18 patients. World Neurosurg. 2014;82:660–71. https://doi.org/10.1016/j.wneu.2013.02.028.
47. Vajkoczy P, Roth H, Horn P, Lucke T, Thomé C, Hubner U, Martin GT, Zappletal C, Klar E, Schilling L, Schmiedek P. Continuous monitoring of regional cerebral blood flow: experimental and clinical validation of a novel thermal diffusion microprobe. J Neurosurg. 2000;93:265–74. https://doi.org/10.3171/jns.2000.93.2.0265.

Vascular Malformation

Taku Sato, Kyouichi Suzuki, Jun Sakuma, and Kiyoshi Saito

Introduction

Cerebral vascular malformation is an abnormal blood vessel formation in the brain, with the following types: brain arteriovenous malformations (bAVMs), arteriovenous fistula, cavernous malformation, and venous malformation.

bAVM surgeries are one of the most difficult to perform because they required considerable surgical skills and identification of feeding vessels to prevent passage vessel injuries and preserve draining veins until the final stage of the procedure. Although the treatment for bAVMs was changed due to improvement in endovascular embolization and stereotactic radiotherapy (SRS), microscopic surgery is one of its definitive treatments [1].

Intraoperative adjuncts are necessary to avoid intraoperative complications. Near-infrared (NIR) fluorescence imaging has been more popular in the recent years due to its convenience and accuracy.

This chapter will mainly address the intraoperative applications of NIR fluorescence imaging in bAVM surgeries. In addition, it will describe the intraoperative laser light imaging to simultaneously visualize visible light and NIR fluorescence for indocyanine green (ICG).

Background

bAVMs represent an uncommon central nervous system disease characterized by an arteriovenous shunt with one or multiple arterial pedicles being feed into a vascular nidus, creating early drainage into a venous outflow channel.

These lesions are considered congenital and can be clinically detected in a variety of ways, such as seizure, intracranial hemorrhage, chronic headache, or progressive neurological deficit [2, 3].

bAVMs have a prevalence of detected asymptomatic or symptomatic in the population of 10–18 per 100,000 adults [4, 5].

The Spetzler-Martin (SM) Grading Scale is the most commonly used classification system.

It uses three anatomic factors (nidus size, nidus location relative to the eloquent brain, and pattern of venous drainage) to enumerate five bAVM grades. It is a well-validated tool for estimating the risks of surgical resection [6].

Electronic Supplementary Material The online version of this chapter (https://doi.org/10.1007/978-3-030-38092-2_6) contains supplementary material, which is available to authorized users.

T. Sato (✉) · J. Sakuma · K. Saito
Department of Neurosurgery, Fukushima Medical University, Fukushima, Japan
e-mail: tak-s@fmu.ac.jp

K. Suzuki
Department of Neurosurgery, Japanese Red Cross Fukushima Hospital, Fukushima, Japan

Indication for Surgery

The first randomized trial on the treatment versus conservative management for unruptured bAVM was also reported [7]. Nevertheless, compelling evidence on many treatment decisions that are routinely made for patients with ruptured and unruptured bAVM remains lacking. Patients with bAVM who present with hemorrhage are at a higher risk for re-bleed compared with patients with bAVM detected presymptomatically [8]. Surgery is recommended for the majority of Spetzler-Martin Grade I and II bAVMs (low-grade bAVMs), utilizing conservative embolization as a preoperative adjunct [9]. However, another randomized trial is needed to establish the role of surgery in bAVM management.

Preoperative Evaluation

Digital subtraction angiography (DSA) is the reference standard for the diagnosis of bAVMs. DSA provides the most detailed and accurate information on bAVM angioarchitecture and hemodynamics. It has the highest degree of both spatial and temporal resolution of all diagnostic imaging modalities. The immediate risks of DSA are primarily related to neurological complications such as thrombotic stroke. DSA entails radiation exposure with potential long-term consequences [10].

Treatment

The definitive treatment for bAVMs should be complete elimination of the nidus and the arteriovenous shunt. Therapeutic tools are three. The first is microscopic surgery, which may be performed primarily or after endovascular embolization to reduce bleeding risks intraoperatively and to facilitate complete and uncomplicated removal. The second is SRS, which may also be performed primarily or after embolization to reduce nidal volumes and potentially improve nidal obliteration rates. The final method is endovascular embolization itself. Although this is most often used as a precursor to microsurgery or radiosurgery, some cases may utilize it as a definitive therapy.

Intraoperative Adjuncts

Intraoperative adjuncts are required the safety of complete removal.

Neurophysiological Monitoring

Intraoperative neurophysiological monitoring of motor evoked potential (MEP), somatosensory evoked potential, and visual evoked potential (VEP) is useful for bAVMs. In the case that a bAVM is located near the motor area, MEP mapping and monitoring are used to confirm the motor area and motor function intraoperatively. The risk of intraoperative injury to the motor area can be reduced by identifying its exact location by MEP mapping [11]. However, neurophysiological monitoring cannot confirm the brain function at all.

Evaluation of the Blood Flow

bAVMs require evaluation of the flow before performing the surgical procedures. Feeding vessels that need to be dissected should be identified in order to avoid the passing arteries and preserve the draining veins.

- Doppler ultrasonography

Doppler ultrasonography may be difficult to interpret, particularly with higher flow lesions, and disrupts the workflow during resection of bAVMs.

- Intraoperative DSA

Intraoperative DSA can effectively identify residual bAVMs after the procedure, but it is not easily translatable in the open microsurgical anatomy [1]. Low-grade bAVMs that are relatively easy to treat are often left out during the intraoperative DSA since the resolution is low.

- Fluorescence angiography

The application of ICG and fluorescein angiography in cerebral vascular surgeries is widely performed [12]. They are real-time intraoperative imaging adjunct to identify the vascular structure and flow direction. They allow surgeons to intraoperatively distinguish between arteries and veins or between normal and abnormal vascular components such as bAVM [13, 14].

After an intravenous bolus injection of ICG, the operative field is illuminated using a microscope-integrated light source with a wavelength covering the ICG absorption band (range, 700–850 nm; maximum, 805 nm). Arterial, capillary, and venous flow images are observed on the video screen in real time. The recommended dose of ICG for this type of angiography is 0.2–0.5 mg/kg.

ICG angiography is safe, requires no additional equipment except for image modification software, and can be repeated multiple times throughout the surgical procedure.

ICG angiography cannot visualize the deep-seated feeders, nidus, and drainers that are covered within the parenchyma.

Indications for ICG Angiography
- AVM that have superficial feeders
- All Spetzler-Martin Grade AVMs
- No history of allergic reactions to ICG

Technical Description of the Procedures
1. Perform a craniotomy to obtain adequate exposure to the bAVM, including its arterial feeders and venous outflow.
2. Dissect the arachnoid of the AVM.
3. Isolate and divide its arterial feeders and venous outflow including the sulcus.
4. Inject the ICG for the first evaluation to identify the vascular architecture and flow direction.
5. After clipping the feeders, inject the ICG repeatedly and identify the passing arteries.
6. Coagulate the feeders and dissecting the subpial tissue.
7. Dissect the nidus and coagulate the deep feeders.
8. Inject the ICG after dissecting the nidus and stopping the flow of the drainer.
9. Coagulate the drainers and excise the AVM.
10. Homeostasis

Interpretation
- ICG angiography can visualize the feeders, passing arteries, nidus, and drainers.
- Re-administration of ICG does reveal not only the angioarchitectural structure of the AVM but also the residual flow of the nidus in superficial AVMs.

Pitfalls
- In normal physiological conditions, ICG takes about 10 minutes to be cleared from the body. If another dose was administered before the previous dose been cleared, the fluorescence emission of both doses could overlap and might affect the neurosurgeon assessment [14].
- ICG angiography is less useful with deep-seated lesions. It is a complement rather than a replacement of DSA. Intraoperative DSA in these cases should be performed.
- ICG angiography can visualize the exposed vessels within the operative microscopic field only [15].
- A high-resolution postoperative angiogram must be performed in bAVM surgery and remains the best test to confidently confirm AVM total resection [16].

Semi-Quantitative Analysis for Blood Flow
Specific software integrated in the surgical microscope was developed as an additional analytical imaging tool to analyze blood flow dynamics using an ICG angiography. This technique enables objective and semi-quantitative analyses demonstrated through color map and ICG intensity-time curve.

The analysis of blood flow in the specific software can be used to understand the hemodynamic changes in AVM surgery [17, 18]. However, it cannot quantitatively estimate the blood flow.

Dual-Image Videoangiography (DIVA)

The blood flow of bAVMs in ICG angiography is noticeably shown in white with a black background. ICG flow alone, but not other structures, can be observed using ICG-VA. The newly developed DIVA system can simultaneously visualize both visible light and NIR fluorescence images of ICG-VA (Fig. 6.1) [19]. In the control system, NIR images can be changed to a designated color from a palette of more than 256 visible colors. We selected green as a nonbiological color. In the microscope, light including fluorescence emission from the operative field enters the camera unit mounted to the side viewer of the microscope. The visible light (400–700 nm) and near-infrared fluorescence emission light (800–900 nm) are filtered using a special sensor unit with an optical filter. Visible light is detected using a color imaging process, and NIR fluores-cence emission light is detected by a near-infrared imaging process. Surgeons can also switch between a white-light binocular view to a simultaneous right monocular DIVA image and a left monocular white-light image. Thus, performing surgery while simultaneously observing both the light and DIVA-processed images was possible [20].

We also developed a laser light source and integrated it with the DIVA system. The novel laser light source is with four bands at 464 (blue), 532 (green), 640 (red), and 785 nm (near-infrared region) [21]. Laser light has some advantages over xenon light (Table 6.1). The present setup clearly visualized the natural color of the operative field with enhanced blood flow.

The feeding vessels, passing arteries, and draining veins were confirmed to be visualized and detected in arteriovenous malformation surgery (Figs. 6.2 and 6.3). In this setup, a single ICG injection was received at a dose of 0.1 mg/kg as a bolus. This dose is sufficient for the analysis

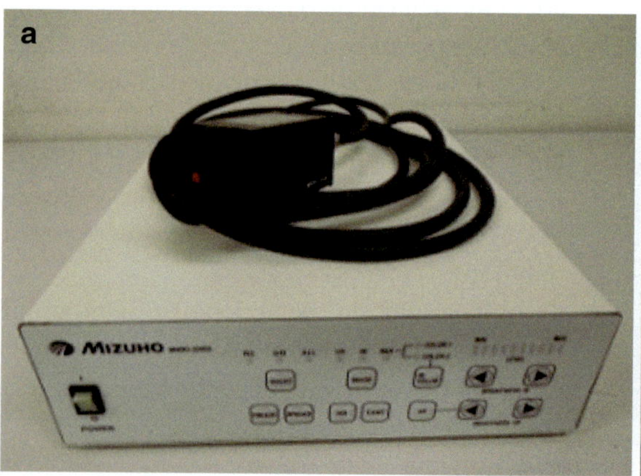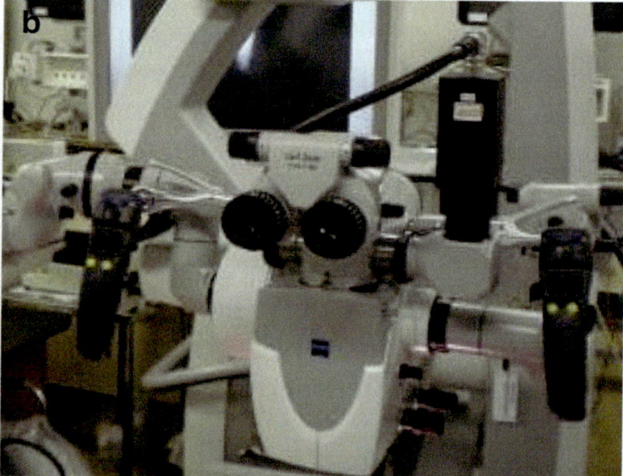

Fig. 6.1 Dual-image videoangiography (DIVA) camera and control unit (**a**). DIVA camera connected to the micro-scope with a C-mount (**b**). (Reprinted with permission from Sato et al. [22])

Table 6.1 Comparison of different light sources

	Halogen	Xenon	LED	Laser
Directivity	Poor	Poor	Poor	Good
Color rendering	Good	Good	Average	Average
Color calibration	Poor	Poor	Average	Good
Energy efficiency	Poor	Poor	Good	Good
Life span	Poor	Poor	Good	Good

From Sato et al. [21]

LED light-emitting diode

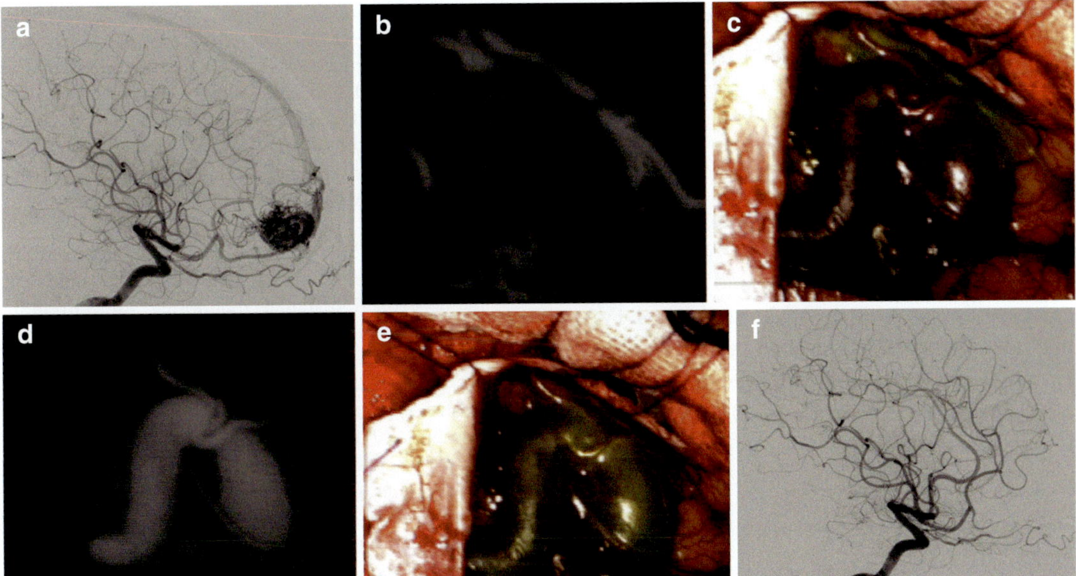

Fig. 6.2 Preoperative angiography (lateral view) showing Grade I arteriovenous malformation (AVM) in the right frontal lobe (**a**). Intra-arterial injection of indocyanine green shows feeding arteries (**b**, **c**) and a draining vein (**d**, **e**). Dual-image videoangiography visualizes the anatomical relationship between the feeders, passing arteries (**c**), and drainer (**e**). Postoperative angiography (lateral view) shows disappearance of the AVM (**f**). (Reprinted with permission from Sato et al. [19])

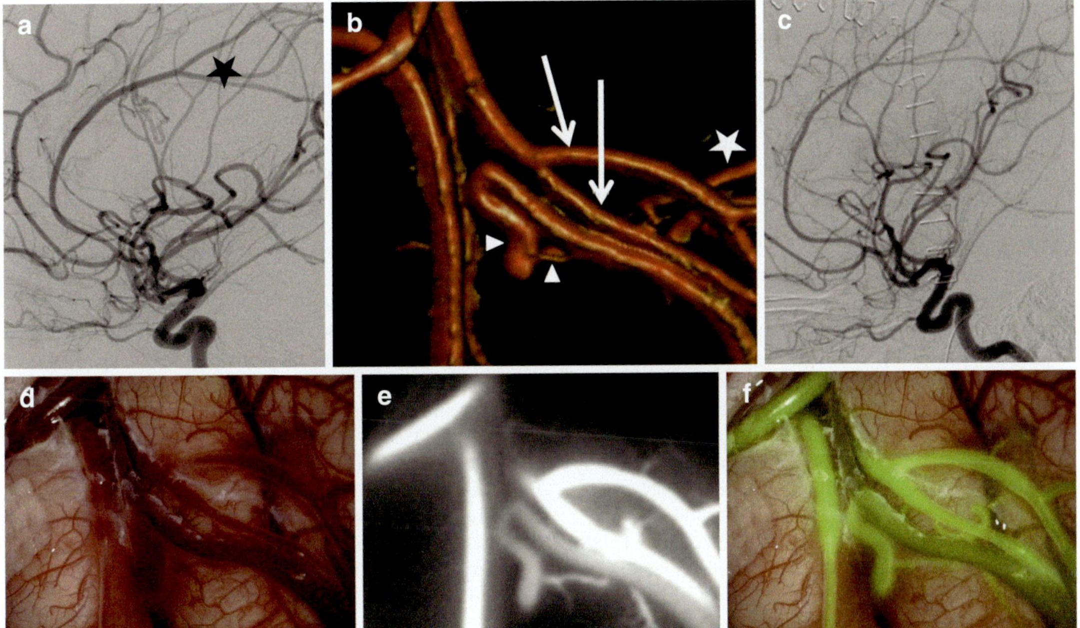

Fig. 6.3 Preoperative angiography (lateral view) showing Grade II arteriovenous malformation (AVM) (star) in the left frontal lobe (**a**). Preoperative angiography showing the nearby passing arteries (arrow), nidus (star), and drainers (arrowhead) (**b**). Postoperative angiography showing disappearance of the AVM (**c**). Microscopic view of the AVM (**d**). Standard indocyanine green videoangiography shows the feeders, nearby passing arteries and drainers. It is difficult to recognize nonvascular structures (**e**). Dual-image videoangiography shows the anatomical relationship between the feeders, nearby passing arteries, drainers, and nonvascular structures (**f**). (Reprinted with permission from Sato et al. [22])

even though it is lower than those in other published reports [12, 14] (see Video 6.1).

Conclusion

ICG angiography is an essential intraoperative adjunct in order to distinguish between arteries and veins or between normal and abnormal vascular components in bAVM surgeries. DIVA, a high-resolution intraoperative imaging system to simultaneously visualize both visible light and NIR fluorescence images of ICG angiography, would be useful in bAVM surgeries.

References

1. Zaidi HA, Abla AA, Nakaji P, Chowdhry SA, Albuquerque FC, Spetzler RF. Indocyanine green angiography in the surgical management of cerebral arteriovenous malformations: lessons learned in 130 consecutive cases. Neurosurgery. 2014;10(Suppl 2):246–51; discussion 251.
2. Brown RD Jr, Wiebers DO, Forbes G, O'Fallon WM, Piepgras DG, Marsh WR, et al. The natural history of unruptured intracranial arteriovenous malformations. J Neurosurg. 1988;68:352–7.
3. Brown RD Jr, Wiebers DO, Torner JC, O'Fallon WM. Frequency of intracranial hemorrhage as a presenting symptom and subtype analysis: a population-based study of intracranial vascular malformations in olmsted country, Minnesota. J Neurosurg. 1996;85:29–32.
4. Al-Shahi R, Fang JS, Lewis SC, Warlow CP. Prevalence of adults with brain arteriovenous malformations: a community based study in Scotland using capture-recapture analysis. J Neurol Neurosurg Psychiatry. 2002;73:547–51.
5. Arteriovenous Malformation Study G. Arteriovenous malformations of the brain in adults. N Engl J Med. 1999;340:1812–8.
6. Spetzler RF, Martin NA. A proposed grading system for arteriovenous malformations. J Neurosurg. 1986;65:476–83.
7. Mohr JP, Parides MK, Stapf C, Moquete E, Moy CS, Overbey JR, et al. Medical management with or without interventional therapy for unruptured brain arteriovenous malformations (Aruba): a multicentre, non-blinded, randomised trial. Lancet. 2014;383:614–21.
8. Kim H, Al-Shahi Salman R, McCulloch CE, Stapf C, Young WL, Coinvestigators M. Untreated brain arteriovenous malformation: patient-level meta-analysis of hemorrhage predictors. Neurology. 2014;83:590–7.
9. Potts MB, Lau D, Abla AA, Kim H, Young WL, Lawton MT, et al. Current surgical results with low-grade brain arteriovenous malformations. J Neurosurg. 2015;122:912–20.
10. Alexander MD, Oliff MC, Olorunsola OG, Brus-Ramer M, Nickoloff EL, Meyers PM. Patient radiation exposure during diagnostic and therapeutic interventional neuroradiology procedures. J Neurointerv Surg. 2010;2:6–10.
11. Ichikawa T, Suzuki K, Sasaki T, Matsumoto M, Sakuma J, Oinuma M, et al. Utility and the limit of motor evoked potential monitoring for preventing complications in surgery for cerebral arteriovenous malformation. Neurosurgery. 2010;67:ons222–8; discussion ons228.
12. Raabe A, Nakaji P, Beck J, Kim LJ, Hsu FP, Kamerman JD, et al. Prospective evaluation of surgical microscope-integrated intraoperative near-infrared indocyanine green videoangiography during aneurysm surgery. J Neurosurg. 2005;103:982–9.
13. Hänggi D, Etminan N, Steiger HJ. The impact of microscope-integrated intraoperative near-infrared indocyanine green videoangiography on surgery of arteriovenous malformations and dural arteriovenous fistulae. Neurosurgery. 2010;67:1094–103; discussion 1103–94.
14. Killory BD, Nakaji P, Gonzales LF, Ponce FA, Wait SD, Spetzler RF. Prospective evaluation of surgical microscope-integrated intraoperative near-infrared indocyanine green angiography during cerebral arteriovenous malformation surgery. Neurosurgery. 2009;65:456–62; discussion 462.
15. Khurana VG, Seow K, Duke D. Intuitiveness, quality and utility of intraoperative fluorescence videoangiography: Australian neurosurgical experience. Br J Neurosurg. 2010;24:163–72.
16. Bilbao CJ, Bhalla T, Dalal S, Patel H, Dehdashti AR. Comparison of indocyanine green fluorescent angiography to digital subtraction angiography in brain arteriovenous malformation surgery. Acta Neurochir. 2015;157:351–9.
17. Fukuda K, Kataoka H, Nakajima N, Masuoka J, Satow T, Iihara K. Efficacy of flow 800 with indocyanine green videoangiography for the quantitative assessment of flow dynamics in cerebral arteriovenous malformation surgery. World Neurosurg. 2015;83:203–10.
18. Kamp MA, Slotty P, Turowski B, Etminan N, Steiger HJ, Hanggi D, et al. Microscope-integrated quantitative analysis of intraoperative indocyanine green fluorescence angiography for blood flow assessment: First experience in 30 patients. Neurosurgery. 2012;70:65–73; discussion 73–4.
19. Sato T, Suzuki K, Sakuma J, Takatsu N, Kojima Y, Sugano T, et al. Development of a new high-resolution intraoperative imaging system (dual-image videoangiography, DIVA) to simultaneously visualize light and near-infrared fluorescence images of indocyanine green angiography. Acta Neurochir. 2015;157:1295–301.

20. Sato T, Bakhit M, Suzuki K, Sakuma J, Fujii M, Murakami Y, Ito Y, Sure U, Saito K. A novel intraoperative laser light imaging system to simultaneously visualize visible light and near-infrared fluorescence for indocyanine green videoangiography. Cerebrovasc Dis Extra. 2018;8:96–100.

21. Sato T, Bakhit MS, Suzuki K, Sakuma J, Fujii M, Murakami Y, et al. Utility and safety of a novel surgical microscope laser light source. PLoS One. 2018;13:e0192112.

22. Sato T, Sakuma J, Suzuki K, Oda K, Kuromi Y, Yamada M, et al. Usefulness of a new high-resolution intraoperative imaging system to simultaneously visualize visible light and near-infrared fluorescence for indocyanine green angiography. Surg Cereb Stroke. 2016;44:362–6. (in Japanese).

Part III

Applications in Cardiothoracic Surgery

Derek Muehrcke

Indications

Coronary artery bypass graft patency is the major predictor of long-term survival after coronary artery bypass grafting (CABG) surgery [1]. Technical anastomotic problems are a major source of early graft closure [2, 3]. The ability to reliably assess the patency of coronary artery bypass grafts using intraoperative fluorescence imaging (IFI) has been shown to improve short-term patient outcomes after coronary artery bypass grafting [4] and to reduce hospital cost of CABG [5, 6]. Several techniques have been used to assess intraoperative graft flow and patency. Most have had drawbacks limiting their use. These have been reviewed previously by Balacumaraswami and Taggert [7]. Electromagnetic flowmetry, based on principles of electromagnetic induction, can quantitate blood flow accurately under experimental conditions where it assumes laminar flow. However, in the clinical setting, flow values fluctuate with movement and changing hematocrit, and consequently, its use has been short-lived [8, 9]. Continuous-wave (CW) and pulsed-wave (PW) Doppler velocity measurements have been used to assess intraoperative graft patency. Although, easy to use, continuous-wave (CW) and pulsed-wave (PW) Doppler velocity measurements are based on the principle of a change in Doppler velocity, but detectors have no range resolution and PW Doppler systems were affected by the angle of insonation [10]. Epicardial ultrasound scanning [11] uses an epicardial probe, which provides satisfactory images of coronary stenosis and graft anastomoses but does not provide real-time angiographic images. Thermal coronary angiography, based on the creation of thermal images with an infrared camera, depends on the temperature difference between the myocardium and the coronary arteries generated with the use of cold or warm saline or cardioplegic injections. Although this provides images of graft, function resolution varies depending on temperature differences [12]. None of these techniques produce reliable or consistent results.

Intraoperative Techniques of Graft Patency Assessment

There are three currently used popular methods of measuring graft patency in CABG surgery. The best but most expensive method is coronary angiography. It does represent the gold standard

Electronic Supplementary Material The online version of this chapter (https://doi.org/10.1007/978-3-030-38092-2_7) contains supplementary material, which is available to authorized users.

D. Muehrcke (✉)
Department of Cardiothoracic Surgery, Flagler Hospital, Saint Augustine, FL, USA

© Springer Nature Switzerland AG 2020
E. M. Aleassa, K. M. El-Hayek (eds.), *Video Atlas of Intraoperative Applications of Near Infrared Fluorescence Imaging*, https://doi.org/10.1007/978-3-030-38092-2_7

to determine graft patency. Coronary angiography provides a clear multiplane visual assessment of all proximal and distal anastomoses. It is however invasive, expensive, and difficult to perform after heart surgery without having a cardiologist and cardiac catheterization lab available.

Transit-time flowmetry (TTFM) and intraoperative fluorescence imaging (IFI) are currently the two most popular methods of assessing intraoperative coronary artery bypass graft patency. Both are relatively inexpensive, are easy to perform, and can provide real-time intraoperative assessment of graft patency. Below, we will discuss both of these techniques: their methodology, current experience, results, and limitations.

Transit-Time Flowmetry (TTFM)

Transit-time flowmetry (Medistim ASA, Norway) is a technique based on the principle of transit-time ultrasound technology. It uses a perivascular flow probe, which consists of two ultrasonic transducers and a fixed acoustic reflector, which holds the graft perpendicular to the position of the transducers and the reflector. The transit time taken from the wave of ultrasound to travel from one transducer to another is derived by the flow meter and provides an accurate measure of flow volume [13].

Technique

The flow probes require the use of an ultrasound gel applied to the lumen of the flow probe. It is important to ensure the graft occupies at least 75% of the area within the probe to get an accurate reading (Fig. 7.1). The coupling agent (gel) improves ultrasound imaging. Results are quantitatively reported as mean graft flow and a flow waveform is generated. In addition to the flow waveform, the systems provide various calculated derivatives such as mean graft flow (MGF), pulsatile index (PI), and diastolic flow index (DFI).

Mean graft flow is expressed as ml/min, which indicates the quantity of graft flow at the time of the measurement. Mean graft flow values above 40 ml/min indicate satisfactory flow, and values less than 5 ml/min are considered unsatisfactory, prompting revision [14]. When mean graft flow values between 5 ml/min and 40 ml are obtained, interpretation depends on certain derived values such as PI and DFI. PI is expressed as an absolute number of the value obtained by the dips between the maximum flow and the minimum flow divided by the mean flow. It gives an estimate of the resis-

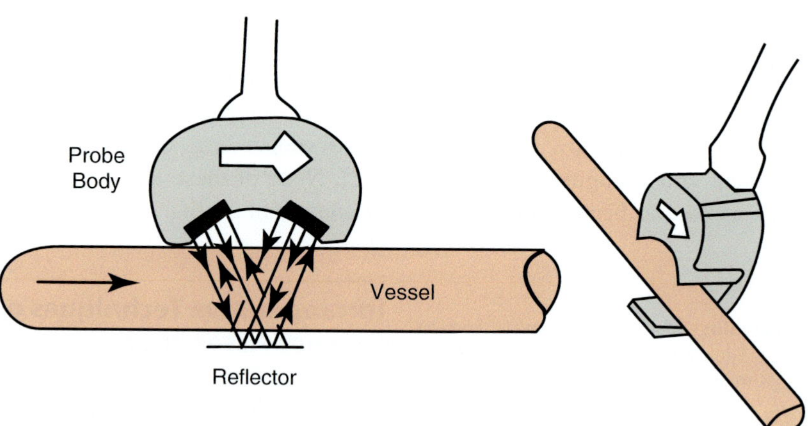

Fig. 7.1 TTFM flow probe with bypass graft inserted for reading of flow expressed as ml/min. The ultrasound flow meter measures the velocity of a fluid with ultrasound to calculate volume flow. Using ultrasound transducers, the flow meter can measure the average velocity along the path of an emitted beam of ultrasound, by averaging the difference in measured transit time between the pulses of ultrasound propagating into and against the direction of flow

tance to graft flow. Generally, a PI value of more than 5 is considered to indicate unsatisfactory graft flow [15], and revision should be considered; however, PI alone cannot be used to determine graft revision. DFI is expressed with the percentage of total graft flow which occurs during diastole. A predominant diastolic flow in the graft with a DFI that is more than 50 is considered normal, similar to the native coronary blood flow [13]. A DFI less than 50 is cause for concern. Unfortunately, there are no images of graft flow produced using this technique to help validate visually marginal or concerning derived values.

Current Experience and Results

Several groups have reported the clinical usefulness of TTFM to assess graft patency.

D'Ancona et al. reported the need to revise 37 of 1147 graft (3%) in 33 of 409 off-pump coronary artery bypass grafts (8%). They emphasize the reliance on correct analysis of TTFM flow patterns to correct the abnormalities, since interpretation of the derived values is variable and may be inconclusive [13].

Likewise, Taggert's group [16] has used TTFM in over 100 patients, and it was found to be useful in confirming graft patency in the majority of patients with good mean graft flow values. Using both TTFM and intraoperative fluorescence imaging (IFI) modalities in the same patient, they found that in the majority of grafts, both TTFM and IFI reliably confirmed graft patency. However, in 3.8% of grafts (10% of patients) with low mean graft flow situations, where TTFM indicated the need to revise the grafts, IFI confirmed satisfactory visual antigrade flow. Because the flow through the grafts could be visualized, no revisions were performed. Taggert expressed concerns that TTFM may overestimate the need for graft revision.

TTFM has been used in the assessment of graft patency with a greater degree of accuracy compared with other flow measurement modalities, such as electromagnetic flowmetry, which varies with movement and hematocrit, and Doppler flowmeters, which vary with the angle of insonation [17]. It has correctly identified occluded grafts when other tests suggested a patent graft. This includes situations where a pulse was felt in an occluded graft (as a tactile pulse can be felt in occluded grafts which can be misinterpreted as "flow"). TTFM can detect graft occlusion even when the ECG remains normal and echocardiography identifies normal wall motion. Jakobsen noted only one of the five cases with TTFM documented graft occlusion was the graft impairment reflected in abnormal ECG findings [18]. Walpoth and colleagues describe two cases in which TTFM detected graft occlusion despite adequate perfusion of the graft assessed by the surgeon's fingers, which was corrected on the operating room table [19].

TTFM, unfortunately, does not always reliably predict graft or anastomotic stenosis as reported by several groups. Hirotani and colleagues evaluated TTFM measurements in a series of 291 in situ internal mammary artery grafts and 190 saphenous vein grafts in 171 patients. They compared the intraoperative measurements with postoperative coronary angiogram performed before hospital discharge [20]. They found that mean graft flow, as measured by TTFM, failed to predict stenosis or partially occluded grafts on postoperative angiograms. Jakobsen and Kjergard reported 1.8% graft revision rate in a series of 280 CABG patients [18].

Limitations

In the major of patients with good MGF (>40 ml/min), TTFM reliably indicates graft patency. However, in low mean graft flow situations, interpretation of PI and DFI values is arbitrary, and there is considerable uncertainty regarding adequacy of graft patency. Transit-time flowmetry is a very easy device to use; however, it does not show a visual image of the graft. When the graft is subjected to spasm, or the stenosis of the native coronary artery is not very severe, flow measurement data may not be diagnostic.

Intraoperative Fluorescence Imaging (IFI) System

Principle

SPY intraoperative fluorescence imaging received FDA 510(K) clearance in 2005 as a system to assess graft patency after CABG surgery.

The IFI system SPY™ (Stryker Corporation, Kalamazoo, MI) depends on the fluorescent properties of indocyanine green (ICG) dye. ICG rapidly binds to the plasma proteins when injected intravenously and is therefore confined to the intravascular compartment. Indocyanine green is excreted unchanged by the liver with a half-life of 3–5 min; thus, there is no potential for nephrotoxic effects for those patients with compromised renal function. The dye also has an excellent safety profile. The incidence of allergic reactions to ICG is approximately 1 in 40,000, and it has been reported mainly in patients with an allergy to iodine [21]. The risk of allergic reactions is strongly dose dependent, being greatest with a dose in excess of 0.5 mg/kg weight. A lower-density laser with a total output of 2.7 w spread over an area of 7.5 × 7.5 cm at a distance of 30 cm has a depth of penetration of about 1–2 mm to avoid thermal damage. ICG fluoresces when illuminated with a laser light of 806 nm and emits light at the longer wavelength at 830 nm. The imaging camera head is a charge-coupled device video camera and is positioned over the exposed heart, and the laser is activated before the first pass of a bolus of ICG through the field of view. Images of the coronary arteries and bypass grafts are acquired at a rate of 30 frames/s and may be viewed in real time. The near-infrared light can maximally penetrate 1–2 mm of soft tissue. The fluorescence sequentially shows illumination of the graft or coronary artery lumen, a blush of the epicardium occurs as the dye passes through the microcirculation, and finally, washout as the dye enters the coronary veins.

The ICG dye transmission time is dependent on various factors including the systemic arterial pressure, competitive native coronary blood flow on the severity of native proximal coronary stenosis, distal coronary vascular resistance, and conduit diameter. The proximal target coronary artery snaring with a silastic sling facilitates anastomotic visualization and largely eliminates competitive flow [13]. Skeletonized internal thoracic artery (ITA) and radial artery (RA) conduit provide better visualization than pedicle ones. The appearance of fluorescent images, as the dye passes through the bypass graft, confirms graft patency.

Technique

There are three different techniques we use to visualize CABG grafts. We only perform coronary artery bypass grafting using the cardiopulmonary bypass machine with the heart arrested. We feel this technique allows us to bypass more vessels, improves long-term graft patency, and improves long-term survival than off-pump bypass techniques (Video 7.1, 00:01). However, the techniques can easily be used with off-pump bypass grafting. A direct handheld injection of ICG down the individual vein grafts is used to assess each vein graft distal anastomosis and to assess perfusion of the heart (Video 7.1, 00:49). Imaging of each graft takes only 2–3 min (Video 7.1, 1:13). Typically, we perform our vein graft anastomoses first followed by the IMA to LAD anastomosis. Each distal vein graft anastomosis can be tested by injecting 10 ccs of contrast down the vein graft (or free arterial graft) through a syringe (Video 7.1, 1:41). The concentration we use is made up by placing 0.5 cc of ICG (concentration 2.5 mg/mi) into 500 cc of normal saline. Of this solution, 30 cc is mixed with 10 cc of heparinized blood. Of the final mixture, 10 cc is injected down the vein graft as images are acquired, and then the graft is flushed with heparinized blood (Video 7.1, 2:14). Care must be taken not to inject air down the grafts, especially when performing off-pump bypass grafting. We specifically look for flow through the vein graft, the anastomosis (Video 7.1, 2:48), and the epicardial artery. The tactile response of how hard or easy it is to inject the solution gives feedback as to the flow in the bypassed vessel. The rate of hand-injected flow is determined by several factors including the diameter of the vein, the size of the anastomosis, the size of the epicardial artery grafted, and the resistance in the vascular bed distal to the anastomosis. Moreover, we look for the three phases of fluorescence. The first is the arterial phase, where the vein graft, anastomosis, and artery illuminate. The second phase is where the myocardial surface illuminates, and the third phase is the venous phase when the veins on the heart are imaged.

An injection of the ICG into the heart-lung machine is used to assess IMA to coronary artery flow when the cross-clamp is on, as the in situ graft is the only source of blood flow to the heart with the cross-clamp on (Video 7.1, 3:10). Flow through the in situ IMA graft is evaluated by injecting 1 cc of undiluted ICG dye (2.5 mg) into the heart-lung machine. Imaging will take 10–15 seconds to occur. There should be a brisk transition from the IMA graft into the left anterior descending coronary artery (Video 7.1, 3:54).

At the end of the procedure after performing the proximal anastomoses, all proximal anastomoses are assessed simultaneously by injecting 0.5 ccs of undiluted ICG into the central line (Video 7.1, 4:23). This is followed by a 10-cc flush of normal saline. Visualization of the proximal anastomoses will take 10–15 seconds to appear as the dye works its way through the heart to the aorta. Revisions are based on the findings of the gross blood flow images. The images are then recorded on a computer hard drive. Repeated

ICG injections can be administered at short intervals, which generate excellent image quality.

It is also possible to assess the presence of competitive flow through the important IMA to LAD anastomosis if one calculates the pixel intensity to the anterior wall using qualification hardware. With the cross-clamp off, serial central line injections of ICG with the IMA occluded using a soft vascular clap first and then subsequently with the IMA not occluded are used to generate pixel intensity grafts. The difference represents the flow to the anterior wall of the heart provided by the IMA graft (Fig. 7.2). The additional flow to the anterior wall from the IMA blood supply can be quantitated by subtracting these two values. Obviously, separate images are recorded for each injection and compared. The lack of increased flow may be a sign of competitive flow due to a non-physiologic proximal coronary artery stenosis.

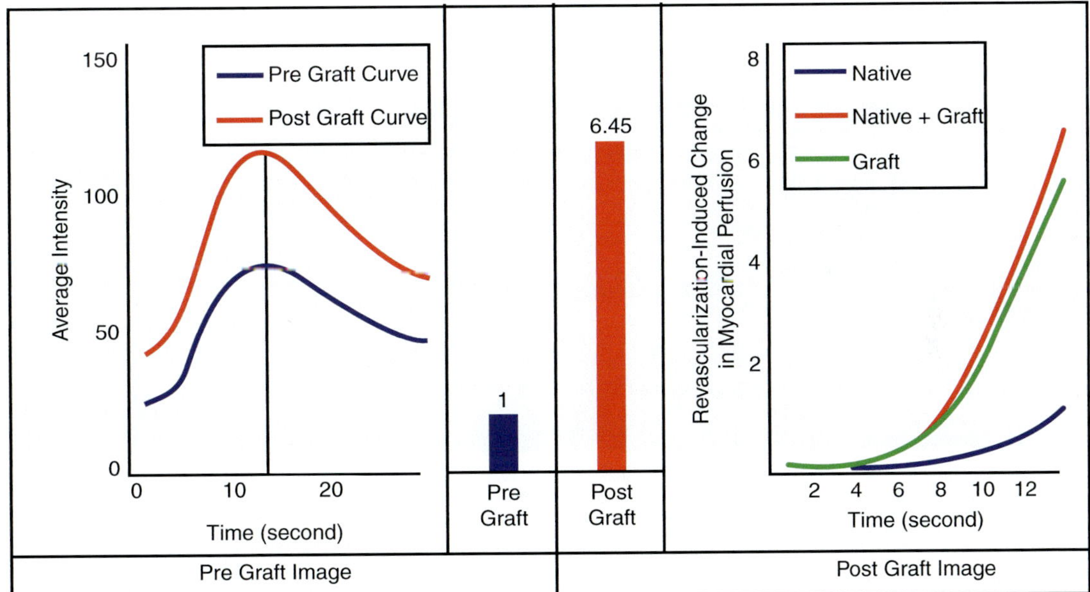

Fig. 7.2 Pixel intensity measurements approximate myocardial blood flow using the SPY Q analysis program. Measurements are made with the cross-clamp off. In the left panel, the blue represents anterior wall pixel intensity (blood flow) to the native myocardium (pre-grafting; IMA occluded). The red line represents the average pixel intensity after grafting with the IMA (post-grafting; IMA graft open). If the native flow is normalized to a value of 1 (middle panel), then the increased flow with the new IMA graft is quantitated to 6.45 times the blood flow. The right panel shows myocardial perfusion the native vessel (blue), the improved flow with a new IMA graft (red), and the flow added to the anterior wall (green) [30]

Validation Studies

Takahashi and associates [22] were one of the first authors to compare IFI with TTFM in off-pump cases in Japan. Each patient served as their own control. They demonstrated high-quality IFI images in 290 grafts of 72 off-pump CABG cases (mean of 4.0 grafts per patient). Four anastomoses (1.4%), including two proximal and two distal, were revised because of defects detected by SPY images. In one case (Fig. 7.3), the SPY system revealed no blood flow in a radial sequential graft, although transit-time flow measurements taken on the sequential portion of the bypass graft showed a diastolic dominant pattern with intermediate flow of 24 ml/min. SPY images revealed the proximal portion of the radial artery graft, between the aorta and the obtuse marginal artery, to be non-patent, allowing them to revise the graft while the patient was still on the operating table. After revision, slide B on the right demonstrates IFI imaging showing both the aorta to obtuse marginal 1 graft and the sequential obtuse

marginal 1 to obtuse marginal 2 graft the be patent. The TTFM flow increased from 22 to 55 ml/min in the sequential portion of the graft. The authors concluded that using the SPY system, technical failures could be completely resolved during surgery. They stated that the use of the SPY system for intraoperative graft validation during off-pump CABG may become the gold standard for surgical management in the near future. Importantly, Takahashi was able to demonstrate a significant flaw in TTFM analysis, namely, the inability to visually assessment of the bypass grafts. He demonstrated two cases were sequential grafts were used where TTFM was unable to identify graft closure correctly.

In another patient depicted in Fig. 7.4, an in situ internal mammary artery has been used as a sequential graft between the diagonal and the left anterior descending artery. Intraoperative fluorescence imaging reveals the sequential portion between the diagonal and the LAD is occluded despite the TTFM flow measuring a flow of 22 ml/min, when measured in the IMA to diago-

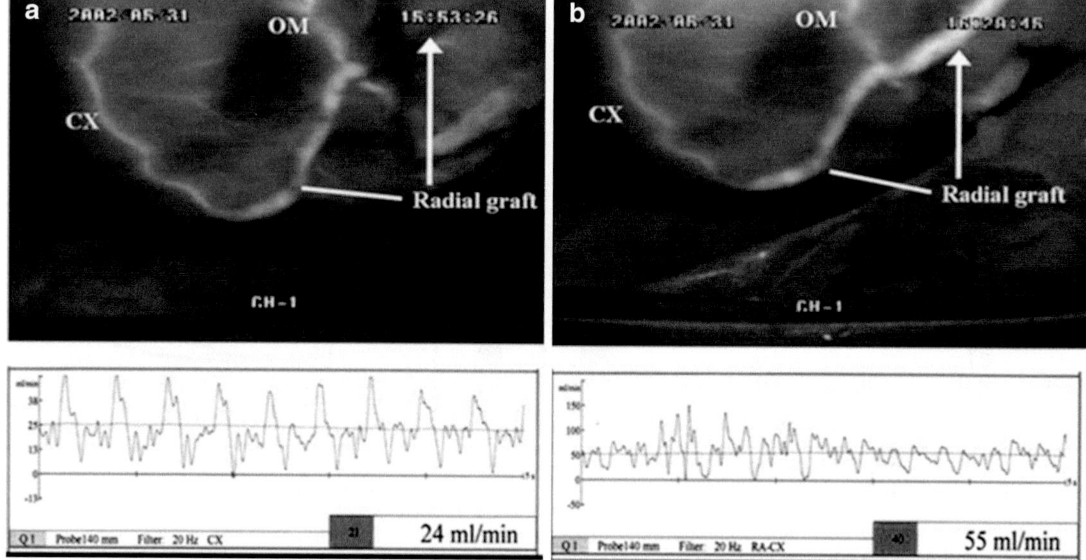

Fig. 7.3 Slide A represents the IFI images of a radial sequential graft from the circumflex obtuse marginal 1 to the circumflex obtuse marginal 2. By IFI, the free radial graft from the aorta to the obtuse marginal 1 is occluded; however, the flow measured on the sequential obtuse marginal 1 to obtuse marginal 2 reveals a flow of 24 ml/min. After revision, slide B on IFI imaging shows both the aorta to obtuse marginal 1 graft and the sequential obtuse marginal 1 to obtuse marginal 2 graft to be patent. The TTFM flow increased from 22 ml/min to 55 ml/min [31]. (From Takahashi et al. [22])

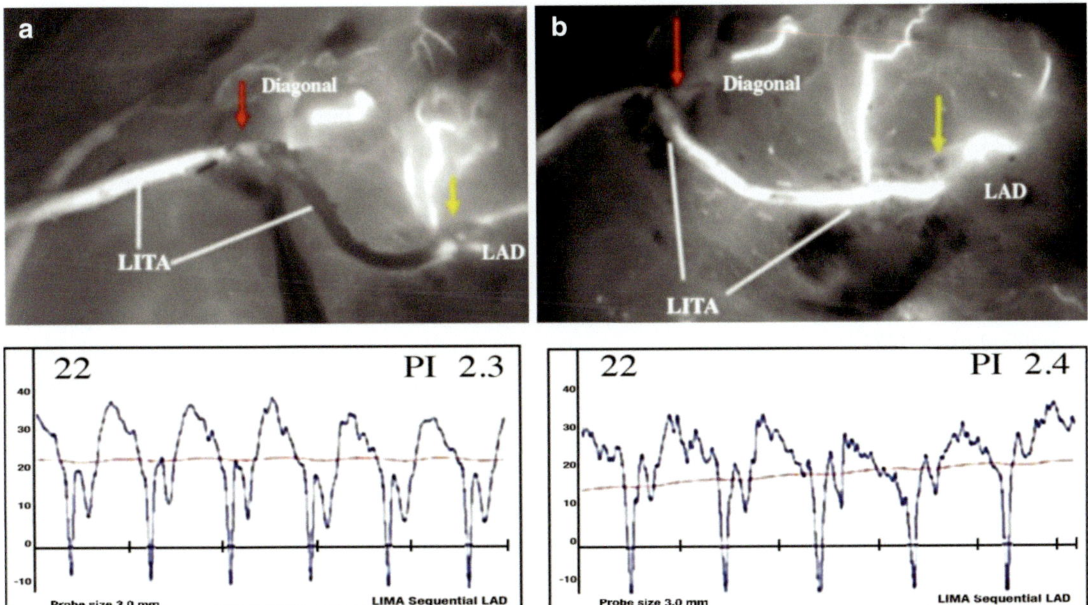

Fig. 7.4 Sequential IMA to diagonal and LAD graft. On the left, the diagonal to LAD sequential graft is occluded by IFI; however, TTFM measured a flow of 22 ml/min. After revision, IFI shows the entire sequential graft to be patent; however, there was no change in the TTFM flow of 22 ml/min [31]. (From Takahashi et al. [22])

nal graft. The images on the right were taken after the graft was revised in the operating room. It demonstrates excellent flow through both anastomoses of the sequential diagonal to LAD graft. The TTFM flow was unchanged (22 ml/min) after revision. In both cases presented, the TTFM was not helpful in detecting a significant intraoperative graft occlusion because of a lack of visual assessment of the graft.

Desai and colleagues [23] also noted that early CABG failures may be corrected if identified intraoperatively. These researchers like Takahashi compared the diagnostic accuracy of transit-time ultrasound flow measurement and ICG fluorescent-dye graft angiography. Both imaging studies were performed in each patient, as they acted as their own control. Virtually all cases were performed with cardioplegic arrest on the cardiopulmonary bypass machine. Patents undergoing isolated CABG with no contraindications for postoperative angiography were enrolled in the study. Patients were randomly assigned to be evaluated with either ICG angiography (ICG) and then transit-time ultrasonic flow measurement or transit-time flow and then ICG angiography. Interestingly, all patients underwent X-ray angiography on postoperative day 4. The primary end point of the trial was to determine the sensitivity and specificity of the two techniques versus standard X-ray angiography to detect graft occlusion or greater than 50% stenosis in the graft or peri-anastomotic area. A total of 106 patients were enrolled, and X-ray angiography was performed in 46 patients. In total, 139 grafts were reviewed with all three techniques, and 12 grafts (8.2%) were demonstrated to have greater than 50% stenosis or occlusion by the reference standard. The sensitivity and specificity of ICG to detect greater than 50% stenosis or occlusion were 83.3% and 100%, respectively. The sensitivity and specificity of transit-time ultrasonic flow measurement to detect greater than 50% stenosis or occlusion were 25% and 98.4%, respectively. The *p* value for the overall comparison of sensitivity and specificity between ICG and transit-time flow ultrasonography was 0.011. The difference between sensitivity for ICG and transit-time flow measurement was 58% with a 95% confidence interval (CI) of 30–86%, $p = 0.023$. The authors concluded that ICG provided a better diagnostic method of detecting clinically significant graft errors than did transit-time ultrasound flow measurement. They also had patients, who had marginal TTFM graft flows (5–40 ml/min) but had occluded grafts when visualized using ICG.

In a separate study, Waseda and associates [24] evaluated the intraoperative fluorescence imaging (IFI) system in the real-time assessment of graft patency during off-pump CABG. Patients undergoing off-pump CABG received IFI analysis, intraoperative transit-time flowmetry, and postoperative X-ray angiography. A total of 507 grafts in 137 patients received underwent analysis. Of all the IFI analyses, 379 (75%) grafts were visualized clearly up to the distal anastomosis. With regard to anastomosis location, anterior location was associated with a higher percentage of fully analyzable images (90%). More than 80% of images were analyzable, irrespective of graft type; six grafts with acceptable transit-time flowmetry results were diagnosed with graft failure by IFI, which required on-site graft revision. All revised grafts' patency was confirmed by postoperative X-ray angiography. Conversely, 21 grafts with unsatisfactory transit time flowmetry results demonstrated acceptable patency with IFI. Graft revision was considered unnecessary in these grafts, and 20 grafts (95%) were patent by postoperative X-ray angiography. Compared with slow washout, fast washout was associated with a higher preoperative ejection fraction, use of internal mammary artery grafts, and anterior anastomosis location. The authors concluded that the IFI system enabled on-site assessment of graft patency, providing both morphologic and functional information. They concluded that this technique may help reduce procedure-related, early graft failures in off-pump bypass patients.

Interpretation

Several researchers have attempted to quantitate myocardial perfusion or graft flow using IFI. None have been able to quantitate myocardial blood flow reliably using the pixel intensity measurements which are used in assessing graft patency. It is important to understand that as a result of the low energy used in the laser to obtain images using IFI, only 2 mm of the myocardial surface can be imaged. Therefore, any quantitative analysis presumes that myocardial blood flow is universal through the entire thickness of the ventricular wall. This obviously may not be true and represents a potential inaccuracy of this methodology. Nonetheless, Detter [25] has shown myocardial blood flow is reduced in a steplike fashion with greater degrees of coronary stenosis. Moreover, Yamamoto [26] has shown a similar association looking at the flow in the vessel itself, not the myocardium. Both attempted to assess myocardial flow by measuring peak pixel intensity and time to peak pixel intensity.

Detter et al. [25] attempted to quantify the blood supply to the heart by measuring the maximum pixel intensity of the myocardium and time to maximum intensity during the myocardial phase of IFI. They evaluated the ability of IFI to quantitatively assess the effect of coronary stenosis of variable severity on myocardial perfusion using two separate methods. They compared the effect of variable coronary artery stenosis in vivo (coronary stenosis of 25%, 50%, 75%, and 100% flow restriction) using IFI compared to the gold standard assessment using the fluorescent microsphere method. Using open-chest pigs, graded stenosis and total occlusion of the left anterior descending coronary artery were created. They showed that increasing graded stenosis and total vessel occlusion reduced normalized background-subtracted peak fluorescence intensity (BSFI) and the slope of fluorescence intensity significantly. Moreover, background-subtracted peak fluorescence intensity and slope of fluorescence intensity (analyzed by ICG) demonstrated good linear correlation with fluorescent microsphere-

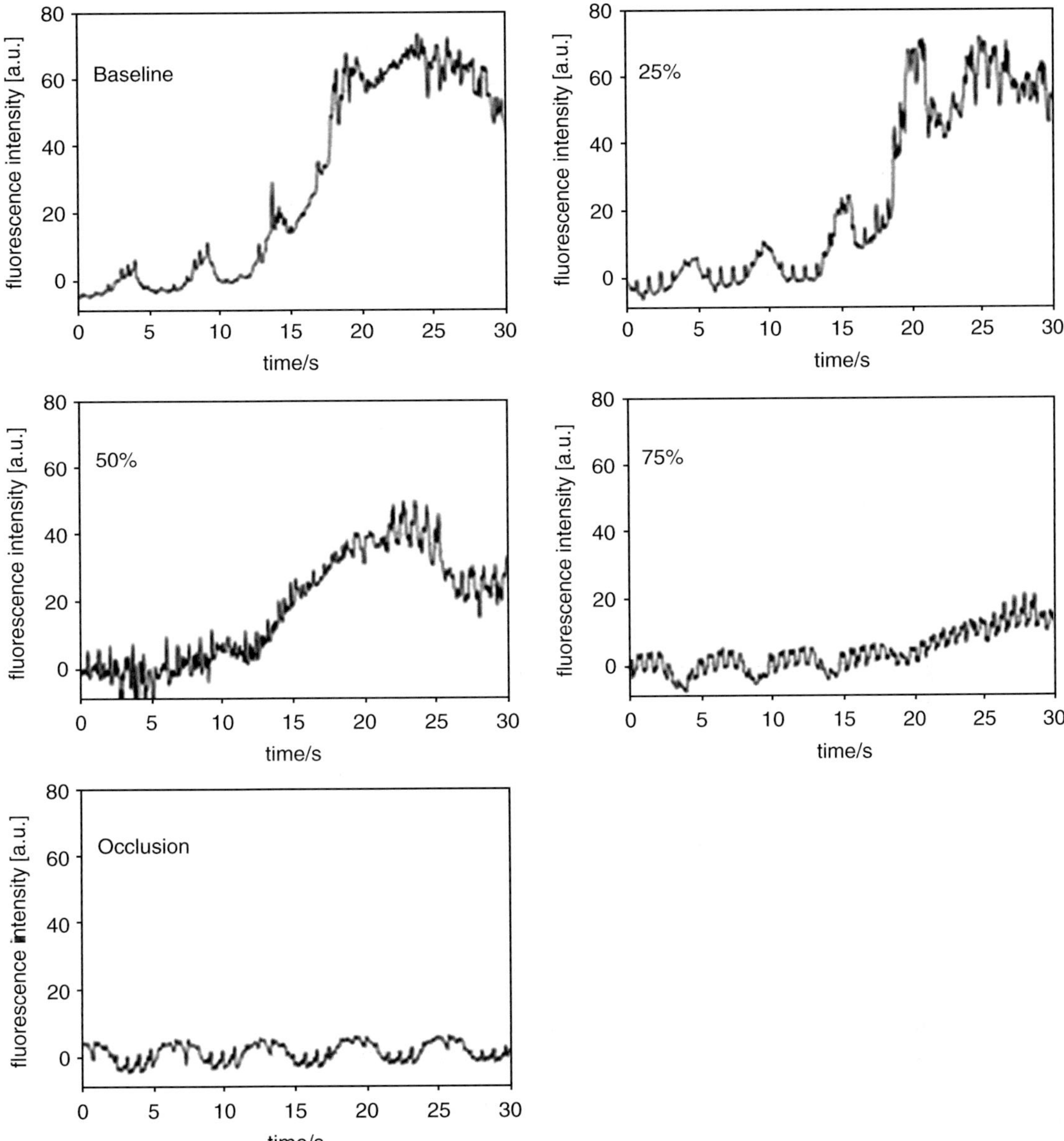

Fig. 7.5 Time-intensity curves of the left ventricular anterior wall analyzed by slope of fluorescence intensity (SFI) in a representative experiment at baseline and four graded coronary stenosis (25%, 50%, 75%, and 100% flow restriction). a.u. equals arbitrary units. One can see the diminished intensity of the fluorescence with increasing degrees of vessel stenosis. (Reproduced with permission: Detter et al. [25])

derived myocardial blood flow. These quantitative assessments of myocardial blood flow using IFI are mostly used to show an increase or no change in myocardial blood flow following bypass grafting (Figs. 7.5 and 7.6). They concluded that the impairment of myocardial perfusion in response to increased coronary stenosis severity and total vessel occlusion can be quantitatively assessed by ICG and correlates well with results obtained by fluorescent microsphere assessment.

Ferguson et al. have also reported that the change in fluorescence intensity is a direct indicator of the change in the myocardial perfusion

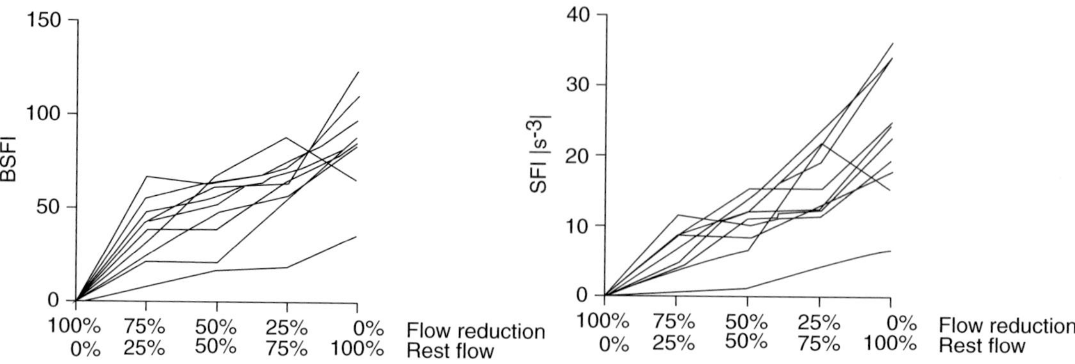

Fig. 7.6 Background-subtracted peak fluorescence intensity (BSFI) (left) and slope of fluorescence intensity (SFI) (right) obtained at baseline and four graded coronary stenosis (25%, 50%, 75%, and 100% flow restriction) in 11 animals. (Reproduced with permission: Detter et al. [25])

using perfusion pixel analysis [27]. Using this methodology, his group has used IFI to assess competitive flow after bypass grafting. He has shown that when there is no increase in myocardial perfusion after grafting, the native vessel stenosis is likely not physiologically significant despite how tight the native vessel stenosis appeared visually. This may help reduce the incidence of early graft closure by better understanding which types of grafts are more prone to competitive flow after they are constructed. Looking at 167 bypass patients with 359 grafts (53% arterial), all grafts were widely patent by IFI, and 24% of the arterial and 22% of the saphenous vein grafts showed no regional myocardial perfusion change in response to bypass grafting, consistent with competitive flow. In 165 in situ internal mammary grafts to the left anterior descending artery (>70% visual stenosis on preoperative angiogram), 40 had no change in regional myocardial perfusion, and 32 of the 40 had competitive flow imaged. They concluded that an important number of angiographic patient bypass grafts demonstrated no change in regional myocardial perfusion suggesting anatomical, but nonfunctional, stenosis in the target vessel epicardial coronary arteries. In in situ arterial grafts imaged, competitive flow was associated with nonfunctional stenosis in the target vessel epicardial coronary artery. During the discussion of this paper [28], it was pointed out that the surgeon only finds out that graft has competitive flow

after the graft has been performed, thereby limiting the usefulness of the technique. Moreover, as the IFI in this study was not performed under stress, the physiologic importance of the epicardial stenosis may have been underestimated. Moreover, Sabik pointed out that there is likely a benefit to bypassing coronary arteries without significant fraction flow reserve numbers as 80% of the grafts remain patient at a year, and the long-term effect is likely beneficial to the patient as their disease is likely to progresses.

While some authors have found IFI helpful in evaluating stenosis at the anastomosis [23, 29], direct assessment of the severity of vessel stenosis by IFI can be limited. While the previously mentioned studies have illustrated that the extent of changes in ICG fluorescence intensity of the myocardial wall is useful, the human myocardium is often covered with an epicardial fat pad that limits ICG fluorescence imaging, thereby making analysis often times inaccurate.

Therefore, Yamamoto et al. [30], using an ex vivo model, studied the effect of vessel stenosis on the maximum intensity and time to maximum intensity in the vessels only, not the myocardium. During near-infrared (NIR) angiography, the fluorescence intensity was calculated during pre- and post-stenosis in an artificial ex vivo circuit. They measured the time to maximum fluorescence intensity and the absolute maximum intensity. They found that severe stenosis (greater than 75%) attenuated the increase in ICG fluorescence intensity in the vessel but not the time to maximum fluorescence. The conventional visual qualitative NIR angiographic assessment may produce a false result due to the human eye not being able to perceive a difference in the intensity of the fluorescence. The anastomoses may appear normal as the flow rate (time to peak intensity) is not affected by greater degrees of stenosis. The surgeon is likely to see flow through the anastomosis but not perceive a diminished intensity of the fluorescent dye. The estimation is made worse by the fact that the time to maximal intensity if one looks at the flow through the vessel only is the same whether there is a tight stenosis at the anastomosis or not. This technique cannot detect small differences over time [31]. Since arterial stenosis attenuates increases in ICG fluorescence intensity through vessels, quantitative analysis using NIR angiography could predict vessel stenosis. This quantitative assessment may provide a more precise evaluation of vessel stenosis or graft complications, as this ex vivo study was able to detect vessel stenosis exceeding 75%.

Clinical Results

The ability to reliably assess the patency of coronary artery bypass grafts using intraoperative fluorescence imaging has been shown to improve short-term patient outcomes after coronary artery bypass grafting [4] and to reduce hospital cost of CABG [5, 6].

SPY imaging has been the topic of a substantial body of evidence supporting its use in CABG surgery. In 2009, cardiac surgeon researchers presented results from 350 patients undergoing CABG including SPY imaging enrolled in the VICTORIA Multicenter Registry. VICTORIA data showed that the complication rates, including reoperation and long length of stay, were 50% lower than expected compared to similar patients enrolled in the Society of Thoracic Surgeons' (STS) national cardiac database. The STS database is one of the longest standing and largest existing medical datasets that exists today [4].

The Centers for Medicare and Medicaid Services independently studied cost data in 2008 and 2009 and concluded that the use of SPY in CABG resulted in average cost reductions of $2000–$4000 per patient (Table 7.1). In today's health-care environment, cost savings resulting from reductions in complications are critical to achieving the goals of health-care reform. Moreover, an improvement in graft patency will likely lead to a reduced readmission rate and hospital reimbursement penalties. This represented a 10% decrease in cost for the average CABG patient after the cost of the procedure was included [5]. Similar results were reported by the Sentara Heart Hospital [6].

A Sentara Heart Hospital independent study of more than 700 patients undergoing CABG demonstrated that total costs of CABG were 4.2% lower and average length of stay is 6–16% lower in 358 patients where the CABG procedure included SPY imaging versus the 225 cases performed without SPY.

The above improved clinical results and cost reductions using IFI during CABG surgery have helped to make a strong case for the use of IFI in all CABG cases.

Table 7.1 Results of a study performed by the Centers for Medicaid and Medicare Services to determine the cost saving associated with the use of SPY angiography

MS-DRG	Number of cases	Average length of stay	Average cost
Bypass + CATH + MCC with SPY	88	9.82	$29,258
Bypass + CATH+ MCC without SPY	10,224	11.14	$33,886
Other cardiac procedures + MCC with SPY	159	6.3	$22,342
CABG with CATH with SPY	60	12.82	$38,842
CABG with CATH without SPY	17,393	13.55	$41,207
CABG w/o CATH with SPY	69	8.75	$25,308
CABG w/o CATH without SPY	26,934	8.7	$29,334

On average, patients having IFI during CABG surgery realized a 10% hospital cost savings [12]. These savings occurred after taking into consideration the cost of performing the angiography

Pitfalls

This technology had several drawbacks. First, IFI does not provide an exact graft flow quantity measurement. Quantitative graft flow measurement software is currently being investigated but not accurate enough to be clinically useful. Second, the laser light source is of relatively low power to ensure safe clinical use. However, this limited the penetration of the light through tissue to about 2 mm. Thus, clear images could not be obtained when the coronary artery has a deep intramyocardial location or is covered by epicardial fat. The pedicled conduits with significant amounts of overlying tissue were also less well visualized. However, these investigators believed that full skeletonizing of the arterial conduits is a very useful and important technique for complete arterial revascularization of all the coronary vascular regions. The technique allows direct illumination of all bypass grafts (potentially difficult on the back of the heart). The entire graft often cannot be imaged in the same sequence by a single central injection. As a result of these drawbacks, Waseda et al. found that only 75% of the grafts were completely visualized [24]. While it appears IFI has an advantage over TTFM in sensitivity, it is also more cumbersome, time-consuming, and expensive.

The official position of The American College of Cardiology Foundation/American Heart Association guideline on "Coronary artery bypass graft surgery" [32] is "Over the past 20 years, the patency rate of all graft types has improved gradually, so that the present failure rate of LIMA grafts at 1 year is about 8 % and of SVGs roughly 20 %." Many patients being referred for CABG nowadays have far advanced CAD, which is often diffuse and exhibits poor vessel runoff. Technical issues at the time of surgery may influence graft patency, and intraoperative imaging may help to delineate technical from nontechnical issues. Because coronary angiography is rarely available intraoperatively, other techniques have been developed to assess graft integrity at this time, most often the transit-time flow and intraoperative fluorescence imaging. The transit-time flow is a quantitative volume-flow technique that cannot define the severity of graft stenosis or discriminate between the influence of the graft conduit and the coronary arteriolar bed on the mean graft flow. Intraoperative fluorescence imaging, which is based on the fluorescent properties of indocyanine green, provides a "semiquantitative" assessment of graft patency with images that provide some details about the quality of coronary anastomoses. Although both methods are valuable in assessing graft patency, neither is sufficiently sensitive or specific to allow identification of more subtle abnormalities. It is hoped that such imaging may help to reduce the occurrence of technical errors.

Conclusions

Intraoperative fluorescent imaging is a helpful technique to visualize coronary artery bypass grafts in real time. The technique has several drawbacks which are important to recognize; however, when used correctly, it is associated with improved clinical results and cost savings. Future research may allow more accurate myocardial blood flow quantification and recognize situations of competitive flow.

References

1. Desai ND, Miwa S, Kodama D, et al. Improving the quality of coronary bypass surgery with intraoperative angiography: validation of a new technique. J Am Coll Cardiol. 2005;46:1521–5.
2. Puskas JD, Williams WH, Mahoney EM, et al. Off-pump vs conventional coronary artery bypass grafting: early and 1-year graft patency, cost, and quality-of-life outcomes: a randomized trial. JAMA. 2004;291:1841–9.
3. Khan NE, De SA, Mister R, et al. A randomized comparison of off-pump and on-pump multivessel coronary-artery bypass surgery. N Engl J Med. 2004;350:21–8.
4. Ferguson TB, et al. Intra-operative angiography in CABG as a quality metric: the Victoria registry. Poster presented at the American Heart Association Meeting, Nov 2009.
5. Department of health and human Centers for Medicare & Medicaid Services 42 CFR Parts 412, 413, 415, and 489, [CMS-1406-P] RIN 0938-AP39, *Medicare Program; Proposed Changes to the*

Hospital Inpatient Prospective Payment Systems for Acute Care Hospitals and Fiscal Year 2010 Rates and to the Long-Term Care Hospital Prospective Payment System and Rate Year 2010 Rates, Sept 2009.

6. Data on File at Sentara Heart Hospital and NOVADAQ (Stryker, Kalamazoo Mich).

7. Balacumaraswami L, Taggert DP. Digital tools to facilitate intraoperative coronary artery bypass graft patency assessment. Semin Thorac Cardiovasc Surg. 2004;16:266–71.

8. Louagie YA, Haxhe JP, Buche M, et al. Intraoperative electromagnetic flowmeter measurements in coronary artery bypass grafts. Ann Thorac Surg. 1994;57:357–64.

9. Dennis J, Wyatt DG. Effects of hematocrit value upon electromagnetic flowmeter sensitivity. Circ Res. 1969;24:875–86.

10. Beard JD, Evans JM, Skidmore R, et al. A Doppler flowmeter for use in theatre. Ultrasound Med boil. 1986;12:883–9.

11. Haaverstad R, Vitale N, Williams RI, et al. Epicardial colour-Doppler scanning of coronary artery stenosis and graft anastomoses. Scand Cardiovasc J. 2002;36:95–9.

12. Falk V, Walther T, Philippi A, et al. Thermal coronary angiography for intraoperative patency control of arterial and saphenous vein coronary artery bypass grafts: results in 370 patients. J Card Surg. 1995;10:147–60.

13. D'Ancona G, Karamanoukian H, Ricci M, et al. Intraoperative graft patency verification in cardiac and vascular surgery. 1st ed. Armonk: Futura Publishing Company; 2001.

14. Mindich BP, BE, Rubinstein M, Urrutia CO, et al. Reduction of technical graft problems utilizing ultrasonic flow measurements. Presented at NY Thorac Society, 17 May 2001.

15. D'Ancona G, Karamanoukian H, Ricci M, et al. Myocardial revascularization on the beating heart after recent acute myocardial infarction. Heart Surg Forum. 2001;4:74–9.

16. Taggart DP, Choudhary B, Anastasiadis K, et al. Preliminary experience with a novel intraoperative fluorescence imaging technique to evaluate the patency of bypass grafts in total arterial revascularization. Ann Thorac Surg. 2003;75:870–3.

17. Canver CC, Dame NA. Ultrasonic assessment of internal thoracic artery graft flow in the revascularized heart. Ann Thorac Surg. 1994;58:135–8.

18. Jakobsen HL, Kjergard HK. Severe impairment of graft flow without electrocardiographic changes during coronary artery bypass grafting. Scand Cardiovasc J. 1999;33:157–9.

19. Walpoth BH, Bosshard A, Kipfer B, et al. Failed coronary artery bypass anastomosis detected by intraoperative coronary flow measurement. Eur J Cardiothorac Surg. 1998;14(Suppl 1):576–81.

20. Hirotani T, Kameda T, Shirota S, et al. An evaluation of the intraoperative transit time measurements of coronary bypass flow. Eur J Cardio Thorac Surg. 2001;19:848–52.

21. Speich R, Saesseli B, Hoffman U, et al. Anaphylactic reaction after indocyanine-green administration. Ann Intern Med. 1988;109:345–6.

22. Takahashi M, Ishikawa T, Higashidani K, Katoh H. SPY: an innovative intra-operative imaging system to evaluate graft patency during off-pump coronary artery bypass grafting. Interact Cardiovasc Thorac Surg. 2004;3:479–83.

23. Desai ND, Miwa S, Kodaama D, et al. A randomized comparison of intraoperative indocyanine green angiography and transit-time flow measurement to detect technical errors in coronary artery bypass grafts. J Thorac Cardiovasc Surg. 2006;132:585–94.

24. Waseda K, Ako J, Hasegawa T, et al. Intraoperative Fluorescence imaging system for on-site assessment of off-pump coronary artery bypass graft. J Am Coll Cardiol Img. 2009;2:604–12.

25. Detter C, Wipper S, Russ D, Iffland A, Burdorf L, Thein E, et al. Fluorescent cardiac imaging: a novel intraoperative method for quantitative assessment of myocardial perfusion during graded coronary artery stenosis. Circulation. 2007;116(9):1007–14.

26. Yamamoto M, Orihashi K, Nishimori H, Wariishi S, Fukutomi T, Kondo N, et al. Indocyanine green angiography for intra-operative assessment in vascular surgery. Eur J Vasc Endovasc Surg. 2012;43(4):426–32.

27. Ferguson TB Jr, Chen C, Babb JD, et al. Fractional flow reserve-guided coronary artery bypass grafting: can intraoperative physiologic imaging guide decision making? J Thorac Cardiovasc Surg. 2013;146(4):824–35.

28. Sabik J. Discussion to: Ferguson TB Jr, Chen C, Babb JD, et al. Fractional flow reserve-guided coronary artery bypass grafting: can intraoperative physiologic imaging guide decision making? J Thorac Cardiovasc Surg. 2013;146(4):824–35.

29. Yamamoto M, Sasaguri S, Sato T. Assessing intraoperative blood fow in cardiovascular surgery. Surg Today. 2011;41(11):1467–74.

30. Yamamoto M, Orihashi K, Nishimori H, Handa T, Kondo N, Fukutomi T, et al. Efficacy of intraoperative HyperEye Medical System angiography for coronary artery bypass grafting. Surg Today. 2015;45(8):966–72.

31. Benson RC, Kues HA. Fluorescence properties of indocyanine green as related to angiography. Phys Med Biol. 1978;23(1):159–63.

32. Hills KD, Smith PK, Bittl JL, et al. 2100 ACCF/AHA Guidelines for coronary artery bypass graft surgery. A report of the American College of Cardiology Foundation/American Heart Association task force on practice guidelines. Developed in collaboration with the American Association for Thoracic Surgery. Society of Cardiovascular Anesthesiologist, and Society of Thoracic Surgeons. J Am Coll Cardiol. 2011;58(24):e 123–210.

Lung Segmentation: The Combination of Lung Volume Analyzer VINCENT for Measuring Resection Margin and ICG Anatomical Segmentectomy

Yasuo Sekine

Indication

Operative indications are as follows:

- Early-stage lung cancer, defined as a maximum diameter of tumor consolidation of 2 cm or shorter in the peripheral region without any evidence of nodal and distant metastasis (c-stage IA1 or IA2) (active limited resection)
- Metastatic lung tumor amenable to sublobar resection
- Benign diseases such as suspected benign tumor in the intermediate portion
- A lung cancer patient at high risk due to exacerbated cardiopulmonary function or poor general condition who is not a candidate for lobectomy (c-stage IA1 to IA3) (passive limited resection).
- Exclusion criteria are a history of iodine allergy and patient refusal.

Electronic Supplementary Material The online version of this chapter (https://doi.org/10.1007/978-3-030-38092-2_8) contains supplementary material, which is available to authorized users.

Y. Sekine (✉)
Department of Thoracic Surgery, Tokyo Women's Medical University Yachiyo Medical Center, Yachiyo, Chiba, Japan
e-mail: sekine.yasuo@twmu.ac.jp

Technical Description of the Procedure

Creation of Virtual Segmentectomy

Before surgery, high-resolution CT, three-dimensional (3D) pulmonary angiography and virtual bronchoscopy are performed to confirm tumor location and associated vessels and bronchi. Several simulated sublobar resections are performed in order to determine the appropriate tumor resection margin. In detail, subjects undergo multislice enhanced CT, using 320-slice scanners to create pulmonary angiography and virtual bronchoscopy, to simulate anatomical sublobar resection, and to measure lung volume by the volume analyzer Synapse 3D VINCENT (Fujifilm Co., Tokyo, Japan) for planning sublobar resection before operation. The shortest distance from the tumor to the resection margin is measured by VINCENT, and the most appropriate area of sublobar resection is selected based on the following criteria: resection margin approximately 2 cm from the tumor or greater than the tumor diameter (Fig. 8.1).

Transbronchial ICG Injection

After induction of general anesthesia, a single-lumen endotracheal tube or laryngeal mask is introduced for transbronchial ICG instillation.

© Springer Nature Switzerland AG 2020
E. M. Aleassa, K. M. El-Hayek (eds.), *Video Atlas of Intraoperative Applications of Near Infrared Fluorescence Imaging*, https://doi.org/10.1007/978-3-030-38092-2_8

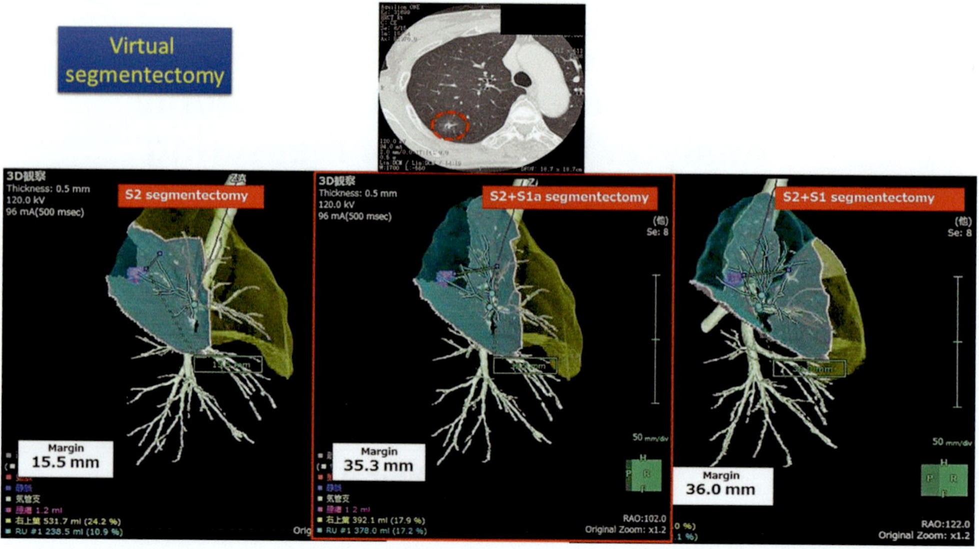

Fig. 8.1 Construction images of virtual segmentectomy. The most appropriate segmentectomy with enough margin can be selected

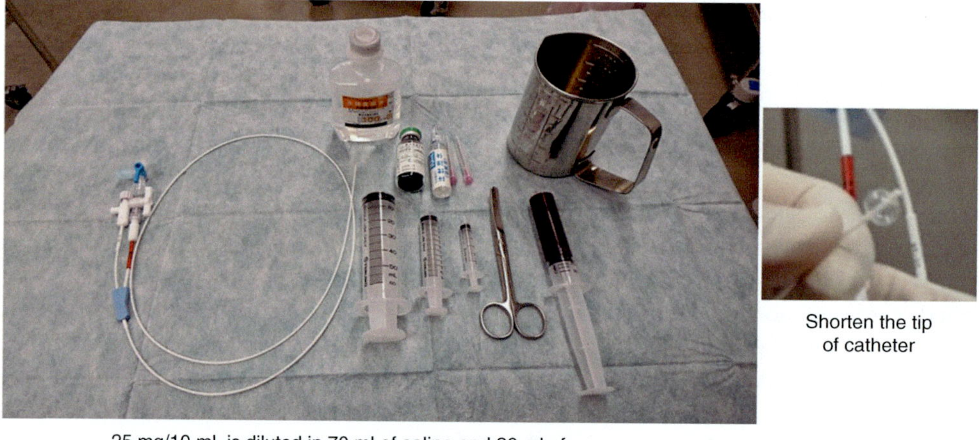

Fig. 8.2 Preparation for transbronchial instillation of ICG

ICG, 25 mg/10 ml, is diluted in 70 ml of saline and 20 ml of autologous blood (AB) for a tenfold diluted ICG solution (Fig. 8.2) because adsorption of ICG to human serum albumin can increase its fluorescence intensity (Video 8.1).

With the patient in a supine position, a thin bronchoscope (BF-P260F, Olympus Medical Co., Tokyo, Japan) is inserted into the targeted bronchus. A bronchial catheter with balloon (Olympus disposable balloon catheter B5-2C/2LA, Olympus Medical Co., Tokyo, Japan) is inserted, and the balloon is inflated at the orifice of the bronchus. Ten millimeter of the tenfold saline-AB-diluted ICG is instilled into each target subsegmental bronchus, and 300–400 ml of air is then directed into the bronchus to distribute ICG to the peripheral regions. During this maneuver, the bronchoscope is fitted over the balloon to prohibit ICG leakage and to visualize the tip of the catheter over the balloon (Video 8.2). After ICG instillation, a double-lumen Broncho-Cath tube is introduced, and 5 cm H_2O

of positive end-expiratory pressure ventilation is maintained until the start of the operation. The approximate time from the ICG instillation to the start of operation is 20–30 minutes.

Anatomical Sublobar Resection

At the beginning of the operation, a near-infrared (NIR) thoracoscope (PINPOINT, Stryker, MI, USA) is used to visualize the intersegmental lines and planes. The visceral pleura is marked using electrocautery along the border of the ICG fluorescence. Simultaneous vascular and bronchial division and segmental division can be performed based on the initial identification of segmental planes. Finally, the intersegmental planes are divided by electrocautery and/or endo-staplers to complete the sublobar resection. After complete resection, the infrared thoracoscope can identify that no residual tissues should be resected. Sufficient distance from the tumor to the resection margin is measured on the resected specimen (Figs. 8.3, 8.4, and 8.5; Video 8.3). The types of segmentectomy include the following: subsegmental resection; simple segmentectomy,

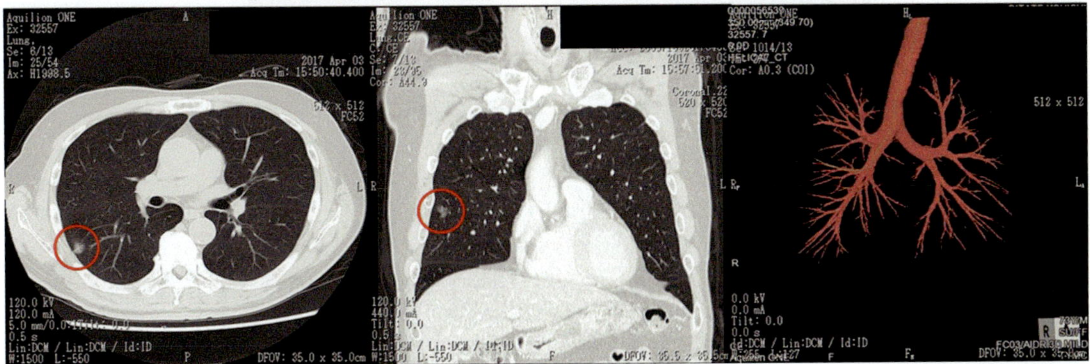

Fig. 8.3 Preoperative CT image: 77-year-old male; right S6b primary lung cancer (consolidation 6 mm, consolidation tumor ratio = 73%)

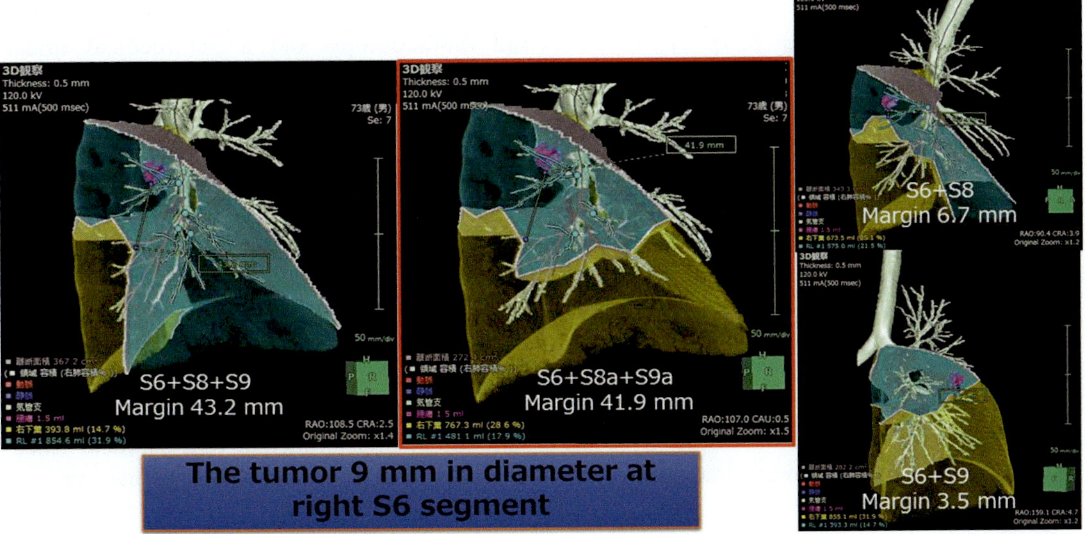

Fig. 8.4 Simulation of lung segmentectomy by 3D-CT image analyzer VINCENT

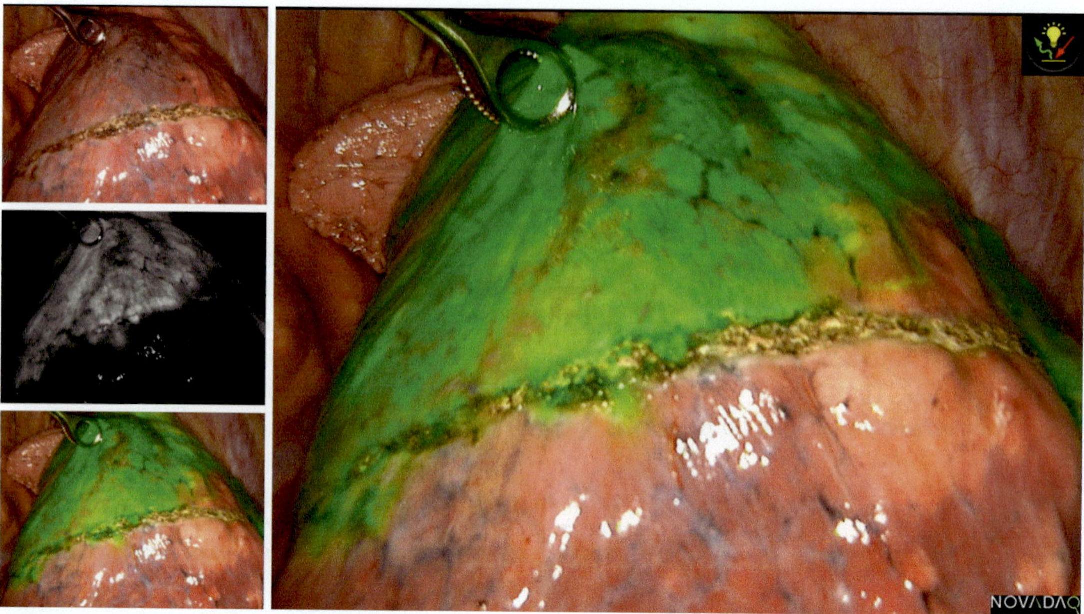

Fig. 8.5 Intraoperative fluorescence image. A clear border can be identified

defined as a simple plane cut with the pulmonary division, i.e., S6; basal, left lingual, and left upper division segmentectomy; complex segmentectomy, defined as multiple planes of the pulmonary division; and extended segmentectomy, defined as segmentectomy with adjacent subsegmental resection.

Interpretation

We previously developed and reported a novel approach for performing segmentectomy by using infrared thoracoscopy with transbronchial instillation of indocyanine green (ICG) [1] and have since improved upon this method. The advantages of this method are as follows:

1. Applicability to any type of sublobar resection
2. Initial determination of resection area at operation
3. Possible anatomical partial resection of the lung (APaRL) with enough margin without individual broncho-vascular transection (Figs. 8.6 and 8.7)
4. Only transection of vessels and bronchi heading for resected lung
5. Long identification of fluorescence
6. Possible operability in case of COPD, interstitial pneumonia, reoperation, and adhesions.

On the other hand, the limitations of this method include (1) the necessity of near-infrared thoracoscopy and a 3D medical image analyzer, (2) knowledge of precise bronchial anatomy, (3) advanced bronchoscopy skills, and (4) initial nonuniform distribution of ICG and distribution of ICG into adjacent areas with the passage of time.

Volume analyzer Synapse 3D VINCENT is a highly advanced technology for visualizing 3D organ structures [2]. It allows physicians to perform a simulation before the operation and minimize excision volume. However, it can be difficult to precisely match the operation with the simulation. Transbronchial ICG-sublobar resection is an ideal procedure to bridge this gap.

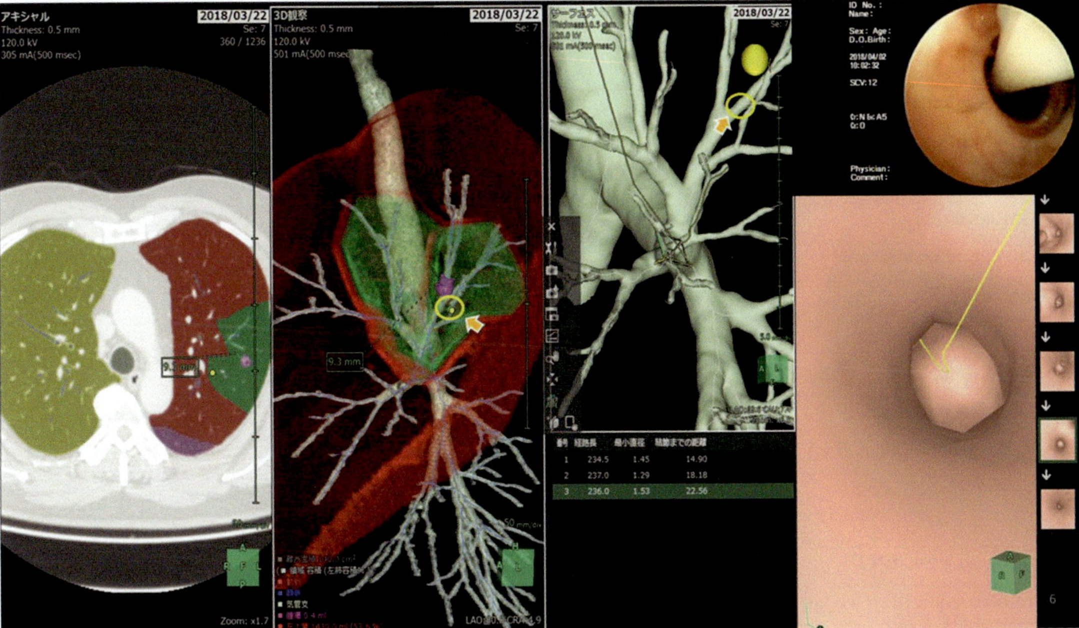

Fig. 8.6 The preoperative image of anatomical partial resection of the lung (APaRL). The yellow circle indicates the position of virtual bronchoscope and matched with the vision of real scope

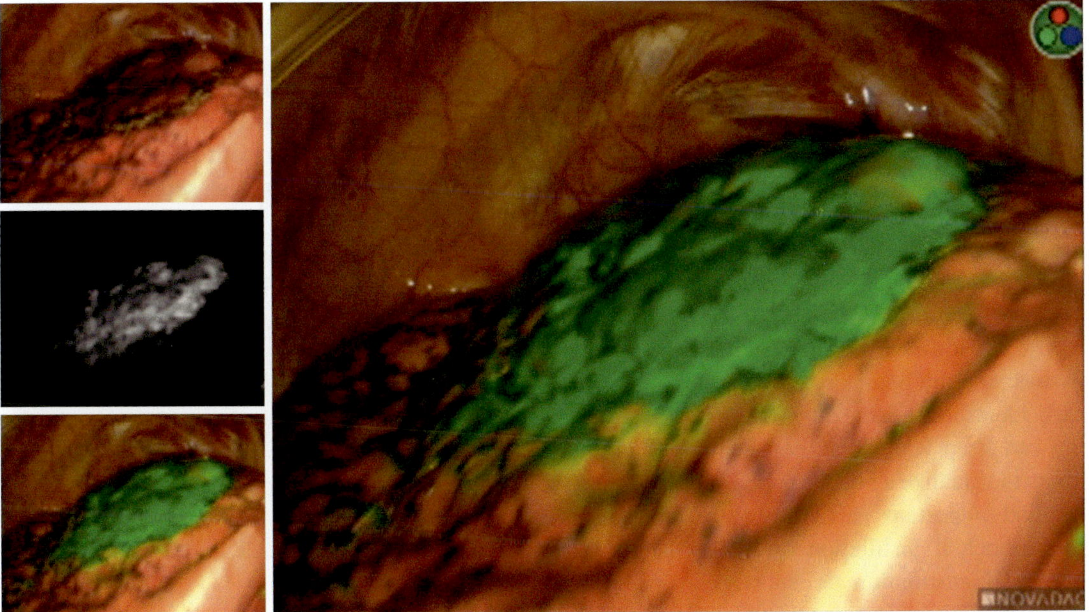

Fig. 8.7 Intraoperative fluorescence image of APaRL. A clear border can be identified, and the image is well matched with the simulation

Table 8.1 Comparison between intravenous and transbronchial injection of ICG

	Intravenous (negative staining)	Transbronchial (positive staining)
Easy manipulation	◎	△
Clear visibility	◎	◎~○
Stable technique	◎	◎~△
Low invasiveness	◎	○
Easy to define transactable vessels and bronchus	○	◎
Uniformity of ICG	◎	◎~△
Duration of fluorescence	△	◎
Operation time	◎	○
Repeated ICG injection	◎	×
Apply for the complicated segmentectomy	○~△	◎
COPD/IP/reop/adhesion	△	◎
Cost	○	△
Affinity with VINCENT	○	◎
Anatomical super deep wedge resection (ASDWR)	×	◎

◎ highly applicable, ○ well applicable, △ not so satisfied, × not suitable

The use of ICG and an infrared thoracoscope in order to identify the borderline of lung resection has been reported by several authors [3, 4]. Since these methods are mainly intravenous injection of ICG, we compared between negative staining by intravenous injection and positive staining by transbronchial instillation (Table 8.1). Negative staining is an easy manipulated, clearly visible, stable technique with low invasiveness because of one intravenous injection of ICG. Although the visibility of the boundary line continues for a short time, ICG injection can be repeated. However, this method stains all body tissues, and the boundary line cannot be specifically identified. On the other hand, positive staining can keep ICG fluorescence for a couple of hours to visualize a boundary line. The most critical and important part of positive staining is transbronchial instillation of ICG. Once transbronchial instillation is successful, the ICG boundary line is continuously visible, and complicated sublobar resection can be made easier. Furthermore, when we hesitate to decide whether small vessels and bronchi should be transected, we can only treat them with heading for resection tissue. This is a significant advantage in compli-cated sublobar resection. However, if ICG is instilled into the wrong bronchus, surgery may be confusing because rechallenge is impossible.

Anatomical partial resection of the lung (APaRL) is a novel concept and approach for a small lung nodule which is defined as a deep partial lung resection along with subsegmental septum. Each subsegment is separated by an intersegmental septum, and pulmonary vessels and bronchi do not cross the septum. Therefore, when the intersegmental plane is given bilateral tractions and cut by electrocautery, the lung is naturally divided along to the plane. Minimal bleeding and air leak are observed in such cases. The associated small vessels and bronchi can be stapled at the deepest portion. Therefore, APaRL along to the septum is possible (Video 8.4).

Pitfalls

Pitfalls include (1) the necessity of a near-infrared thoracoscopy and 3D medical image analyzer, (2) knowledge of precise bronchial anatomy, (3) advanced manipulation skills of bronchoscopy, and (4) initial nonuniform distribution of ICG and distribution of ICG into the adjacent area with the passage of time.

If ICG is instilled into the wrong bronchus, surgery may be difficult and confusing because rechallenge is impossible. To reduce this problem, we apply precise virtual bronchoscopy to identify bronchi into which we should inject ICG and a bronchial balloon catheter to prohibit ICG leakage.

Summary

In summary, the combination of virtual sublobar resection and ICG-guided sublobar resection using transbronchial ICG injection is applicable to any type of sublobar resection. This technique is an advancement over current techniques because of the additional improvements such as the injection technique and intraoperative confirmation of the ICG injection areahis technique is an advancement over current techniques because of the additional improvements such as the injection technique and intraoperative confirmation of the icg injection area.

References

1. Sekine Y, Koh E, Oishi H, Miwa M. A simple and effective technique for identification of intersegmental planes by infrared thoracoscopy after transbronchial injection of indocianine green. J Thorac Cardiovasc Surg. 2012;143:1330–5.
2. Oshiro Y, Ohkohchi N. Three-dimensional liver surgery simulation: computer-assisted surgical planning with three-dimensional simulation software and three-dimensional printing. Tissue Eng Part A. 2017;23:474–80.
3. Misaki N, Chang SS, Gotoh M, Yamamoto Y, Satoh K, Yokomise H. A novel method for determining adjacent lung segments with infrared thoracoscopy. J Thorac Cardiovasc Surg. 2009;138:613–8.
4. Mun M, Nakao M, Matsuura Y, Ichinose J, Nakagawa K, Okumura S. Thoracoscopic segmentectomy for small-sized peripheral lung cancer. J Thorac Dis. 2018;10:3738–44.

Part IV

Applications in Foregut Surgery

Juliana de Paula Machado Henrique,
Fernando Dip, Emanuele Lo Menzo,
and Raul J. Rosenthal

Introduction

Since the first description of esophagectomy, many different technical variations have been described in order to decrease the frequently associated complications [1]. Among these complications, the most dreaded remains anastomotic leakage. Based on the technique utilized, the anastomosis leakage can occur either in the thorax or in the neck, with different outcomes and prognosis. Often, anastomotic leaks increase hospital stay and mortality [2]. Several factors contribute to the high leakage rate after esophagectomies. Among these, we can identify patient-specific, anatomical, and technical factors. Often, patients undergoing esophageal surgery are more likely to have significant comorbidities (especially cardiopulmonary) secondary also to lifestyle habits, such as smoking and drinking. Furthermore, these patients typically present feeding difficulties due to the primary disease and the abovementioned lifestyle habits. The presence of malnutrition associated with high-grade dysphagia or in association with side effects of neoadjuvant radiation and chemotherapy is also considered one of the major risk factors for anastomotic leakage. The anatomical peculiarities of this operation also contribute significantly to the high incidence of leakage at the anastomosis, in particular the often tenuous blood supply of the gastric pull up and remaining esophagus [3, 4]. The introduction of minimally invasive approaches to esophagectomies, on the one hand, has reduced many of the comorbidities associated with this procedure, but on the other hand, it has not improved the incidence of leaks [5]. For many years, surgeons have relied on subjective ways to assess blood supply of the organs before and after an anastomosis. However, these methodologies are often imprecise and cumbersome. More recently, the introduction of fluorescence in the assessment of organ and anastomotic perfusion has gained popularity based on its safety and reliability.

Electronic Supplementary Material The online version of this chapter (https://doi.org/10.1007/978-3-030-38092-2_9) contains supplementary material, which is available to authorized users.

J. de Paula Machado Henrique · E. Lo Menzo
R. J. Rosenthal (✉)
Department of General Surgery, The Bariatric and Metabolic Institute, Cleveland Clinic Florida, Weston, FL, USA
e-mail: ROSENTR@CCF.ORG

F. Dip
Hospital de Clinicas Jose de San Martin, Buenos Aires, Argentina

Background

Fluorescence imaging (FI) is widely used in biomedical science for the visualization of cells and tissues, both in vivo and in vitro. This method gives accurate anatomic and qualitative information of the visualized tissue. Besides its easy applicability and safety, the FI techniques are inexpensive and do not present a steep learning curve. The FI techniques are based on the premise of emission of different wavelengths of light by the injected substances as compared to the background [6]. In this regard, many substances with the characteristics of emitting different wavelength light after being excited with infrared light (fluorophores) have been used. Among these, indocyanine green (ICG) remains the most commonly used since its first approval for clinical use in 1959. In fact, ICG has been routinely used for several clinical applications, from the measurement of cardiac and hepatic flow in the 1950s to retinal angiography in the 1970s.

ICG angiography (ICGA) FI is based on the principle that when the tissue containing the fluorophore is illuminated with near-infrared light (NIR wavelength of 750–800 nm), it emits fluorescence at a higher wavelength (over 800 mm) that can be captured with a filtered camera. The current availability of several cameras and video systems with the capability of filtering the light, for both open and laparoscopic surgery, has contributed to the more widespread application of the technique [6]. ICG has the characteristic of binding to plasma proteins and can quickly reach organs via the bloodstream. ICG is also well tolerated by patients and has a short lifetime in blood circulation, allowing repeat injections. However, since ICG is exclusively extracted by the liver into the bile, it is contraindicated in patients with severe liver dysfunction. Also, ICG is normally combined with sodium iodide to improve its solubility; therefore, it is contraindicated in patients with iodine allergy. An iodine-free version of ICG, named infracyanine green (IFCG) (SERB Laboratories, Paris, France), also known as *IFC green*, is thought to be less cytotoxic than ICG in macular applications and could be used for those patients with an allergy to iodine [6].

ICG Applications in Surgery

There are several ICG perfusion and imaging applications in the surgical field, ranging from assessment of liver and cardiac function to lym-

phography in cancer [6]. Among the several applications of ICG, the assessment of tissue perfusion has been the area with the most expansion. Perfusion evaluation with ICG is performed via intravenous injection prior to surgery, at the time of anesthesia induction, or a few seconds before the assessment, based on the organ to visualize. The intramucosal injection, instead, is utilized for lymph node identification. In neuroscience, ICG FI has been used as a complement for the identification of cerebral aneurysms [7–9]. Recently, near-infrared incisionless fluorescent cholangiography (NIFC) is emerging as a promising tool to enhance the visualization of extrahepatic biliary structures during laparoscopic cholecystectomies. Dip et al. conducted a randomized controlled trial with 649 patients in which NIFC was statistically superior to white light alone in visualizing extrahepatic biliary structures [10]. Also, FI has been proven to be an effective tool to assess anastomotic perfusion and seems to reduce anastomotic leakage rates following colorectal surgery for cancer [11, 12]. Shimada et al. performed an evaluation of ICG fluorescence method of harvesting lymph nodes (LNs) from resected specimens. Fluorescence allowed easy, highly sensitive, and real-time imaging-guided sentinel lymph node mapping in patients with colorectal cancer. Fluorescence-labeled LNs were found even when ICG solution was injected ex vivo and observed in paraffin-embedded specimens that provided precise evaluation of the LNs' pathological status, including sentinel LNs after surgery [12].

Esophagectomy: Surgical Options

The esophagus uniquely occupies three different anatomic areas—the neck, thorax, and abdomen. Also, its histological characteristic of lacking serosa and the potentially tenuous blood supply make it a challenging organ to reconstruct. Several esophagectomy techniques have been described over the years; however, the two most commonly employed open techniques are transhiatal esophagectomy (THE) and Ivor Lewis esophagectomy (ILE) [5]. In spite of some differences between the two options, significant morbidity and mortality are described for both. Orringer et al. published a review on a 30-year experience with 2007 THE performed at a single institution. In the series, the stomach was the esophageal substitute in 97% of the cases. The hospital mortality rate has steadily fallen as the volume of THE operations increased. Early mortality rate was 10% from 1978 to 1982, with an average of 23 THE operations annually, to 1%, with more than 100 THE operations annually [13]. Sauvanet et al. reported data collected on 1192 patients who underwent surgery for gastroesophageal junction adenocarcinoma from 1985 to 2000. Operative mortality rates decreased with time: 11% from 1985 to 1990 to 6% from 1996 to 2000. At least one complication (including death) occurred in each of 423 patients (35%). Anastomotic leakage was diagnosed in 104 patients (9%) and 22 of those patients have died (21%) [5, 14]. The transthoracic esophagectomy (TTE) is a less performed option, secondary due to its potentially added morbidity and mortality of the chest portion of the approach. The 2001 meta-analysis of 7527 patients undergoing either THE or TTE (Ivor Lewis esophagectomy/Sweet procedure) for carcinoma between 1990 and 1999 documented a statistically significant difference favoring THE over TTE in terms of hospital mortality, blood loss, pulmonary complications, chylothorax, intensive care unit (ICU) stay, and hospital stay. However, TTE patients had lower anastomotic leak rates than THE patients and a lower incidence of vocal cord paralysis [15]. Other less utilized esophagectomy techniques include left thoracoabdominal approach or three-incision McKeown-type esophagectomy [5].

Minimally Invasive Esophagectomy (MIE)

In an effort to reduce the morbidity of esophagectomy, minimally invasive esophagectomy (MIE) methods began to be increasingly utilized in the 1990s [5]. A multicenter randomized trial comparing traditional versus minimally invasive esophagectomy (TIME-Trial) was published in 2011 by Biere et al. As expected, the MIE group had fewer pulmonary complications [16]. In a recent meta-analysis comparing open and minimally invasive approaches, MIE was found to be superior to open esophagectomy, secondary to fewer perioperative complications and lower in-hospital mortality [17]. As previously stated, however, the anastomotic leakage rate remains significantly higher than in other gastrointestinal procedures.

Anastomotic Perfusion: Before ICG

The effect of ischemia on anastomotic dehiscence rates is well documented [3, 18–20]. The tenuous blood supply to the gastric conduit constitutes one of the major risk factors for anastomotic leakage after esophagectomy. Over the years, several attempts were made to increase the vascular supply of the conduit. Similar to the application in other procedures (i.e., liver resections), the idea of an ischemic conditioning by ligating the left gastric and short gastric vessels at the time of staging laparoscopy or pretreatment jejunostomy placement was developed [21, 22]. Nguyen et al. studied 81 patients who underwent laparoscopic staging with gastric ischemic conditioning. Despite the limitations of the study, the results support that gastric ischemic conditioning probably does not play a major role in the clinical reduction of postoperative leaks and strictures [23].

Several techniques have been described to assess the blood supply of organs and anastomosis intraoperatively. Among these are polarographic measurement of oxygen tension, visible light spectroscopy, Doppler ultrasound, radioisotope studies, laser Doppler flowmetry, and others, but only visible light spectroscopy and laser Doppler flowmetry were largely studied in human subjects [24–26].

ICG and Esophagectomy

The evaluation of the microcirculation in gastrointestinal organs has only been recently studied. In fact, Okamoto et al. published preliminary experiments in swine, and one of the first clinical evaluations of ICG perfusion was conducted in 20 patients with esophageal varices [27, 28]. Shimada et al. presented a series of 40 consecutive esophagectomies with the use of ICG FI to visualize the blood supply of the anastomosis [26]. Shimada concluded that ICG could detect organ blood flow before reconstruction and assist in evaluating the appropriate anastomotic sites. However, he found that the incidence of anastomotic leakage was not reduced (7.5%) [26]. Additional case series or case reports were then published correlating gastric pull up necrosis with areas of ICG-visualized ischemia [29, 30]. At this point, it was clear that ICG angiography could distinguish the ischemic and nonischemic areas. Murawa et al., in their retrospective study, concluded that ICG angiography for evaluation of gastric conduit perfusion during esophagectomy is a simple, safe, inexpensive, and expeditious technique [31]. With the increase in popularity of ICG FI among researchers, several larger additional reports were published [32–36]. The ability of ICG to assess perfusion was then utilized for more accurate and extensive evaluations during esophagectomies.

A prospective cohort study from Japan assessed the hemodynamics of the gastroepiploic vessels in 20 patients undergoing esophagectomy, distinguishing between good blood flow and sparse blood flow. They also calculated the median time to perfusion of the tip of the gastric tube between both groups. Overall, there were no statistically significant differences in postoperative leaks in the two groups. Nevertheless, despite the low number of cases, there was an important outcome: two patients had necrosis of the gastric tube with the flow time to the tip around 103 and 141 seconds [33]. This was the first attempt to analyze flow time and correlate it to ischemia. In a larger prospective cohort study by Zehetner et al. including 150 patients, the perfusion of the gastric graft was assessed and correlated to subsequent anastomotic leak after esophagectomy. The overall leakage rate was 16.7%, but only 2% occurred in the group considered with good perfusion, whereas a 45% leakage rate was found in the less robust perfusion group [37]. Campbell

et al. published a similar outcome regarding anastomotic leaks. This retrospective cohort study came about with 90 patients who underwent esophagectomy with gastric conduit reconstruction. ICG FI contributed to an unexpected absence of leakage in the experimental group versus a 20% leakage rate in the control group [38]. At the same time, Kamiya et al., in a retrospective series of 26 cases of pharyngolaryngoesophagectomy, reported that the quantitative analysis of ICG fluorescence angiography was useful in detecting venous anastomotic failure of free jejunal graft. None of the patients had anastomotic leaks, although two of them progressed to graft necrosis. According to the authors, these findings were due to venous thrombosis after the surgery [39].

In another prospective cohort study on the rate of perfusion of the gastric conduit of 40 patients, Koyanagi et al. found that neither the dose of ICG injected nor the arterial blood pressure during ICG FI was associated with the flow speed of ICG fluorescence. In this study, the number of leaks in the group with simultaneous flow of both the gastric wall and the greater curvature vessels was zero, whereas seven leaks occurred in the delayed flow group [40]. More recently, Degett et al. conducted a systematic review of all clinical trials on fluorescent perfusion assessment during esophagectomy (214 patients) and concluded that leaks tend to be lower in the well-perfused area of the anastomosis [41]. Noma et al., in a single-center retrospective cohort trial of 285 subjects, showed that the objective perfusion evaluation of the reconstructed conduit using ICG FI reduces the risk and degree of anastomotic complication [42]. This result is in agreement with the study by Ohi et al., in which the lack of ICG imaging was an independent risk factor for anastomotic leakage (p value <0.01) [43].

ICG angiography in the assessment of gastric conduit perfusion has been used not only for qualitative analysis but also for quantitative measures, based on the time of perfusion. In fact, Kumagai et al. hypothesized that the risk of anastomotic leakage might be minimized if the anastomosis was performed in the area that was enhanced within 60 seconds of ICG injection

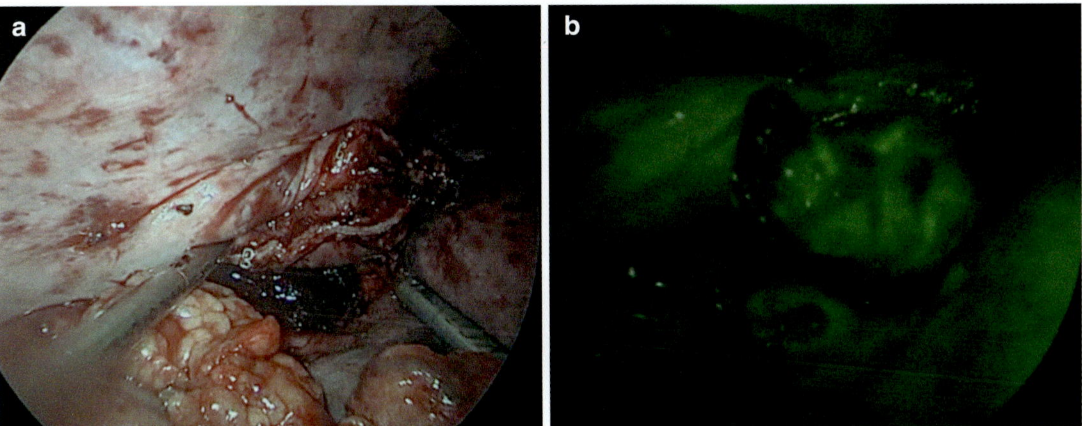

Fig. 9.1 Esophageal stump in the thorax, before (**a**) and after (**b**) ICG fluorescence imaging, during minimally invasive Ivor Lewis esophagectomy

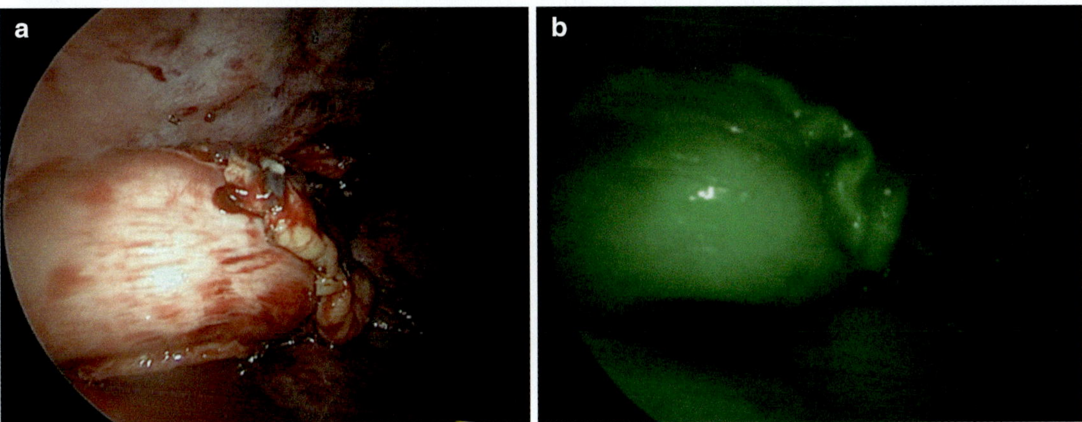

Fig. 9.2 Gastric stump in the thorax, before (**a**) and after (**b**) ICG fluorescence imaging, during minimally invasive Ivor Lewis esophagectomy

[44]. Also, the visualization of the esophageal stump perfusion is important for a successful anastomosis (Fig. 9.1a, b). This area can be visualized during the first ICG injection, or during required additional ones. Repeating the ICG evaluation after the completion of the gastro-esophageal anastomosis could help surgeons verify if the perfusion assessment of the organ is still adequate and comparable to before the anastomosis [26, 29, 45, 46].

Finally, a recent meta-analysis of 17 studies by Ladak et al. found a leakage rate of 5.7% (15/261) in the ICG group vs. 22.9% (89/388) in the control group. This represents an absolute risk reduction of 69 [47].

Technical Description of the Procedure

The evaluation of the perfusion is initially conducted on the gastric pull-up. This evaluation can be performed either while the gastric conduit still resides in the abdominal cavity or at its final location (thorax or neck) (Fig. 9.2a, b). Before the anastomosis, ICG is injected intravenously. The operating room lights are then dimmed. Depending on the approach used, open vs. minimally invasive, the appropriate camera device is used to excite the fluorophore with near-infrared light. The devices designed for open surgery must be held between 20 and

30 cm above the target. If a minimally invasive procedure is conducted, the camera system must have the capability to emit the near-infrared light and capture images in the adequate wavelength. This is usually done by use of a pedal that shifts from the white light to the near-infrared light (Video 9.1).

Near-infrared perfusion assessment has been reported in robotic assisted minimally invasive esophagectomy [34]. Currently, there is no consensus on the ideal ICG dosage. In fact, in reviewing 30 published articles regarding ICG and esophagus, from 2005 to 2019, the dose ranged between 1.25 and 25 mg. In three studies, the dosages were expressed in mg/kg (0.1 and 0.5 mg/kg) [32, 48, 49]. In 11 of them, the ICG dose was 2.5 mg [26, 30, 33, 35, 37, 40, 41, 43, 44, 50, 51]. Within a short period of time, the intravascular fluorescence becomes visible. Obviously, the non-perfused area will remain dark.

Pitfalls

Overall, ICG angiography results in accurate assessment of organ perfusion. However, several pitfalls and unanswered questions remain. Obesity, especially the visceral type, might reduce the ability of visualizing the perfusing vessels, due to limited penetration of the near-infrared light [34]. Other factors that might contribute to inaccurate assessment of the perfusion are venostasis, tension at the anastomosis, variation in systemic arterial pressure, and intramural ecchymosis [26, 35, 36, 49, 52]. ICG FI has not been proven to identify venous poor outflow. Also, venous thrombosis can occur after adequate flow shown intraoperatively [39]. Furthermore, the optimal dose of ICG remains undetermined. It is possible that the change in dose might influence the visual results of perfusion. Lastly, the interpretation of ICG perfusion remains mostly dependent on the subjective evaluation of the surgeon. An objective quantitative analysis of the perfusion is necessary in order to achieve more accurate and reproducible results.

Conclusion

Near-infrared ICG FI is a novel technique that may guide surgeons to perform a safer anastomosis. However, lack of objective quantification is of critical importance. Based on the safe, practical, and inexpensive characteristics of this technique, it is feasible to foresee wider acceptance in the near future.

References

1. Turner GG, Grey Turner G. Carcinoma of the (esophagus the question of its treatment by surgery). Lancet. 1936;227:130–4.
2. Wright CD, Kucharczuk JC, O'Brien SM, Grab JD, Allen MS, Society of Thoracic Surgeons General Thoracic Surgery Database. Predictors of major morbidity and mortality after esophagectomy for esophageal cancer: a Society of Thoracic Surgeons General Thoracic Surgery Database risk adjustment model. J Thorac Cardiovasc Surg. 2009;137:587–95; discussion 596.
3. Thompson SK, Chang EY, Jobe BA. Clinical review: healing in gastrointestinal anastomoses, part I. Microsurgery. 2006;26:131–6.
4. Lorentz T, Fok M, Wong J. Anastomotic leakage after resection and bypass for esophageal cancer: lessons learned from the past. World J Surg. 1989;13:472–7.
5. Kim T, Hochwald SN, Sarosi GA, Caban AM, Rossidis G, Ben-David K. Review of minimally invasive esophagectomy and current controversies. Gastroenterol Res Pract. 2012;2012:683213.
6. Alander JT, Kaartinen I, Laakso A, Pätilä T, Spillmann T, Tuchin VV, Venermo M, Välisuo P. A review of indocyanine green fluorescent imaging in surgery. Int J Biomed Imaging. 2012;2012:1–26.
7. Kato Y, Balamurugan S, Agrawal A, Sano H. Intraoperative indocyanine green video-angiography in cerebrovascular surgery: an overview with review of literature. Asian J Neurosurg. 2011;6:88.
8. Roessler K, Krawagna M, Dörfler A, Buchfelder M, Ganslandt O. Essentials in intraoperative indocyanine green videoangiography assessment for intracranial aneurysm surgery: conclusions from 295 consecutively clipped aneurysms and review of the literature. Neurosurg Focus. 2014;36:E7.
9. Catapano G, Sgulò F, Laleva L, Columbano L, Dallan I, de Notaris M. Multimodal use of indocyanine green endoscopy in neurosurgery: a single-center experience and review of the literature. Neurosurg Rev. 2018;41:985–98.
10. Dip F, LoMenzo E, Sarotto L, et al. Randomized trial of near-infrared incisionless fluorescent chol-

angiography. Ann Surg. 2019;270:992. https://doi.org/10.1097/SLA.0000000000003178.

11. Blanco-Colino R, Espin-Basany E. Intraoperative use of ICG fluorescence imaging to reduce the risk of anastomotic leakage in colorectal surgery: a systematic review and meta-analysis. Tech Coloproctol. 2018;22:15–23.

12. Shimada S, Ohtsubo S, Kusano M. Applications of ICG fluorescence imaging for surgery in colorectal cancers. In: Fluorescence imaging for surgeons; 2015. p. 203–8.

13. Orringer MB, Marshall B, Chang AC, Lee J, Pickens A, Lau CL. Two thousand transhiatal esophagectomies: changing trends, lessons learned. Ann Surg. 2007;246:363–72; discussion 372–4.

14. Sauvanet A, Mariette C, Thomas P, et al. Mortality and morbidity after resection for adenocarcinoma of the gastroesophageal junction: predictive factors. J Am Coll Surg. 2005;201:253–62.

15. Hulscher JB, Tijssen JG, Obertop H, van Lanschot JJ. Transthoracic versus transhiatal resection for carcinoma of the esophagus: a meta-analysis. Ann Thorac Surg. 2001;72:306–13.

16. Biere SS, Maas KW, Bonavina L, et al. Traditional invasive vs. minimally invasive esophagectomy: a multi-center, randomized trial (TIME-trial). BMC Surg. 2011;11:2.

17. Yibulayin W, Abulizi S, Lv H, Sun W. Minimally invasive oesophagectomy versus open esophagectomy for resectable esophageal cancer: a meta-analysis. World J Surg Oncol. 2016;14:304.

18. Enestvedt CK, Kristian Enestvedt C, Thompson SK, Chang EY, Jobe BA. Clinical review: healing in gastrointestinal anastomoses, part II. Microsurgery. 2006;26:137–43.

19. Briel JW, Tamhankar AP, Hagen JA, DeMeester SR, Johansson J, Choustoulakis E, Peters JH, Bremner CG, DeMeester TR. Prevalence and risk factors for ischemia, leak, and stricture of esophageal anastomosis: gastric pull-up versus colon interposition. J Am Coll Surg. 2004;198:536–41; discussion 541–2.

20. Schröder W, Stippel D, Gutschow C, Leers J, Hölscher AH. Postoperative recovery of microcirculation after gastric tube formation. Langenbeck's Arch Surg. 2004;389:267–71.

21. Pham TH, Melton SD, McLaren PJ, Mokdad AA, Huerta S, Wang DH, Perry KA, Hardaker HL, Dolan JP. Laparoscopic ischemic conditioning of the stomach increases neovascularization of the gastric conduit in patients undergoing esophagectomy for cancer. J Surg Oncol. 2017;116:391–7.

22. Veeramootoo D, Shore AC, Wajed SA. Randomized controlled trial of laparoscopic gastric ischemic conditioning prior to minimally invasive esophagectomy, the LOGIC trial. Surg Endosc. 2012;26:1822–9.

23. Nguyen NT, Nguyen X-MT, Reavis KM, Elliott C, Masoomi H, Stamos MJ. Minimally invasive esophagectomy with and without gastric ischemic conditioning. Surg Endosc. 2012;26:1637–41.

24. Miyazaki T, Kuwano H, Kato H, Yoshikawa M, Ojima H, Tsukada K. Predictive value of blood flow in the gastric tube in anastomotic insufficiency after thoracic esophagectomy. World J Surg. 2002;26:1319–23.

25. Ikeda Y, Niimi M, Kan S, Shatari T, Takami H, Kodaira S. Clinical significance of tissue blood flow during esophagectomy by laser Doppler flowmetry. J Thorac Cardiovasc Surg. 2001;122:1101–6.

26. Shimada Y, Okumura T, Nagata T, Sawada S, Matsui K, Hori R, Yoshioka I, Yoshida T, Osada R, Tsukada K. Usefulness of blood supply visualization by indocyanine green fluorescence for reconstruction during esophagectomy. Esophagus. 2011;8:259–66.

27. Okamoto K, Muguruma N, Kimura T, et al. A novel diagnostic method for evaluation of vascular lesions in the digestive tract using infrared fluorescence endoscopy. Endoscopy. 2005;37:52–7.

28. Sader AA. Esophagectomy with gastric reconstruction for achalasia. J Thorac Cardiovasc Surg. 2000;119:194–5.

29. Saito T, Yano M, Motoori M, Kishi K, Fujiwara Y, Shingai T, Noura S, Ohue M, Ohigashi H, Ishikawa O. Subtotal gastrectomy for gastric tube cancer after esophagectomy: a safe procedure preserving the proximal part of gastric tube based on intraoperative ICG blood flow evaluation. J Surg Oncol. 2012;106:107–10.

30. Ishiguro T, Kumagai Y, Ono T, et al. Usefulness of indocyanine green angiography for evaluation of blood supply in a reconstructed gastric tube during esophagectomy. Int Surg. 2012;97:340–4.

31. Murawa D, Hünerbein M, Spychala A, Nowaczyk P, Potom K, Murawa P. Indocyanine green angiography for evaluation of gastric conduit perfusion during esophagectomy—first experience. Acta Chir Belg. 2012;112:275–80.

32. Kubota K, Yoshida M, Kuroda J, Okada A, Ohta K, Kitajima M. Application of the HyperEye Medical System for esophageal cancer surgery. a preliminary report. Surg Today. 2013;43:215–20.

33. Kumagai Y, Ishiguro T, Haga N, Kuwabara K, Kawano T, Ishida H. Hemodynamics of the reconstructed gastric tube during esophagectomy: assessment of outcomes with indocyanine green fluorescence. World J Surg. 2014;38:138–43.

34. Sarkaria IS, Bains MS, Finley DJ, Adusumilli PS, Huang J, Rusch VW, Jones DR, Rizk NP. Intraoperative near-infrared fluorescence imaging as an adjunct to robotic-assisted minimally invasive esophagectomy. Innovations. 2014;9:391–3.

35. Rino Y, Yukawa N, Sato T, Yamamoto N, Tamagawa H, Hasegawa S, Oshima T, Yoshikawa T, Masuda M, Imada T. Visualization of blood supply route to the reconstructed stomach by indocyanine green fluorescence imaging during esophagectomy. BMC Med Imaging. 2014;14:18.

36. Pacheco PE, Hill SM, Henriques SM, Paulsen JK, Anderson RC. The novel use of intraoperative laser-induced fluorescence of indocyanine green tissue

angiography for evaluation of the gastric conduit in esophageal reconstructive surgery. Am J Surg. 2013;205:349–52. discussion 352–3

37. Zehetner J, DeMeester SR, Alicuben ET, Oh DS, Lipham JC, Hagen JA, DeMeester TR. Intraoperative assessment of perfusion of the gastric graft and correlation with anastomotic leaks after esophagectomy. Ann Surg. 2015;262:74–8.

38. Campbell C, Reames MK, Robinson M, Symanowski J, Salo JC. Conduit vascular evaluation is associated with reduction in anastomotic leak after esophagectomy. J Gastrointest Surg. 2015;19:806–12.

39. Kamiya K, Unno N, Miyazaki S, Sano M, Kikuchi H, Hiramatsu Y, Ohta M, Yamatodani T, Mineta H, Konno H. Quantitative assessment of the free jejunal graft perfusion. J Surg Res. 2015;194:394–9.

40. Koyanagi K, Ozawa S, Oguma J, Kazuno A, Yamazaki Y, Ninomiya Y, Ochiai H, Tachimori Y. Blood flow speed of the gastric conduit assessed by indocyanine green fluorescence: new predictive evaluation of anastomotic leakage after esophagectomy. Medicine. 2016;95:e4386.

41. Degett TH, Andersen HS, Gögenur I. Indocyanine green fluorescence angiography for intraoperative assessment of gastrointestinal anastomotic perfusion: a systematic review of clinical trials. Langenbeck's Arch Surg. 2016;401:767–75.

42. Noma K, Shirakawa Y, Kanaya N, Okada T, Maeda N, Ninomiya T, Tanabe S, Sakurama K, Fujiwara T. Visualized evaluation of blood flow to the gastric conduit and complications in esophageal reconstruction. J Am Coll Surg. 2018;226:241–51.

43. Ohi M, Toiyama Y, Mohri Y, et al. Prevalence of anastomotic leak and the impact of indocyanine green fluorescein imaging for evaluating blood flow in the gastric conduit following esophageal cancer surgery. Esophagus. 2017;14:351–9.

44. Kumagai Y, Hatano S, Sobajima J, Ishiguro T, Fukuchi M, Ishibashi K-I, Mochiki E, Nakajima Y, Ishida H. Indocyanine green fluorescence angiography of the reconstructed gastric tube during esophagectomy: efficacy of the 90-second rule. Dis Esophagus. 2018;31. https://doi.org/10.1093/dote/doy052.

45. Karampinis I, Ronellenfitsch U, Mertens C, Gerken A, Hetjens S, Post S, Kienle P, Nowak K. Indocyanine green tissue angiography affects anastomotic leakage after esophagectomy. A retrospective, case-control study. Int J Surg. 2017;48:210–4.

46. Schlottmann F, Patti MG. Evaluation of gastric conduit perfusion during esophagectomy with indocyanine green fluorescence imaging. J Laparoendosc Adv Surg Tech A. 2017;27:1305–8.

47. Ladak F, Dang JT, Switzer N, Mocanu V, Tian C, Birch D, Turner SR, Karmali S. Indocyanine green for the prevention of anastomotic leaks following esophagectomy: a meta-analysis. Surg Endosc. 2019;33:384–94.

48. Van Daele E, Van Nieuwenhove Y, Ceelen W, et al. Assessment of graft perfusion and oxygenation for improved outcome in esophageal cancer surgery: protocol for a single-center prospective observational study. Medicine. 2018;97:e12073.

49. Yukaya T, Saeki H, Kasagi Y, Nakashima Y, Ando K, Imamura Y, Ohgaki K, Oki E, Morita M, Maehara Y. Indocyanine green fluorescence angiography for quantitative evaluation of gastric tube perfusion in patients undergoing esophagectomy. J Am Coll Surg. 2015;221:e37–42.

50. Nishikawa K, Tanaka Y, Tanishima Y, Akimoto S, Yano F, Mitsumori NNM, Yanaga KK. Comparison of intraoperative evaluation of the gastric conduit perfusion between thermal imaging and indocyanine green fluorescence angiography. J Am Coll Surg. 2018;227:e9.

51. Fikfak V, Gaur P, Kim MP. Endoscopic evaluation of gastric conduit perfusion in minimally invasive Ivor Lewis esophagectomy. Int J Surg Case Rep. 2016;19:112–4.

52. Kitagawa H, Namikawa T, Iwabu J, Fujisawa K, Uemura S, Tsuda S, Hanazaki K. Assessment of the blood supply using the indocyanine green fluorescence method and postoperative endoscopic evaluation of anastomosis of the gastric tube during esophagectomy. Surg Endosc. 2018;32:1749–54.

The Use of Near-Infrared Fluorescence in Sleeve Gastrectomy

Leonard K. Welsh, Jin S. Yoo, and A. Daniel Guerron

Introduction

Obesity is the most prevalent chronic disease and a leading cause of morbidity and mortality in the United States. More than one-third of the population meets criteria for obesity, and the prevalence continues to increase [1, 2]. Bariatric surgery has been proven to be the most effective treatment in achieving significant weight loss and resolution of associated comorbid conditions [3–7]. Laparoscopic sleeve gastrectomy (LSG) has rapidly become the most common bariatric surgery performed in the United States [8] largely due to its technical simplicity, favorable complication profile, and similar weight loss outcomes compared to more complex operations such as Roux-en-Y gastric bypass and biliopancreatic diversion with duodenal switch [9].

Leaks after LSG occur in a relatively low percentage of cases (<0.5–6%) but arguably represent the most serious complications [10–12]. The majority of leaks occur in the proximal third of the stomach near the angle of His with ischemic and mechanical factors as the most likely etiologies [13–17]. The stomach is known to have a redundant blood supply, and ischemia stands as an often overlooked and improperly assessed factor contributing to leaks. Most surgeons preserve the blood supply of the lesser curvature arcade, namely, the right and left gastric arteries, when performing LSG without much regard to other sources of blood supply to the sleeved stomach and gastroesophageal (GE) junction. Previous anatomic studies found that the vascular supply to the proximal stomach is often unequal and can be injured during LSG, resulting in ischemia and thus leaks [18].

Traditionally, surgeons evaluate perfusion based on a wide constellation of clinical signs including serosal color, palpable or visual pulsation, peristaltic movement, and active bleeding from cut margins. These parameters contain a large amount of subjectivity that can contribute to misinterpretation, even by experienced surgeons [19]. Intravenous indocyanine green (ICG) rapidly and extensively binds to plasma proteins and is largely confined to the intravascular compartment before extraction by the liver and ultimate excretion in bile. These properties make ICG an ideal compound to assess tissue perfusion intraoperatively and has found utility in many applications including gastrointestinal surgery [20–29], tissue flaps [30], and neurovascular

Electronic Supplementary Material The online version of this chapter (https://doi.org/10.1007/978-3-030-38092-2_10) contains supplementary material, which is available to authorized users.

L. K. Welsh · J. S. Yoo · A. D. Guerron (✉)
Department of Surgery, Division of Metabolic and Weight Loss Surgery, Duke University, Durham, NC, USA
e-mail: alfredo.guerron-cruz@duke.edu

© Springer Nature Switzerland AG 2020
E. M. Aleassa, K. M. El-Hayek (eds.), *Video Atlas of Intraoperative Applications of Near Infrared Fluorescence Imaging*, https://doi.org/10.1007/978-3-030-38092-2_10

reconstructions [31]. ICG use is safe in patients with decreased liver function and is often used to quantify liver function [32, 33].

Clinical studies suggest that real-time assessment of vascular perfusion with ICG may decrease the potential development of gastrointestinal anastomotic leaks associated with ischemia [24, 34]. ICG fluorescence angiography during LSG can be used intraoperatively to identify the variable blood supply patterns of the GE junction, which will aid in improving surgical technique for preventing ischemia-related sequelae [35].

Indications

As with other bariatric operations, LSG is indicated in patients meeting the National Institutes of Health consensus conference criteria [36] including:

- Body mass index (BMI) $\geq$40 kg/m^2 with or without any associated comorbidities
- BMI between 35 and 40 kg/m^2 with at least one serious weight-related comorbidity

Additionally, LSG is indicated for patients with a BMI between 30 and 35 kg/m^2 with uncontrollable type 2 diabetes or metabolic syndrome [37]. According to a multinational consensus statement released by an expert panel, LSG is safe for patients with inflammatory bowel disease [38] and other high-risk patients such as those with Child's A or B liver cirrhosis or awaiting kidney or liver transplant [39]. Barrett's esophagus and uncontrolled severe gastroesophageal reflux disease (GERD) are commonly accepted relative contraindications; however, others disagree [40]. Performing LSG in patients with known GERD is controversial, with evidence existing for both exacerbation and improvement of GERD symptoms after surgery [41]. LSG is also used as the first step in a staged operative plan for super-morbid- obese patients [42] often paired with subsequent biliopancreatic

diversion with duodenal switch or single-anastomosis duodenoileal bypass [43, 44].

ICG is inert with a highly favorable safety profile. It does contain a small portion (<5.0%) of sodium iodide and should be used with caution in patients with a history of allergy to iodides or iodinated imaging agents and in patients with a history of thyrotoxicosis [32]. The most serious, albeit rare, risk of intravenous ICG is anaphylaxis [24].

Technical Description of Procedure

We typically use an insufflation needle to establish pneumoperitoneum and proceed with a standard four-port technique; however, access can be obtained and ports placed in whichever fashion the surgeon is accustomed. A liver retractor is placed to expose the hiatus.

Classically, the proximal stomach and gastroesophageal (GE) junction derive their blood supply from the left gastric, short gastric, and inferior phrenic arteries [45, 46]. Additionally, an accessory or replaced left gastric artery can be found in the gastrohepatic ligament arising from the left hepatic artery to supply the cardia and fundus [47]. A solution of 25-mg ICG reconstituted in 10 mL of injectable saline is used to better identify these networks and the pattern of blood flow.

Initially, 1 mL ICG solution (2.5 mg) is injected intravenously, and a near-infrared camera system is used to map the blood supply to the stomach. Our practice has been to use the PINPOINT™ Endoscopic Fluorescence Imaging System (Stryker, Kalamazoo, MI, USA), but other systems are available. Three main variations in perfusion patterns have been described [35] and are detailed in Table 10.1 and depicted in Fig. 10.1.

After the vasculature to the GE junction has been mapped, dissection begins by dividing the gastroepiploic and short gastric vessels along the greater curvature of the stomach. Starting a few centimeters from the pylorus, the vessels are divided close to the stomach with a bipolar or

Table 10.1 Blood supply patterns to the GE junction

Pattern	% incidence	Significant blood supply to GE junction
Right-side dominant	20	Left gastric artery
Right-side accessory	36	Accessory artery in the gastrohepatic ligament: Accessory hepatic artery (55%) Accessory gastric artery (45%)
Left-side accessory	34	Tributaries from the left inferior phrenic artery significantly contributing to the right-sided supply
Right- + left-side accessory	10	Accessory gastric artery and tributaries from the left inferior phrenic artery, simultaneously

Used with permission from Ortega et al. [35]. Courtesy of the Society of Laparoendoscopic Surgeons

ultrasonic energy device working cephalad until all the short gastric arteries and the small blood vessels near the left crus are divided. The dissection should be carried very close to the angle of His to avoid leaving a significant portion of the fundus. The vascular supply of the upper part of the gastric tube can be significantly damaged during this portion of the procedure when branches of the left gastric artery are ligated. Likewise, a branch of the left inferior phrenic artery can be inadvertently divided during the left crural dissection (Fig. 10.2). The hazards of this dissection are further compounded if a concurrent hiatal hernia repair is to be performed—a common practice to decrease the risk of postoperative reflux [48], as an accessory gastric artery in the gastrohepatic ligament may be inadvertently coagulated and divided during the repair.

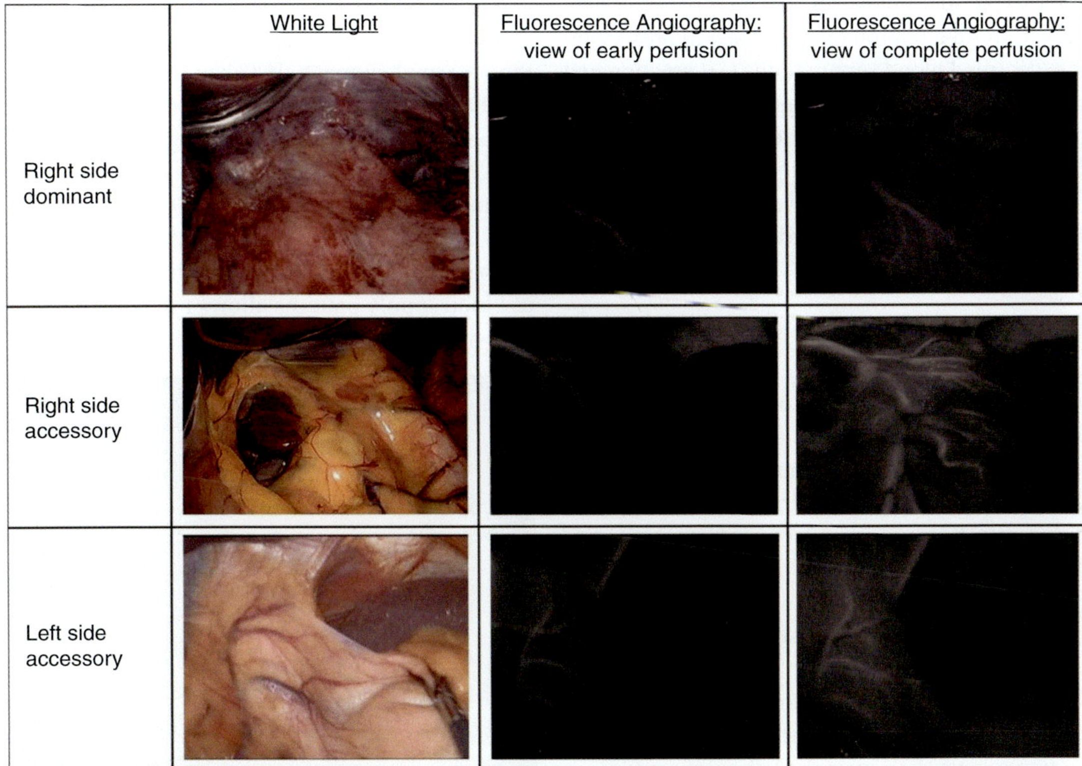

Fig. 10.1 Blood supply patterns before surgical dissection. (Used with permission from Ortega et al. [35]. Courtesy of the Society of Laparoendoscopic Surgeons)

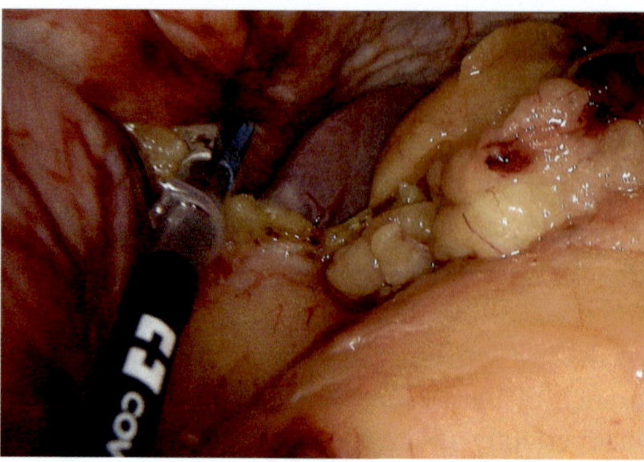

Fig. 10.2 Left crural dissection. Dissection of the angle of His near the left crus of the diaphragm. Inadvertent injury to the left inferior phrenic artery can happen during this portion of the procedure

Next, the sleeve is constructed as the stomach is divided over a bougie dilator using sequential loads of a laparoscopic stapler. Our standard practice is to use tissue reinforcement material with each staple load; however, practice patterns may vary. Careful attention must be used in preserving the identified blood supply to the GE junction and gastric tube as previously mapped with ICG. After completion of the gastrectomy, an additional 3–5 mL ICG solution are injected to ensure that necessary vessels and flow were preserved. These steps are demonstrated in Video 10.1.

Interpretation

Variations in blood supply to the proximal stomach and GE junction create a significant risk for ischemia of the sleeve from dissection-related vascular injuries. In our series, we noted three different patterns of vascular supply to the proximal stomach [35]:

1. Right-side dominant, arising from the left gastric artery
2. Left-side accessory pattern arising from tributaries of the left inferior phrenic artery in addition to perfusion from the left gastric artery
3. Right-side accessory pattern from an accessory hepatic artery or an accessory gastric artery in the gastrohepatic ligament supplementing the main left gastric artery

A right-side dominant pattern is often thought to be the most common pattern based on understanding of the anatomic blood supply of the proximal stomach but is only found in 20% of cases. In patients with a pure right-side dominant pattern, routine LSG dissection can be performed without jeopardizing the blood supply to the proximal stomach. However, in patients with significant contributions from the left inferior phrenic artery, an accessory gastric artery, or both, care must be taken to avoid injuries to these vessels to limit potential ischemic complications. Ten percent of the patients in our prior series had both significant left-side patterns and an accessory gastric artery. In these patients, if we had performed a hiatal hernia repair with sacrifice of the accessory gastric artery for exposure, and also injured the left inferior phrenic artery during the left crural dissection, it is likely that the proximal stomach would be left with compromised perfusion and its consequences.

In addition to evaluating the primary supply to the proximal stomach, ICG can be used to evaluate the perfusion of the remainder of the stomach by assessing flow through the segmental arteries (Fig. 10.3). Often, acute venous congestion and thromboses are identified (Fig. 10.4), which typically are insignificant and resolve over time.

Intraoperative ICG angiography identification of blood supply patterns allows for assessment of

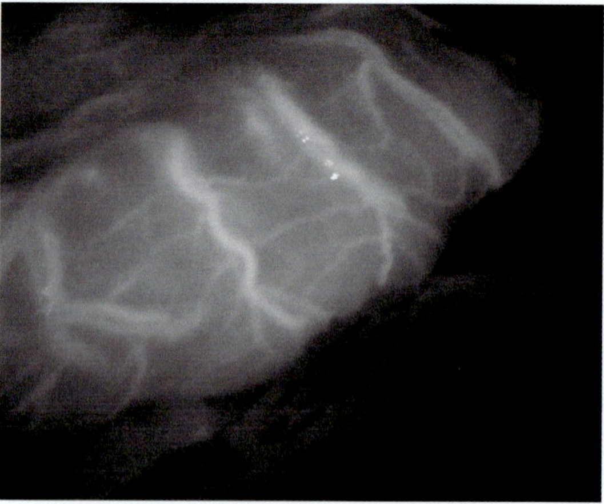

Fig. 10.3 Segmental branches. ICG enhancement of segmental branches after stapling demonstrating perfusion of the sleeve remnant

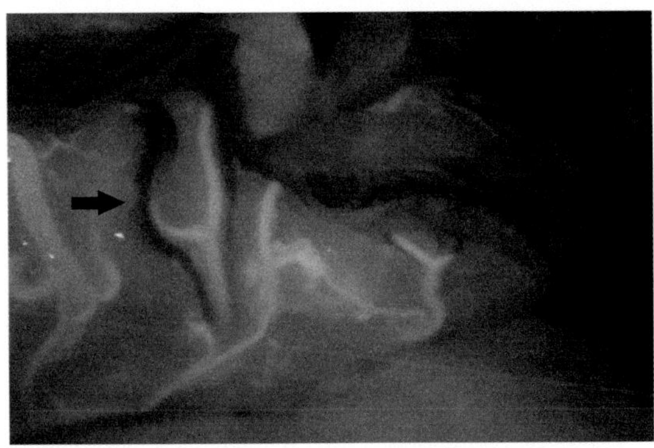

Fig. 10.4 Thrombosed vessels after resection. Non-enhancement of vessels (arrow) to the sleeved stomach indicating venous congestion or thrombosis

the proximal portion of the stomach where mechanical forces and reduced local perfusion make this specific location especially vulnerable to leak [16]. Other potential causes of leaks besides ischemia include increased intragastric pressure secondary to relative stenosis at the incisura angularis, at the pylorus related to decreased gastric volume, or both. It is likely that a combination of both mechanical and ischemic events leads to leaks such as a relatively ischemic area near the GE junction that subsequently perforates from increased luminal pressure from a distal obstruction.

Few studies have been conducted to investigate gastric perfusion as a source of ischemia after LSG. Saber et al. found decreased perfusion at the angle of His using CT imaging in healthy subjects with normal anatomy [49]. Delko et al. performed real-time intraoperative perfusion measurements at multiple locations across the stomach during sleeve gastrectomy. They found significant reduction in perfusion at the most proximal region before mobilization. The group concluded that the reduced post procedure perfusion at this region potentially explains this location as the predominant site of leak formation [17].

ICG fluorescence angiography allows for mapping of the major blood supply to the proximal stomach before any dissection so that unnecessary injury to these vessels during the procedure can be avoided. Furthermore, if an accessory vessel is present in the gastrohepatic ligament, this technology allows for a determination of the direction of the blood flow to assess whether the vessel is an accessory gastric (flow toward the stomach) or an accessory hepatic artery (flow to the liver). ICG injections can be repeated multiple times throughout the procedure, and we typically perform a second injection at the completion of our sleeve gastrectomy to ensure that the blood vessels in question were indeed preserved.

Pitfalls

Pitfalls are commonly related to dosing and administration timing errors. Our experience in the bariatric population is that it usually takes 20–60 seconds after injection to see the desired vessels enhance. Timing depends on several hemodynamics factors such as heart rate, blood pressure, relative intravascular volume, etc. The gauge of the catheter and length of the tubing may also affect lag time. Regardless, it is prudent to be completely ready without distraction once ICG is administered as the vessels may enhance and wash out rapidly if not prepared. Often, the heart can be visualized enhancing through the diaphragm and act as an indicator of the impending vessel enhancement.

Ample time for washout and sequestration in the liver is required before repeat dosing. When redosing, such as when verifying preservation of an artery after stapling, we recommend waiting at least 20–30 minutes from the previous dose and increasing the amount given by two to three times. That is, if the first dose was 2 mL (5 mg ICG), then the second dose should be 5–6 mL (12.5–15 mg ICG). Properly waiting allows for adequate clearance of the previous dose from the target tissue and provides time for the liver to excrete the dye into the bile. Image quality can be hindered by a bright liver and distort the definition required for proper assessment. Increasing the dose amount will assist in providing ample contrast against any residual dye that has yet to clear.

Other factors that can influence the quality of the enhancement and possible lead to false negatives exist. Near-infrared light poorly penetrates tissue, and vessels can be obscured by fat or other tissue and not appear on imaging despite flow.

Simply ensuring that all loose tissue (including the resected portion of the stomach) is clear prior to ICG administration easily corrects this issue.

Conclusion

Fluorescence imaging has multiple applications across many subspecialties of surgery. Intraoperative ICG use in LSG is a simple, real-time method for mapping vascular patterns and assessing tissue perfusion. Confirming adequate perfusion of the sleeved stomach may minimize perfusion compromise and prevent potential serious postoperative complications such as leaks or strictures. ICG can also be used in anastomotic operations such as gastric bypass and biliopancreatic diversion with duodenal switch. Future applications are in development.

References

1. Ogden CL, Carroll MD, Fakhouri TH, Hales CM, Fryar CD, Li X, et al. Prevalence of obesity among youths by household income and education level of head of household - United States 2011–2014. MMWR Morb Mortal Wkly Rep. 2018;67(6):186–9. https://doi.org/10.15585/mmwr.mm6706a3.
2. Hales CM, Carroll MD, Fryar CD, Ogden CL. Prevalence of obesity among adults and youth: United States, 2015–2016. NCHS data brief. 2017;(288):1–8.
3. Currie A, Chetwood A, Ahmed AR. Bariatric surgery and renal function. Obes Surg. 2011;21(4):528–39. https://doi.org/10.1007/s11695-011-0356-7.
4. Nostedt JJ, Switzer NJ, Gill RS, Dang J, Birch DW, de Gara C, et al. The effect of bariatric surgery on the spectrum of fatty liver disease. Can J Gastroenterol Hepatol. 2016;2016:2059245. https://doi.org/10.1155/2016/2059245.
5. Sarkhosh K, Switzer NJ, El-Hadi M, Birch DW, Shi X, Karmali S. The impact of bariatric surgery on obstructive sleep apnea: a systematic review. Obes Surg. 2013;23(3):414–23. https://doi.org/10.1007/s11695-012-0862-2.
6. Tan O, Carr BR. The impact of bariatric surgery on obesity-related infertility and in vitro fertilization outcomes. Semin Reprod Med. 2012;30(6):517–28. https://doi.org/10.1055/s-0032-1328880.
7. Yska JP, van Roon EN, de Boer A, Leufkens HG, Wilffert B, de Heide LJ, et al. Remission of type 2 diabetes mellitus in patients after different types of bariatric surgery: a population-based cohort study in the United Kingdom. JAMA Surg. 2015;150(12):1126–33. https://doi.org/10.1001/jamasurg.2015.2398.
8. Angrisani L, Santonicola A, Vitiello A, Iovino P. Reply to letter to the editor: bariatric surgery and endoluminal procedures: IFSO Worldwide Survey 2014. Obes Surg. 2018;28(1):251–2. United States.
9. Altieri MS, Yang J, Groves D, Obeid N, Park J, Talamini M, et al. Sleeve Gastrectomy: the first 3 years: evaluation of emergency department visits, readmissions, and reoperations for 14,080 patients in New York State. Surg Endosc. 2018;32(3):1209–14. https://doi.org/10.1007/s00464-017-5793-5.
10. Guerron AD, Ortega CB, Portenier D. Endoscopic abscess septotomy for management of sleeve gastrectomy leak. Obes Surg. 2017;10. United States.:2672–4.
11. Aminian A, Brethauer SA, Sharafkhah M, Schauer PR. Development of a sleeve gastrectomy risk calculator. Surg Obes Relat Dis. 2015;11(4):758–64. https://doi.org/10.1016/j.soard.2014.12.012.
12. Takahashi H, Strong AT, Guerron AD, Rodriguez JH, Kroh M. An Odyssey of complications from band, to sleeve, to bypass; definitive laparoscopic completion gastrectomy with distal esophagectomy and esophagojejunostomy for persistent leak. Surg Endosc. 2018;32(1):507–10. https://doi.org/10.1007/s00464-017-5757-9.
13. Ortega CB, Guerron AD, Portenier D. Endoscopic abscess septotomy: a less invasive approach for the treatment of sleeve gastrectomy leaks. J Laparoendosc Adv Surg Tech A. 2018;28(7):859–63. https://doi.org/10.1089/lap.2017.0429.
14. Galloro G, Ruggiero S, Russo T, Telesca DA, Musella M, Milone M, et al. Staple-line leak after sleve gastrectomy in obese patients: a hot topic in bariatric surgery. World J Gastrointest Endosc. 2015;7(9):843–6. https://doi.org/10.4253/wjge.v7.i9.843.
15. Abou Rached A, Basile M, El Masri H. Gastric leaks post sleeve gastrectomy: review of its prevention and management. World J Gastroenterol. 2014;20(38):13904–10. https://doi.org/10.3748/wjg.v20.i38.13904.
16. Sakran N, Goitein D, Raziel A, Keidar A, Beglaibter N, Grinbaum R, et al. Gastric leaks after sleeve gastrectomy: a multicenter experience with 2,834 patients. Surg Endosc. 2013;27(1):240–5. https://doi.org/10.1007/s00464-012-2426-x.
17. Delko T, Hoffmann H, Kraljevic M, Droeser RA, Rothwell L, Oertli D, et al. Intraoperative patterns of gastric microperfusion during laparoscopic sleeve gastrectomy. Obes Surg. 2017;27(4):926–32. https://doi.org/10.1007/s11695-016-2386-7.
18. Perez M, Brunaud L, Kedaifa S, Guillotin C, Gerardin A, Quilliot D, et al. Does anatomy explain the origin of a leak after sleeve gastrectomy? Obes Surg. 2014;24(10):1717–23. https://doi.org/10.1007/s11695-014-1256-4.
19. Karliczek A, Harlaar NJ, Zeebregts CJ, Wiggers T, Baas PC, van Dam GM. Surgeons lack predictive accuracy for anastomotic leakage in gastrointestinal

surgery. Int J Color Dis. 2009;24(5):569–76. https://doi.org/10.1007/s00384-009-0658-6.

20. Betz CS, Zhorzel S, Schachenmayr H, Stepp H, Matthias C, Hopper C, et al. Endoscopic assessment of free flap perfusion in the upper aerodigestive tract using indocyanine green: a pilot study. J Plast Reconstr Aesthet Surg. 2013;66(5):667–74. https://doi.org/10.1016/j.bjps.2012.12.034.

21. Boni L, Fingerhut A, Marzorati A, Rausei S, Dionigi G, Cassinotti E. Indocyanine green fluorescence angiography during laparoscopic low anterior resection: results of a case-matched study. Surg Endosc. 2017;31(4):1836–40. https://doi.org/10.1007/s00464-016-5181-6.

22. Jafari MD, Lee KH, Halabi WJ, Mills SD, Carmichael JC, Stamos MJ, et al. The use of indocyanine green fluorescence to assess anastomotic perfusion during robotic assisted laparoscopic rectal surgery. Surg Endosc. 2013;27(8):3003–8. https://doi.org/10.1007/s00464-013-2832-8.

23. Hellan M, Spinoglio G, Pigazzi A, Lagares-Garcia JA. The influence of fluorescence imaging on the location of bowel transection during robotic left-sided colorectal surgery. Surg Endosc. 2014;28(5):1695–702. https://doi.org/10.1007/s00464-013-3377-6.

24. Jafari MD, Wexner SD, Martz JE, McLemore EC, Margolin DA, Sherwinter DA, et al. Perfusion assessment in laparoscopic left-sided/anterior resection (PILLAR II): a multi-institutional study. J Am Coll Surg. 2015;220(1):82–92.e1. https://doi.org/10.1016/j.jamcollsurg.2014.09.015.

25. Kawada K, Hasegawa S, Wada T, Takahashi R, Hisamori S, Hida K, et al. Evaluation of intestinal perfusion by ICG fluorescence imaging in laparoscopic colorectal surgery with DST anastomosis. Surg Endosc. 2017;31(3):1061–9. https://doi.org/10.1007/s00464-016-5064-x.

26. Hutteman M, van der Vorst JR, Mieog JS, Bonsing BA, Hartgrink HH, Kuppen PJ, et al. Near-infrared fluorescence imaging in patients undergoing pancreaticoduodenectomy. Eur Surg Res. 2011;47(2):90–7. https://doi.org/10.1159/000329411.

27. Shimada Y, Okumura T, Nagata T, Sawada S, Matsui K, Hori R, et al. Usefulness of blood supply visualization by indocyanine green fluorescence for reconstruction during esophagectomy. Esophagus. 2011;8(4):259–66. https://doi.org/10.1007/s10388-011-0291-7.

28. Nachiappan S, Askari A, Currie A, Kennedy RH, Faiz O. Intraoperative assessment of colorectal anastomotic integrity: a systematic review. Surg Endosc. 2014;28(9):2513–30. https://doi.org/10.1007/s00464-014-3520-z.

29. Degett TH, Andersen HS, Gogenur I. Indocyanine green fluorescence angiography for intraoperative assessment of gastrointestinal anastomotic perfusion: a systematic review of clinical trials. Langenbeck's Arch Surg. 2016;401(6):767–75. https://doi.org/10.1007/s00423-016-1400-9.

30. Holm C, Tegeler J, Mayr M, Becker A, Pfeiffer UJ, Muhlbauer W. Monitoring free flaps using laser-induced fluorescence of indocyanine green: a preliminary experience. Microsurgery. 2002;22(7):278–87. https://doi.org/10.1002/micr.10052.

31. Rodriguez-Hernandez A, Lawton MT. Flash fluorescence with indocyanine green videoangiography to identify the recipient artery for bypass with distal middle cerebral artery aneurysms: operative technique. Neurosurgery. 2012;70(2 Suppl Operative):209–20. https://doi.org/10.1227/NEU.0b013e31823158f3.

32. De Gasperi A, Mazza E, Prosperi M. Indocyanine green kinetics to assess liver function: ready for a clinical dynamic assessment in major liver surgery? World J Hepatol. 2016;8(7):355–67. https://doi.org/10.4254/wjh.v8.i7.355.

33. Vos JJ, Wietasch JK, Absalom AR, Hendriks HG, Scheeren TW. Green light for liver function monitoring using indocyanine green? An overview of current clinical applications. Anaesthesia. 2014;69(12):1364–76. https://doi.org/10.1111/anae.12755.

34. Zehetner J, DeMeester SR, Alicuben ET, Oh DS, Lipham JC, Hagen JA, et al. Intraoperative assessment of perfusion of the gastric graft and correlation with anastomotic leaks after esophagectomy. Ann Surg. 2015;262(1):74–8. https://doi.org/10.1097/sla.0000000000000811.

35. Ortega CB, Guerron AD, Yoo JS. The use of fluorescence angiography during laparoscopic sleeve gastrectomy. JSLS. 2018;22(2). https://doi.org/10.4293/jsls.2018.00005.

36. NIH conference. Gastrointestinal surgery for severe obesity. Consensus Development Conference Panel. Ann Intern Med. 1991;115(12):956–61.

37. Mechanick JI, Youdim A, Jones DB, Garvey WT, Hurley DL, McMahon MM, et al. Clinical practice guidelines for the perioperative nutritional, metabolic, and nonsurgical support of the bariatric surgery patient--2013 update: cosponsored by American Association of Clinical Endocrinologists, The Obesity Society, and American Society for Metabolic & Bariatric Surgery. Obesity (Silver Spring, Md). 2013;21 Suppl 1:S1–27. https://doi.org/10.1002/oby.20461.

38. Rosenthal RJ, Diaz AA, Arvidsson D, Baker RS, Basso N, Bellanger D, et al. International sleeve gastrectomy expert panel consensus statement: best practice guidelines based on experience of >12,000 cases. Surg Obes Relat Dis. 2012;8(1):8–19. https://doi.org/10.1016/j.soard.2011.10.019.

39. Borbely Y, Juilland O, Altmeier J, Kroll D, Nett PC. Perioperative outcome of laparoscopic sleeve gastrectomy for high-risk patients. Surg Obes Relat Dis. 2017;13(2):155–60. https://doi.org/10.1016/j.soard.2016.08.492.

40. Gagner M. Is sleeve gastrectomy always an absolute contraindication in patients with Barrett's? Obes Surg. 2016;26(4):715–7. https://doi.org/10.1007/s11695-015-1983-1.

41. Rebecchi F, Allaix ME, Giaccone C, Ugliono E, Scozzari G, Morino M. Gastroesophageal reflux disease and laparoscopic sleeve gastrectomy: a physiopathologic evaluation. Ann Surg. 2014;260(5):909–14; discussion 14–5. https://doi.org/10.1097/sla.0000000000000967.

42. Alexandrou A, Felekouras E, Giannopoulos A, Tsigris C, Diamantis T. What is the actual fate of super-morbid-obese patients who undergo laparoscopic sleeve gastrectomy as the first step of a two-stage weight-reduction operative strategy? Obes Surg. 2012;22(10):1623–8. https://doi.org/10.1007/s11695-012-0718-9.

43. Sanchez-Pernaute A, Rubio MA, Conde M, Arrue E, Perez-Aguirre E, Torres A. Single-anastomosis duodenoileal bypass as a second step after sleeve gastrectomy. Surg Obes Relat Dis. 2015;11(2):351–5. https://doi.org/10.1016/j.soard.2014.06.016.

44. Biertho L, Theriault C, Bouvet L, Marceau S, Hould FS, Lebel S, et al. Second-stage duodenal switch for sleeve gastrectomy failure: a matched controlled trial. Surg Obes Relat Dis. 2018;14(10):1570–9. https://doi.org/10.1016/j.soard.2018.05.008.

45. Panagouli E, Venieratos D, Lolis E, Skandalakis P. Variations in the anatomy of the celiac trunk: a systematic review and clinical implications. Ann Anat. 2013;195(6):501–11. https://doi.org/10.1016/j.aanat.2013.06.003.

46. Loukas M, Hullett J, Wagner T. Clinical anatomy of the inferior phrenic artery. Clin Anat. 2005;18(5):357–65. https://doi.org/10.1002/ca.20112.

47. Tomosugi T, Takahashi T, Kawase Y, Yoshida K, Hayashi S, Sugiyama T, et al. Accessory left gastric artery aneurysms in granulomatosis with polyangiitis: a case report and literature review. Nagoya J Med Sci. 2017;79(1):75–83. https://doi.org/10.18999/nagjms.79.1.75.

48. Boules M, Corcelles R, Guerron AD, Dong M, Daigle CR, El-Hayek K, et al. The incidence of hiatal hernia and technical feasibility of repair during bariatric surgery. Surgery. 2015;158(4):911–6; discussion 6–8. https://doi.org/10.1016/j.surg.2015.06.036.

49. Saber AA, Azar N, Dekal M, Abdelbaki TN. Computed tomographic scan mapping of gastric wall perfusion and clinical implications. Am J Surg. 2015;209(6):999–1006. https://doi.org/10.1016/j.amjsurg.2014.05.023.

Vascular Perfusion in Small Bowel Anastomosis

Shiksha Joshi, Emanuele Lo Menzo, Fernando Dip, Samuel Szomstein, and Raul J. Rosenthal

Introduction

Anastomotic leakage remains one of the most dreaded complications of gastrointestinal surgery. In fact, between 2% and 19.2% of anastomoses will result in a leak. This is not only a source of significant morbidity and costs, but more importantly it has been linked to up to 32% mortality [1]. Bowel perfusion remains a key element in the proper healing of a gastrointestinal anastomosis. Although the perfusion is usually assessed by color of the serosal surface, presence of bowel peristalsis, and pulsation and bleeding from the marginal arteries, these methodologies remain very subjective and, as such, potentially inaccurate. Furthermore, the assessment of perfusion after the completed anastomosis can be more challenging due to the potential presence of vascular congestion.

Bowel ischemia occurs as a result of compromised blood flow in mesenteric vessels with a reported mortality rate of 60% in cases of acute insufficiency [2]. Factors that can determine ischemia of a bowel segment include arterial occlusion, venous congestion or thrombosis, and low flow states. These etiologies of the ischemia determine the clinical course, prognosis, and appearance of the bowel at the time of evaluation. It is common practice to only remove the clearly ischemic and gangrenous portion and plan on a second look to reassess the reminder of the intestine. Many confounding factors, in fact, influence the assessment during the first look, such as resuscitation, hemodynamic status, pressor requirement, body temperature, acidosis, etc. Reexploration in 24–48 hours allows for normalization of some of the abovementioned parameters and for a more definitive assessment of viability.

Electronic Supplementary Material The online version of this chapter (https://doi.org/10.1007/978-3-030-38092-2_11) contains supplementary material, which is available to authorized users.

S. Joshi · S. Szomstein
Department of General Surgery, The Bariatric and Metabolic Institute, Cleveland Clinic Florida, Weston, FL, USA

E. Lo Menzo
Department of General Surgery, The Bariatric and Metabolic Institute, Cleveland Clinic Florida, Weston, FL, USA

F. Dip
Hospital de Clinicas Jose de San Martin, Buenos Aires, Argentina

R. J. Rosenthal (✉)
Department of General Surgery, The Bariatric and Metabolic Institute, Cleveland Clinic Florida, Weston, FL, USA
e-mail: ROSENTR@CCF.ORG

© Springer Nature Switzerland AG 2020
E. M. Aleassa, K. M. El-Hayek (eds.), *Video Atlas of Intraoperative Applications of Near Infrared Fluorescence Imaging*, https://doi.org/10.1007/978-3-030-38092-2_11

The intraoperative assessment of the viability of the bowel is also paramount to accurately determine the margins of resection. Several modalities have been implemented to help assess perfusion and predict viability of the anastomosis or the intestine not resected. Among these are polarographic measurement of oxygen tension, visible light spectroscopy, Doppler ultrasound, radioisotope studies, laser Doppler flowmetry, and others, but only visible light spectroscopy and laser Doppler flowmetry were largely studied in human subjects. These techniques can be used intraoperatively, but they have yet to show accuracy and reproducibility of their results [3].

More recently, immunofluorescence has been used to evaluate intraoperative anatomy, organ perfusion, and lymphatic drainage in both benign and malignant diseases. Most of the current data in cases of small bowel perfusion comes from animal studies, but more data from human studies are now becoming available.

Indications

In general, fluorescence can be used in every case that requires assessment of perfusion of the bowel. This includes after anastomosis of the entire gastrointestinal tract. The following are some of its specific indications.

Bowel Incarceration

Incarcerated hernia requires immediate management in the form of reduction of hernia and its assessment for macroscopic signs of ischemia leading to potential bowel necrosis. However, mucosa of the bowel is the first part to be affected by reduced blood supply, and the superficial serosal layer of the bowel may not show the ischemic changes. Use of ICG angiography in this setting can assist in locating a well-perfused site for resection and anastomosis or assessing viability of the segment itself.

There have been case reports about the use of near-infrared (NIR) ICG angiography after reduction of the incarcerated obturator and umbilical hernias. In both cases, ICG angiography was used to assess viability of the incarcerated segment of bowel after its reduction. The fluorescent modality was able to accurately predict adequate perfusion and prevented unnecessary resection [4, 5].

Mesenteric Ischemia

The decreased blood supply to the intestine can be due to several etiopathogenesis such as arterial occlusion, venous congestion or thrombosis, and low flow states. Although the end result (i.e., bowel ischemia) is the same, the different etiology determines the overall clinical presentation, prognosis, and treatment of the disease. Furthermore, the assessment of bowel perfusion can vary based on the underlying etiology. Fluorescent angiography can be used in the assessment of bowel viability in any of the etiologies; however, scarce data exists.

In nonocclusive mesenteric ischemia (NOMI), there is no evidence of occlusion of the mesenteric vessels. The pathophysiologic mechanism is thought to involve spasm of the mesenteric vessels and low flow states. Moreover, the blood carried by the mesenteric arteries is supplied in the direction of serosa to mucosa. Therefore, the primary ischemic insult to bowel may only be evident in mucosa of the bowel without any changes to the serosa. Since a mesenteric vessel with a reduced blood supply does not show any gross changes, it is difficult to find out the territory of ischemic bowel solely based on clinical examination. The affected bowel segments are often found to be spread in a patchy manner and may be associated with multifocal mucosal segmental necrosis. ICG use in this scenario can help identify individual bowel subsegments with compromised blood supply. A recent study by Nakagawa et al. showed its successful use in a case of advanced gastric cancer post-gastrectomy where the patient developed signs of mesenteric ischemia on postoperative day 4 and was found to have no occlusion in the mesenteric vessel. The ischemic bowel was identified with ICG angiography and resected with no postoperative complication [6]. Similar use of the ICG was also reported by Irie et al. in a case of cervicothoracic esophageal cancer post-esophagectomy [7] and NOMI in a case of prostate cancer on chemotherapy by Nitori et al. [8].

Small Bowel Volvulus

Resection of bowel in cases of volvulus may extend to longer parts of intestine, and Iinuma et al. reported a case in which they used NIR ICG to identify the resection site. ICG showed hypoperfusion in the jejunal stump, but surgeons decided not to resect, relying on the presence of clinical indicators of viability, and completed the anastomosis. However, on postoperative day 22, the patient developed stricture of that anastomotic site. Retrospective review of the ICG perfusion images was done by measuring the pixel intensity, and they found gradual increase in pixel intensity over time at the mesentery, but the distal part of residual jejunum showed no such increment in the pixel intensity. The patient underwent resection of stricture of anastomotic site. After this second surgery, postoperative course was uneventful. This shows ICG use may guide the resection site as clinical assessment may not accurately reflect the perfusion status in the intestine [9].

The attached video illustrates the case of an internal hernia secondary to an adhesion causing volvulus of the small bowel and mesenteric ischemia secondary to acute venous outflow and arterial inflow insufficiency. After removal of the adhesive band and untwisting of the mesentery, the bowel was observed and evaluated with ICG angiography to establish viability (Video 11.1).

Perfusion of Anastomosis

The success of an anastomosis depends on several factors, among which tension and blood supply remain the most critical. Data exists on the use of ICG angiography to assess the perfusion of the bowel ends before and after the anastomosis. This technique has been utilized in anastomosis of the entire gastrointestinal tract, from the esophagus to the colon. Use of ICG in colorectal anastomosis has been well studied. The blood supply to colon is through inferior mesenteric artery, and the end arteries of colon are not densely connected to each other when compared to the blood supply of the small intestine. This increases the risk of anastomotic leaks after resection, and the leak rate has been reported from 3% to 20%. Multiple studies have reported revision of resection site based on the guidance by use of ICG fluorescence, thereby reducing the complication of anastomotic leaks to minimal [10].

Boni et al. studied 107 cases of colorectal anastomosis in which ICG was used to identify the hypoperfused region. Only 4 out of 107 cases showed reduced microcirculation in the bowel. The site of resection was revised prior to anastomosis and none reported a leak [11].

Technique and Description

Angiography and imaging based on fluorescent properties of ICG have been widely described in the literature. The low cost and minimal side effect profile combined with a simple and convenient methodology of using it intraoperatively make it a superior choice.

The ability of ICG to be fluorescent is based on its capability to absorb the higher wavelengths (750–800 nm) in the visible spectrum of the white light. The charged ICG molecule then emits a wavelength higher than 800 nm, which is imaged by the cameras with the ability to capture the NIR waves.

ICG has a good safety profile, and the molecule is largely confined to the circulatory system due to its property to attach to plasma proteins in the blood. The half-life of ICG in plasma is 3–5 minutes, with complete elimination of the drug by liver and its secretion into the bile. This property allows for multiple injections of ICG as required for imaging and analysis [12].

ICG can be injected as a peripheral intravenous injection, or it can directly be injected in an arterial line. A few seconds after the injection, the tissue that needs to be imaged is exposed to the specific bright light source and fluorescent images are captured by the NIR cameras with filters. The combination of such cameras with computers is able to produce a graphic analysis of the image. Multiple images of the same tissue can be acquired with this setup over a period of time to calculate the range of fluorescence intensity. Pixel intensity varies with time, and it can also be different for an individual as it is affected by the individual's hemodynamic status.

These principles can guide surgeons to objectively assess the bowel perfusion [13].

Discussion

The presence of tissue ischemia has been linked to the release of certain biomarkers such as ischemia-modified albumin, intestinal fatty acid binding protein, and D-lactate. None of these biomarkers, however, have been able to provide specific threshold values with accuracy [14].

Fluorescence angiography has been recently utilized as a more practical and useful perfusion assessment. Although the technology has been well documented to assess the intestinal perfusion and anastomosis in colorectal surgery, its utility in the resection and anastomosis of small bowel has mostly been studied in animal models. Behrendt et al. in 2004 measured the fluorescence in rat models after intestinal manipulation at 0 and 24 hours. They found a 29% reduction in perfusion index immediately after the intestinal manipulation and a 59% reduction after 24 hours compared to control group using IC-VIEW and IC-CALC system. Matsui et al. studied small bowel ischemia in experimental porcine models with near-infrared angiography (NIR-AG) and the FLARE (fluorescence-assisted resection and exploration) system in 336 subsegments of small bowel in pigs. Analysis of contrast background ratio (CBR) time graph revealed four patterns. Before occlusion of the mesenteric vessel, all the regions of interest (ROI) showed normal pattern of arterial inflow peak followed by a relatively steady plateau of fluorescence. After creating ischemia, the normal arterial pattern was seen in 177 (52.7%) subsegments. A total of 73 (21.7%)

subsegments showed delayed drainage pattern in which there was arterial inflow peak with fluorescence signal increasing over time. An additional 75 (22.3%) subsegments showed capillary drainage pattern in which there was an absent inflow peak with slow rise of fluorescence over time. Eleven (3.3%) subsegments showed arterial insufficiency pattern in which there was a fixed defect with no change in CBR over time. Capillary and arterial insufficiency patterns were more evident as the distance from normal bowel wall increased. Short-segment ischemia (2–3 cm) did not change the CBR time curve. Arterial peak inflow loss was noticed beyond 4 cm of ischemia [15].

One of the pioneer studies regarding small bowel perfusion was done by Diana et al. They studied bowel perfusion in porcine models with ad hoc imaging software (VR-RENDER), which captures and creates the perfusion map of the tissue and then rebuilds that image over the same laparoscopic image. In this study, they created ischemic segments to mimic mesenteric ischemia in the small bowel of the pigs by clipping the selective mesenteric vessels followed by intravenous ICG 15 minutes later. Based on the perfusion map by the image software, the bowel wall was marked with ROI and named as ischemic, marginal, and vascularized zones (Fig. 11.1).

These ROI were assessed for metabolic markers of ischemia by collecting and comparing capillary lactate levels, mitochondrial respiratory chain assessment, and MR spectroscopy metabolomic measurement. These ischemia markers showed statistical significance when ischemic regions were compared with marginal and vascularized regions, thereby supporting the idea that using fluorescence-based imaging may clearly delineate the ischemic region from well-vascularized ones.

Diana et al. also explored the accuracy of fluorescence-based enhanced reality (FLER) technique by creating ischemia in the small bowel segment of their porcine model for longer hours. Five ROI were marked based on the augmented reality (AR) and addressed as ischemic zone, presumed viable zone, and vascularized zones, respectively. They measured capillary lactate and created the perfusion map of the region

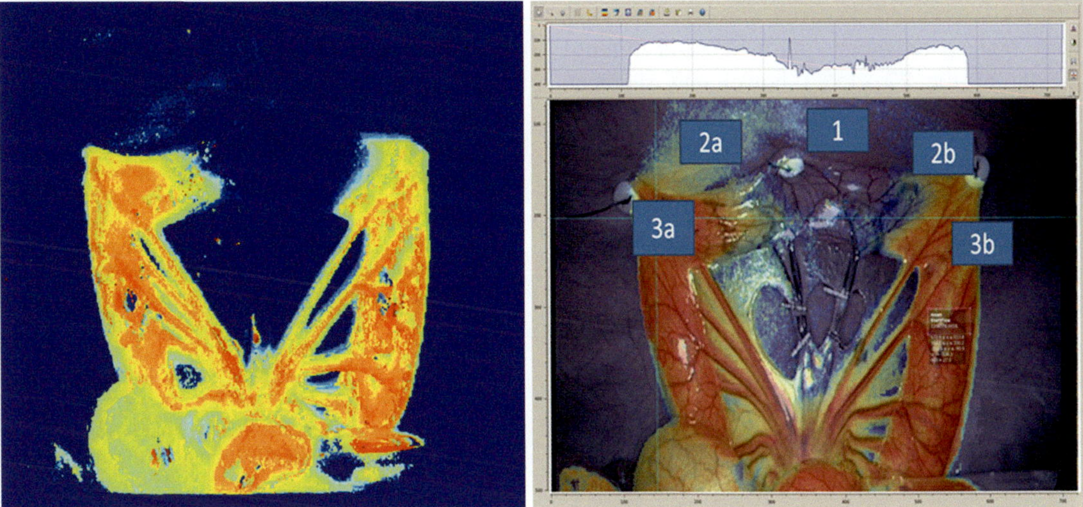

Fig. 11.1 Easy identification of low perfused areas by using ICG. (From Diana et al. [18]; used with permission)

every 2 hours after creating the ischemia in the models. In the presumed viable zone, FLER had concordance with clinical examination in 50% of cases, but the resection margin by clinical assessment was closer to ischemic zone in rest of the cases. The cases not concordant regarding the resection lines had statistically significant capillary lactate levels in the resection margin assumed by clinical exam after 4 hours of ischemia.

This is of great significance because it backs the idea of objective assessment of the small bowel perfusion. In fact, there are several cases to support the fact that clinical assessment of perfusion in small bowel may not accurately reflect the viability of the tissue [13, 16].

In another study with FLER in experimental models, Diana et al. measured the capillary lactate in the ischemic areas of bowel and created a map displaying bowel perfusion in percentages for the same bowel segments. Two groups (25% and 75% perfusion) were created based on assessment by FLER comparison of 100% perfused bowel region. They found that capillary lactate level at the resection line with 75% perfusion was statistically significantly lower when compared to lactate level at resection line with 25% perfusion and similar to tissue with 100% perfusion [15, 17–19].

A healthy and well-perfused tissue depends not only on arterial inflow but also on the venous outflow in order to maintain the circulation in the organ. All of the above studies have presented evidence on the ability of ICG to closely predict the zone of adequate perfusion in the bowels of animal models. A recent study by Bornstein et al. looked at the microvascular perfusion as well as venous drainage in the bowel ends after mesenteric division with both clinical evaluation and fluorescence and measuring pixel intensity with comprehensive angiographic perfusion assessment (CAPA) analysis. This study was performed on 49 consecutive patients. After mesenteric division, they performed surgical visual assessment followed by immediate NIR imaging assessment. The operating surgeon was blinded from the results from NIR imaging and completed the bowel resection surgery based on the clinical assessment. Images were later assessed by an independent operator. A total of 72 bowel segments of 46 patients were analyzed for microvascular perfusion and venous outflow (timing) by measuring the rate of change and duration of intensity curve. Disparity was defined as a difference between surgeon-marked site and site suggested by the fluorescence and CAPA analysis. Single disparity was the difference in one parameter and combined disparity was the difference with both parameters (perfusion and timing). Eleven of the 72 (15%) bowel end segments showed disparity with five (7%) segments showing disparity either in perfusion or timing (single) with median disparity distance being 2.0 cm by perfusion and 4.0 cm by timing. In six (8%) bowel segments, disparity was due to both perfusion and timing (combined) with the median disparity distance of 3.8 cm by perfusion and 3.5 cm by timing. The type of disparity and the disparity distance when compared between small and large bowel were not statistically significant, but the small bowel could be imaged with a 92% success rate.

Therefore, these studies show that objective assessment of blood supply to bowel is feasible intraoperatively with NIR ICG angiography technique and it can guide the decision of resection site. Newer imaging systems are being developed to simplify the analysis and make it cost effective.

Pitfalls

The quality of the perfusion with ICG use is heavily dependent on the imaging device and the technique used. The results may change if the distance between the tissue and camera is not constant. Pixel intensity also varies with time after injection, and it is influenced by patient-related factors such as the hemodynamic status like cardiac output, venous return and tissue edema, local inflammation, and amount of adipose tissue. Finally, the penetrance of the ICG is only of few centimeters, and this might play a role in the identification of perfusion in thick inflamed mesenteries.

Future Direction

The widespread availability and user-friendly characteristics of the fluorescent technology will likely result in expanded applications beyond perfusion. Tumor identification, especially when the fluorescent agent is bound to specific particles, has already been demonstrated in a few studies. Time-based correlation of perfusion with mitochondrial injury may help find the point of no return for ischemic tissue.

References

1. Kudszus S, Roesel C, Schachtrupp A, Höer JJ. Intraoperative laser fluorescence angiography in colorectal surgery: a noninvasive analysis to reduce the rate of anastomotic leakage. Langenbeck's Arch Surg. 2010;395:1025–30.
2. McKinsey JF, Gewertz BL. Acute mesenteric ischemia. Surg Clin N Am. 1997;77:307–18.
3. Urbanavičius L, Pattyn P, Van de Putte D, Venskutonis D. How to assess intestinal viability during surgery: a review of techniques. World J Gastrointest Surg. 2011;3:59–69.
4. Daskalopoulou D, Kankam J, Plambeck J, Ambe PC, Zarras K. Intraoperative real-time fluorescence angiography with indocyanine green for evaluation of intestinal viability during surgery for an incarcerated obturator hernia: a case report. Patient Saf Surg. 2018;12:24.
5. Ryu S, Yoshida M, Ohdaira H, Tsutsui N, Suzuki N, Ito E, Nakajima K, Yanagisawa S, Kitajima M, Suzuki Y. Intestinal blood flow assessment by indocyanine green fluorescence imaging in a patient with the incarcerated umbilical hernia: report of a case. Ann Med Surg (Lond). 2016;8:40–2.
6. Nakagawa Y, Kobayashi K, Kuwabara S, Shibuya H, Nishimaki T. Use of indocyanine green fluorescence imaging to determine the area of bowel resection in non-occlusive mesenteric ischemia: a case report. Int J Surg Case Rep. 2018;51:352–7.
7. Irie T, Matsutani T, Hagiwara N, Nomura T, Fujita I, Kanazawa Y, Kakinuma D, Uchida E. Successful treatment of non-occlusive mesenteric ischemia with indocyanine green fluorescence and open-abdomen management. Clin J Gastroenterol. 2017;10:514–8.
8. Nitori N, Deguchi T, Kubota K, et al. Successful treatment of non-occlusive mesenteric ischemia (NOMI) using the HyperEye Medical System™ for intraoperative visualization of the mesenteric and bowel circulation: report of a case. Surg Today. 2014;44:359–62.
9. Iinuma Y, Hirayama Y, Yokoyama N, Otani T, Nitta K, Hashidate H, Yoshida M, Iida H, Masui D, Manabe S. Intraoperative near-infrared indocyanine green fluorescence angiography (NIR-ICG AG) can predict delayed small bowel stricture after ischemic intestinal injury: report of a case. J Pediatr Surg. 2013;48:1123–8.
10. Keller DS, Ishizawa T, Cohen R, Chand M. Indocyanine green fluorescence imaging in colorectal surgery: overview, applications, and future directions. Lancet Gastroenterol Hepatol. 2017;2:757–66.

11. Boni L, David G, Dionigi G, Rausei S, Cassinotti E, Fingerhut A. Indocyanine green-enhanced fluorescence to assess bowel perfusion during laparoscopic colorectal resection. Surg Endosc. 2016;30:2736–42.
12. Menzo EL, Lo Menzo E, Dip FD, Szomstein S, Rosenthal RJ. Economic impact of fluorescent cholangiography. In: Fluorescence imaging for surgeons. UK: Springer; 2015. p. 99–106.
13. Bornstein JE, Munger JA, Deliz JR, Mui A, Chen CS, Kim S, Khaitov S, Chessin DB, Ferguson TB, Bauer JJ. Assessment of bowel end perfusion after mesenteric division: eye versus SPY. J Surg Res. 2018;232:179–85.
14. Treskes N, Persoon AM, van Zanten ARH. Diagnostic accuracy of novel serological biomarkers to detect acute mesenteric ischemia: a systematic review and meta-analysis. Intern Emerg Med. 2017;12:821–36.
15. Matsui A, Winer JH, Laurence RG, Frangioni JV. Predicting the survival of experimental ischaemic small bowel using intraoperative near-infrared fluorescence angiography. Br J Surg. 2011;98:1725–34.
16. Karampinis I, Keese M, Jakob J, Stasiunaitis V, Gerken A, Attenberger U, Post S, Kienle P, Nowak K. Indocyanine green tissue angiography can reduce extended bowel resections in acute mesenteric ischemia. J Gastrointest Surg. 2018;22:2117–24.
17. Diana M, Agnus V, Halvax P, Liu YY, Dallemagne B, Schlagowski AI, Geny B, Diemunsch P, Lindner V, Marescaux J. Intraoperative fluorescence-based enhanced reality laparoscopic real-time imaging to assess bowel perfusion at the anastomotic site in an experimental model. Br J Surg. 2015;102:e169–76.
18. Diana M, Noll E, Diemunsch P, et al. Enhanced-reality video fluorescence: a real-time assessment of intestinal viability. Ann Surg. 2014;259:700–7.
19. Diana M, Halvax P, Dallemagne B, et al. Real-time navigation by fluorescence-based enhanced reality for precise estimation of future anastomotic site in digestive surgery. Surg Endosc. 2014;28:3108–18.

Part V

Applications in Hepatopancreatobiliary Surgery

Nobuyuki Takemura and Norihiro Kokudo

Introduction

Indocyanine green (ICG) fluorescent imaging was first applied in laparoscopic cholecystectomy in hepatobiliary surgery [1]. Subsequently, it has been applied to detect intra- and extrahepatic liver tumors [2, 3] to confirm hepatic anatomy in the intraoperative bile leak test [4] and during anatomical hepatectomy [5]. Identifying the hepatic segmental boundary is the most effective technique for accurate and safe hepatic resection. ICG fluorescent imaging can help surgeons identify the hepatic segmental boundary not only on the liver surface but also inside the hepatic parenchyma. When diluted ICG is injected intravenously after clumping the hepatic inflow, the ischemic area presents as non-fluorescent region under fluorescent imaging. Another application of ICG fluorescent imaging for the hepatic anatomy identification is the intraoperative cholangi-

ography. ICG is excreted into the bile and becomes fluorescent by binding to serum albumin. This is how it was first applied to laparoscopic cholecystectomy. The same principle is used in intraoperative cholangiography and is applied in determining the bile duct resection line in major hepatectomy.

Detection of the Hepatic Segmental Boundary

Indications

ICG fluorescent imaging is used to determine the hepatic boundaries when performing major hepatectomy, especially in patients with liver surface adhesions or liver cirrhosis with irregularities on the liver surface. This technique is indicated for the removal of hepatic malignancy, hilar bile duct tumor, gall bladder cancer requiring major hepatectomy, and graft harvesting operation for living donor liver transplantation. Anatomical hepatectomy with injecting ICG into the portal branch and fluorescent imaging is described in Chap. 14.

Technical Description of the Procedures

Liver mobilization and cholecystectomy are performed initially, followed by hepatic hilum

---

Electronic Supplementary Material The online version of this chapter (https://doi.org/10.1007/978-3-030-38092-2_12) contains supplementary material, which is available to authorized users.

N. Takemura
Hepat-Biliary Pancreatic Surgery Division,
Department of Surgery, National Center for Global Health and Medicine, Tokyo, Japan

N. Kokudo (✉)
National Center for Global Health and Medicine (NCGM), Tokyo, Japan
e-mail: nkokudo@hosp.ncgm.go.jp

E. M. Aleassa, K. M. El-Hayek (eds.), *Video Atlas of Intraoperative Applications of Near Infrared Fluorescence Imaging*, https://doi.org/10.1007/978-3-030-38092-2_12

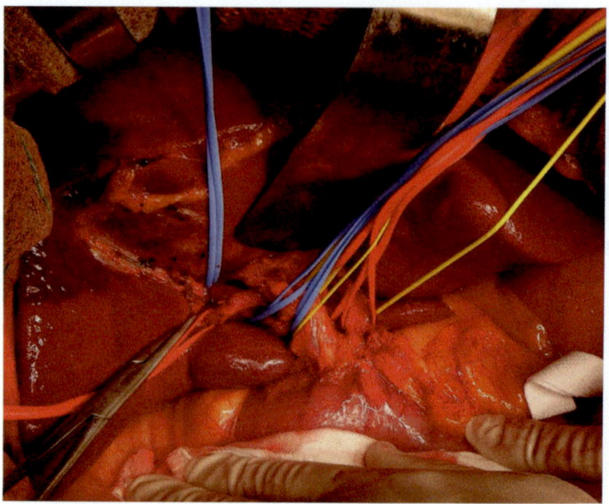

Fig. 12.1 Hilar vessel dissection approach

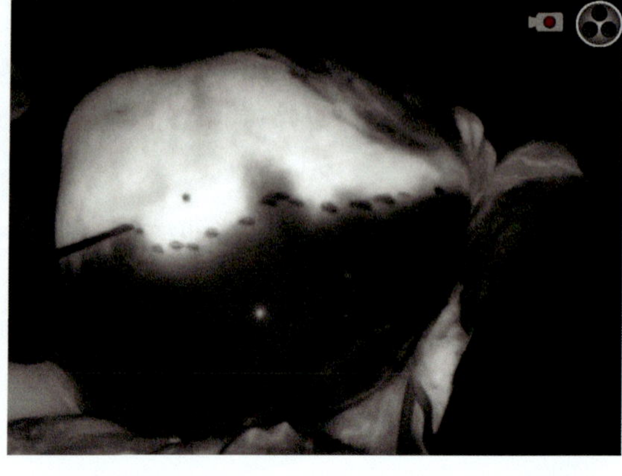

Fig. 12.3 Hepatic segmental boundaries are visualized on the hepatic surface of the liver by fluorescent imaging

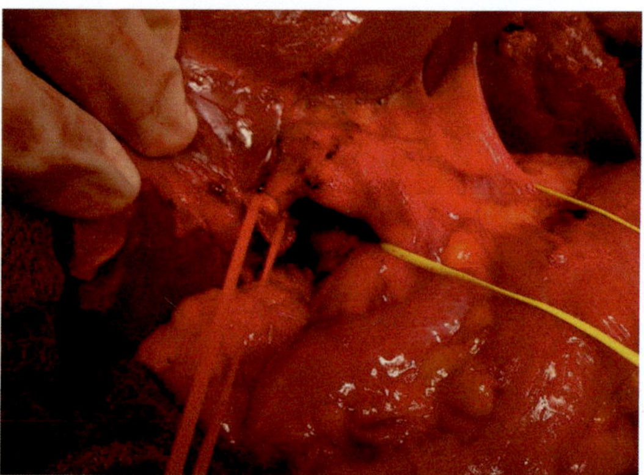

Fig. 12.2 Glissonian pedicle approach

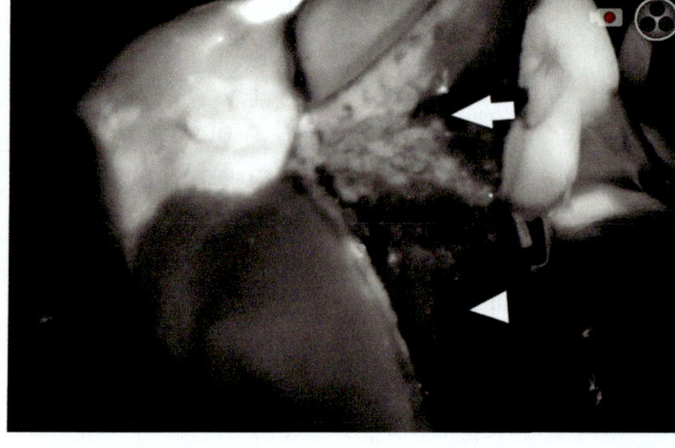

Fig. 12.4 Boundary plane between the stained segment (arrow) and non-stained segment (arrowhead) can be confirmed during the hepatic parenchymal resection

dissection. The portal vein or Glissonian sheath is encircled and clamped with the hilar vessel dissection approach (Fig. 12.1) or the Glissonian pedicle approach (Fig. 12.2), respectively. Subsequently, 2.5 mg diluted ICG is administrated by an intravenous injection. The hepatic segments with functional portal and arterial blood supply illuminate under ICG fluorescent imaging; the ischemic segments are confirmed as a non-illuminated area with ICG fluorescent imaging system (Fig. 12.3 and Video 12.1). This technique visualizes the boundaries of the hepatic segment not only on the surface of the liver but also inside the liver parenchyma during parenchymal dissection (Fig. 12.4 and Video 12.2).

Interpretation

To minimize postoperative complications after hepatectomy, it is essential for the hepatic surgeons to accurately recognize the segmental hepatic boundaries. Incorrect determination of the hepatic anatomy might cause remnant hepatic parenchymal necrosis, unnecessary hepatic venous congestion, or bile duct injury. As the systemically circulating ICG is taken up by the hepatocytes, the hepatic ischemic area is clearly visualized as a non-illuminated area in contrast with the illuminated area where the portal and arterial blood supply are maintained.

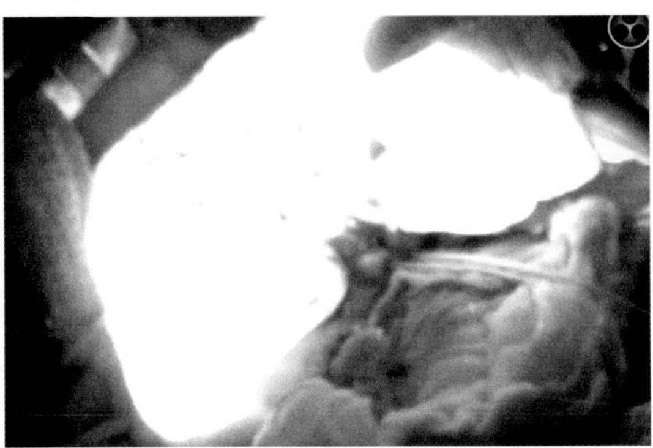

Fig. 12.5 Whole liver fluorescent due to the incomplete hepatic inflow occlusion

Pitfalls

ICG stays in the hepatic parenchyma for a few hours after the intravenous injection. Incomplete hepatic inflow occlusion might make the whole liver fluorescent (Fig. 12.5). Once the whole liver is illuminated, further examination with ICG fluorescent imaging becomes impossible, including anatomical staining, tumor detection, and ICG fluorescent cholangiography. It is important to abstain from liver function testing using ICG within a few days before surgery, which also makes whole liver fluorescent.

Intraoperative ICG Fluorescent Cholangiography

Indications

ICG fluorescent cholangiography was first applied in a clinical setting for laparoscopic cholecystectomy by Ishizawa et al. [1]. Later, its use has been extended to intraoperative cholangiography during hepatectomy and the bile leakage test [4]. The anatomy of the bile duct has some variations such as a right posterior bile duct confluence to the left bile duct, and ligation of the intrahepatic left or right bile ducts might make a stricture on the confluence of the opposite side of the hepatic duct. Therefore, the surgeon should constantly pay attention to the variation of the bile duct and

ensure that the point of the bile duct ligation does not injure the remnant bile duct during hemi-hepatectomy. After the dissection of the hepatic hilum, the anatomy of the bile duct around hepatic hilum can be visualized using ICG fluorescent cholangiography during hepatectomy. Applications of intraoperative ICG cholangiography for laparoscopic cholecystectomy is described in Chap. 14.

Technical Description of the Procedures

Cholecystectomy is done before the liver parenchymal transection. A tube for intraoperative cholangiography is inserted through the cystic duct. After more than half of the transection of the hepatic parenchyma and the dissection of the hepatic hilum are done, 3–5 ml of ICG diluted solution (2.5 ml of ICG in 100 ml saline) is injected through the tube to confirm the confluence point and the anatomy of the right and left hepatic ducts before bile duct resection so that the remnant hepatic duct is not injured (Video 12.3, Fig. 12.6). The best timing of ICG fluorescent cholangiography is before hepatic duct resection.

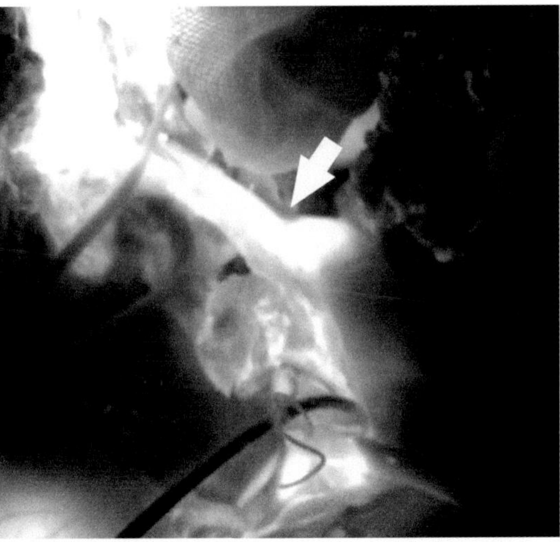

Fig. 12.6 Bifurcation of the right and left hepatic ducts (arrowhead) can be confirmed after the hepatic parenchymal resection

Interpretation

ICG injected directly into the bile duct binds with bile proteins and becomes fluorescent. This method uses direct local administration into the bile; hence, if the concentration of ICG is not reduced, the fluorescence may become excessively strong, making it difficult to identify the bile duct.

Pitfalls

The use of ICG should be restricted to cholangiography, if it is planned to be performed during hepatectomy. Once ICG is injected intravenously to detect the hepatic segmental boundary, the recirculating ICG might make the whole liver fluorescent even after the left or right portal vein ligation as there is vascular communication around the hepatic hilum. The tissue permeability of ICG is low (about 1 cm). If ICG fluorescent cholangiography is performed before liver transection, the left or right hepatic duct is covered with liver parenchyma and cannot be identified under ICG fluorescent imaging. Therefore, it is better to check the anatomy of the bile duct by ICG fluorescent cholangiography just before bile duct resection.

References

1. Ishizawa T, Bandai Y, Kokudo N. Fluorescent cholangiography using indocyanine green for laparoscopic cholecystectomy: an initial experience. Arch Surg. 2009;144:381–2. https://doi.org/10.1001/archsurg.2009.9.
2. Ishizawa T, Fukushima N, Shibahara J, Masuda K, Tamura S, Aoki T, et al. Real-time identification of liver cancers by using indocyanine green fluorescent imaging. Cancer. 2009;115:2491–504. https://doi.org/10.1002/cncr.24291.
3. Satou S, Ishizawa T, Masuda K, Kaneko J, Aoki T, Sakamoto Y, et al. Indocyanine green fluorescent imaging for detecting extrahepatic metastasis of hepatocellular carcinoma. J Gastroenterol. 2013;48:1136–43. https://doi.org/10.1007/s00535-012-0709-6.
4. Kaibori M, Ishizaki M, Matsui K, Kwon AH. Intraoperative indocyanine green fluorescent imaging for prevention of bile leakage after hepatic resection. Surgery. 2011;150:91–8. https://doi.org/10.1016/j.surg.2011.02.011.
5. Aoki T, Yasuda D, Shimizu Y, Odaira M, Niiya T, Kusano T, et al. Image-guided liver mapping using fluorescence navigation system with indocyanine green for anatomical hepatic resection. World J Surg. 2008;32:1763–7. https://doi.org/10.1007/s00268-008-9620-y.

Identification of Liver Segments Guided by Indocyanine Green Fluorescence Imaging During Anatomical Liver Resections

Takeshi Aoki, Doaa A. Mansour,
Tomotake Koizumi, and Masahiko Murakami

Introduction

Anatomical liver resections (ALR) including segmentectomy or subsegmentectomy have been established as standard operations for hepatocellular carcinoma. They require an in-depth understanding of liver anatomy regarding the variations in blood vessel and biliary tract bifurcation. Couinaud [1] classified liver segments according to portal vein anatomy, and in 1985, Makuuchi et al. introduced intraoperative ultrasonography (IOUS)-guided indigo carmine injection into the portal branch supplying the tumor segment [2]. Dye injection, leading to staining of the liver surface outlining the target segment, combined with IOUS can be considered as the preliminary version of a real-time intraoperative navigation system. This method for anatomical resection of liver cancer resulted in reduced blood loss and prevention of biliary fistula formation which remarkably improved the safety and postoperative outcome [3].

However, the early washout of indigo carmine and its suboptimal delineation of intersegmental planes prompted the development of the current generation real-time intraoperative navigation system consisting of indocyanine green (ICG) fluorescence and a near infrared (NIR) imaging system.

ICG has an excitation wavelength in the NIR spectrum (760 nm) and it emits fluorescent light of 830 nm. NIR light can penetrate deep into the tissue as compared to other types of light. This property is being applied clinically as an intraoperative NIR navigation system for identification of sentinel lymph nodes in digestive cancer and other cancers, evaluation of graft blood flow for cardiovascular surgery and organ transplantation, and tumor [4] and bile duct [5] imaging in the field of liver surgery. Pathological cells as in HCC and CRLM take up ICG but do not secrete it into bile and can therefore be detected by their retention of ICG.

In 2008, we were the first to report the applicability of ICG fluorescence as intraoperative identification tool for liver segments during ALR [6]. The continuously expanding use of laparoscopy in ALR triggered attempts to introduce ICG fluorescence imaging to the laparoscopic setting [7]. Thus, this chapter focuses on the improvements and challenges of laparoscopic ALR with ICG fluorescence imaging for segment identification

Electronic Supplementary Material The online version of this chapter (https://doi.org/10.1007/978-3-030-38092-2_13) contains supplementary material, which is available to authorized users.

T. Aoki (✉) · T. Koizumi · M. Murakami
Division of Gastroenterological and General Surgery,
Department of Surgery, Showa University,
Tokyo, Japan
e-mail: takejp@med.showa-u.ac.jp

D. A. Mansour
Division of Gastroenterological and General Surgery,
Department of Surgery, Showa University,
Tokyo, Japan

General Surgery Department, Cairo University
Hospitals, Cairo, Egypt

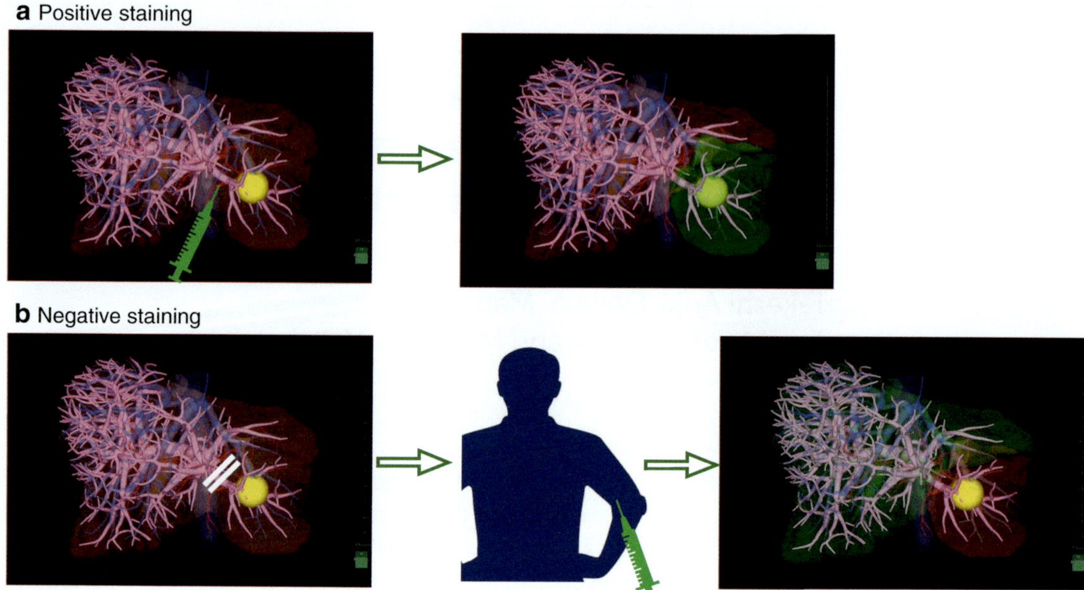

Fig. 13.1 Preoperative simulation of hepatic subsegment staining using indocyanine green (ICG) fluorescence method. (**a**) Positive staining method: identification of the portal vein to the tumor-bearing segment, determination of the exact injection point, and visualization of the esti- mated staining volume. (**b**) Negative staining method: identification of the portal vein to the tumor-bearing seg- ment, determination of the point of planned occlusion before intravenous injection, and estimation of the non- staining volume

even though the same principles perfectly apply to open ALR.

Preoperative Diagnostic Workup and ICG Segmental Staining Simulation for Laparoscopic Liver Subsegmentectomy

As part of the planning for laparoscopic liver sub- segmentectomy, preoperative B-mode ultrasonog- raphy, magnetic resonance imaging-ethoxybenzyl (MRI-EOB), and dynamic computed tomography (CT) are performed to determine the exact tumor location and its relevant arterial, portal venous, and hepatic venous relationship. The preoperative CT imaging protocol involved a multi-detector CT scan with nonionic intravenous contrast agent at a rate of 4 mL/s with the following parameters: 100 kV, 400 mAs, and section thickness/collima- tion = 0.75 mm/0.7 mm [8].

CT volume data is fed to an image analysis workstation (Synapse VINCENT, Fujifilm Medical, ZioStation2, Amin Co., Ltd.) to create a 3D reconstruction liver map. This map can be used by the surgical team for preoperative simula- tion of the intervention, identification of the can- cer-bearing Glissonian vessel, decision on the exact ICG injection point, and the resultant esti- mated stained liver volume (Fig. 13.1). Finally, the designated portal branch is confirmed by B-mode ultrasonography to evaluate accessibility to the determined injection point prior to surgery.

This comprehensive simulated surgical strategy design for laparoscopic liver resection enhances the surgical team understanding of detailed anat- omy and consequently the safety of intervention.

Staining of Liver Segments Using ICG Fluorescence Method

Liver segment staining with ICG fluorescence can be achieved through the following two meth- ods. In *positive staining*, ICG is injected directly into the segmental portal branch under ultrasound guidance, and the target segment is identified through its ICG luminescence. If the segmental portal branch cannot be punctured directly, or the tumor-bearing segment is supplied by multiple portal veins, the counterstaining method can be used, in which portal branches to the adjacent segments are selectively punctured and stained instead. Thus, the segment to be resected appears as a non-fluorescent area bounded by the adjacent fluorescent segments [3].

In *negative staining,* the portal vein to the cancer-bearing segment is occluded, and ICG is administered intravenously. The target area for resection is identified by its lack of ICG fluorescence as compared to the rest of the liver.

These two methods are very useful intraoperative real-time navigation tools during ALR or subsegmentectomy. The specialized laparoscope camera with built-in NIR light functionality used for laparoscopic operations can provide superb intraoperative real-time display of ICG fluorescence for clear segment identification (Table 13.1) [6, 7, 9–18].

Liver Segment Identification Using ICG Fluorescence Method During Laparoscopic Liver Segmentectomy: Negative Staining Method

Several reports exist on the application of the negative ICG fluorescence staining method for hepatic segment identification during laparoscopic segmentectomy. Portal flow occlusion to the cancer-bearing parenchyma is performed as in open surgery, i.e., Glissonian pedicle approach [19]. After portal occlusion and intravenous ICG injection, parenchymal fluorescence demarcation does not only appear on the liver surface as in standard liver segmentectomy procedures, but the segmental boundaries of the whole volume to be resected is visualized in real-time 3D view.

Case Report: Negative Staining Method

During laparoscopic S6 subsegmentectomy for a liver hemangioma, the boundaries of the lesion, the right hepatic vein, and the dominant portal vein branches (P6a + b) were identified via IOUS. After clipping and separation of the portal branches, 2.5 mg/ml of ICG are injected intravenously. Two minutes later, NIR light function of the laparoscopic camera revealed a distinct lack of ICG fluorescence in the area fed by P6a + b. The boundaries of the segment are marked on the surface of the liver. During parenchymal transection, an interface between fluorescent and non-fluorescent areas could be clearly observed and defined the transection plane. An additional portal branch (P6c) to S6 exhibiting ICG fluorescence was encountered. It was ligated and separated. In this way, anatomical segmentectomy was carried out under the guidance of ICG fluorescence imaging (Fig. 13.2).

Liver Segment Identification Using ICG Fluorescence Method During Laparoscopic Liver Segmentectomy: Positive Staining Method

Similarly, various reports on positive ICG fluorescence in laparoscopic segmentectomy exist. Laparoscopic IOUS-guided direct puncture of the dominant portal pedicle is accomplished in a fashion similar to open surgery [7]. The target segment appears as a selectively fluorescent area. However, laparoscopic liver segmentectomy bears its specific challenges during laparoscopic IOUS-guided portal puncture. The laparoscopic IOUS probe offers less freedom of angulation and movement compared to open surgery especially after its introduction through a port fixed in position. Furthermore, the integration of the image of the target portal branch depicted on the IOUS monitor with the image on the laparoscopic screen during the puncture is technically quite demanding.

Therefore, the authors introduced a simpler method for positive staining during laparoscopic liver segmentectomy. After anesthesia and before pneumoperitoneum induction, an abdominal US-guided percutaneous puncture of the designated portal vein is performed. This method provides clear staining of the hepatic segment to be resected (Fig. 13.3).

Table 13.1 Near-infrared fluorescence imaging for liver segmentation

Study	Liver segmentation	Surgical approach	Imaging system	Injection site	Blood flow clamping	Dosage of ICG	Accuracy (%)	Reference
Aoki 2008	Positive staining	Open	PDE	Portal vein	Pringle	5 mg	94.3	[6]
Uchiyama 2011	Negative staining	Open	PDE	i.v.	Segmental PV	0.5 mg/kg body weight	100	[9]
Ishizawa 2012	Positive/negative staining	Lap	Not reported	Portal vein/i.v.	HA/segmental PV	0.025 mg / 2.5 mg	100	[7]
Sakoda 2014	Positive staining	Lap	IRI	Portal vein	None	5 mg	100	[10]
Inoue 2015	Positive/negative staining	Open	HyperEye Medical System	Portal vein/i.v.	HA/segmental PV	2.5 mg / 2.5 mg	95.8	[11]
Miyata 2015	Positive staining	Open	PDE-neo	Portal vein	HA	0.25 mg	100	[12]
Mizuno 2017	Negative staining	Lap	SPY	i.v.	Segmental PV	Not reported	100	[13]
Kobayashi 2017	Positive/negative staining	Open	PDE	Portal vein/i.v.	None/segmental PV	0.25 mg / 2.5 mg	100	[14]
Terasawa 2017	Negative staining	Lap	SPY	i.v.	Segmental PV	1.25 mg	100	[15]
Ueno 2018	Positive staining	Lap	SPY	Arterial branch	Artery embolization (IVR)	0.25 mg	100	[16]
Peyrat 2018	Negative staining	Open	Fluobeam	i.v.	Segmental PV	0.625–1.25 mg	80	[17]
Nishino 2018	Negative staining	Open	Medical imaging projection system	i.v.	Segmental PV	0.25 mg	91.3	[18]

ICG Indocyanine green, *PDE* Photodynamic eye, *Lap* Laparoscopic surgery, *HA* Hepatic artery, *PV* Portal vein *i.v.;* intravenous injection

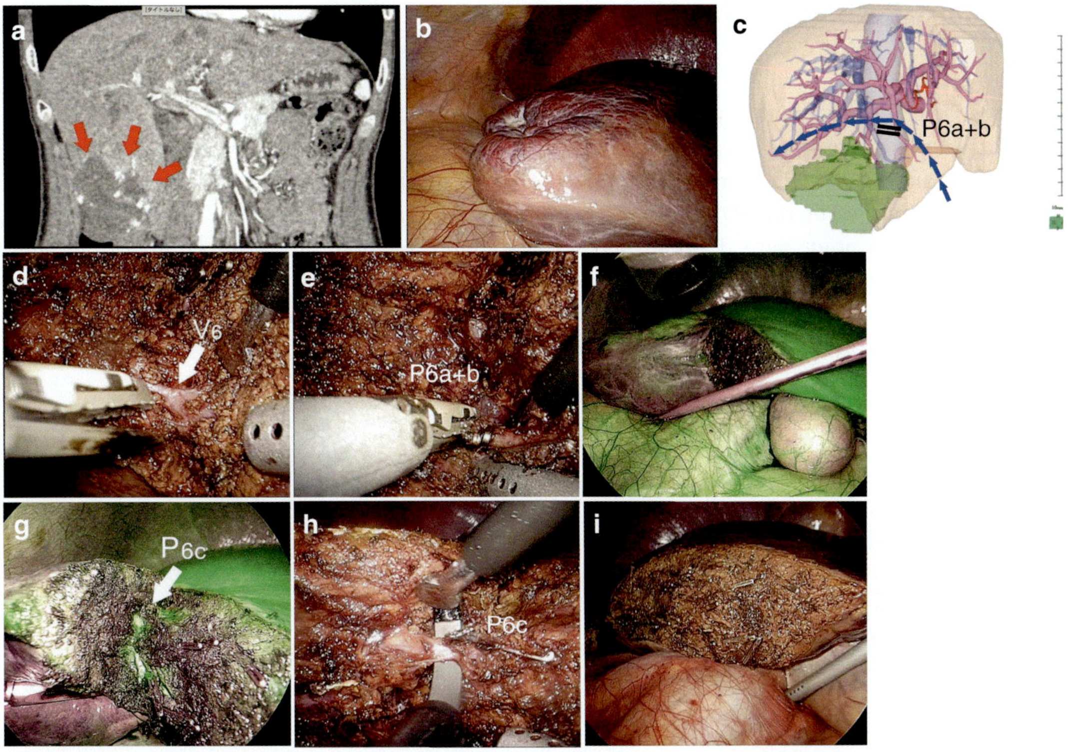

Fig. 13.2 Laparoscopic S6 subsegmentectomy guided by ICG fluorescence method (negative staining). Laparoscopic S6 liver segmentectomy performed on a 42-year-old woman with an S6 hepatic hemangioma. (**a**) Identification of the hepatic S6 tumor on a CT scan (marked with a red arrow). (**b**) Hepatic S6 tumor intraoperative findings. (**c**) Identification of the cancer-bearing Glissonian vessel (P6a + b), simulation of the point of vessel occlusion, and the resultant estimated non-staining area. (**d**) Dissection of the hepatic vein (V6), which appeared in the liver transection plane. (**e**) Identified cancer-bearing Glissonian vessel (P6a + b) as seen in the liver transection plane. The vessel has been clipped. (**f**) Intravenous injection of 2.5 mg/ml of ICG following ligature application and separation of the cancer-bearing Glissonian vessel (P6a + b) (negative staining method). (**g**) During liver transection, another portal vein (P6c) was observed feeding into the S6 hepatic segment as a blood vessel displaying ICG fluorescence. (**h**) Ligation and dissection of P6c (**i**) Liver transection plane after the completion of the laparoscopic S6 subsegmentectomy

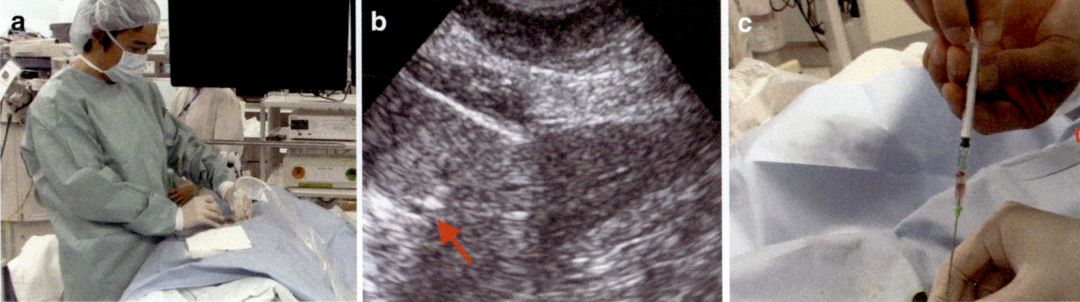

Fig. 13.3 Actual application of percutaneous ultrasound-guided portal vein puncture using ICG fluorescence (positive staining). (**a**) Immediately prior to surgery and following general anesthesia induction, an 18-G needle was used to puncture the designated portal vein under transabdominal US guidance. (**b**) Ultrasound-guided puncture of the cancer-bearing portal vein (red arrow marks the tip of the needle penetrating the portal vein). (**c**) 0.025 mg/ml of ICG is injected

Case Report: Positive Staining Method

A laparoscopic S2 resection for a localized hepatocellular carcinoma was performed as follows. The Glissonian vessel to the tumor-bearing segment S2 was identified on the 3D simulation liver map, the injection point agreed upon, and the expected staining volume determined. Accessibility to the injection point via transabdominal US was confirmed prior to operation.

Immediately after general anesthesia induction, an 18-G needle was inserted percutaneously to puncture the portal vein branches feeding S2 under external ultrasound guidance, and 0.025 mg/ml ICG were injected. S2 boundaries could be clearly visualized on the liver surface as an ICG fluorescent area. Similar to the negative staining method, the parenchymal transection plane was driven by the interface between fluorescent and non-fluorescent parenchyma (Fig. 13.4 and Video 13.1).

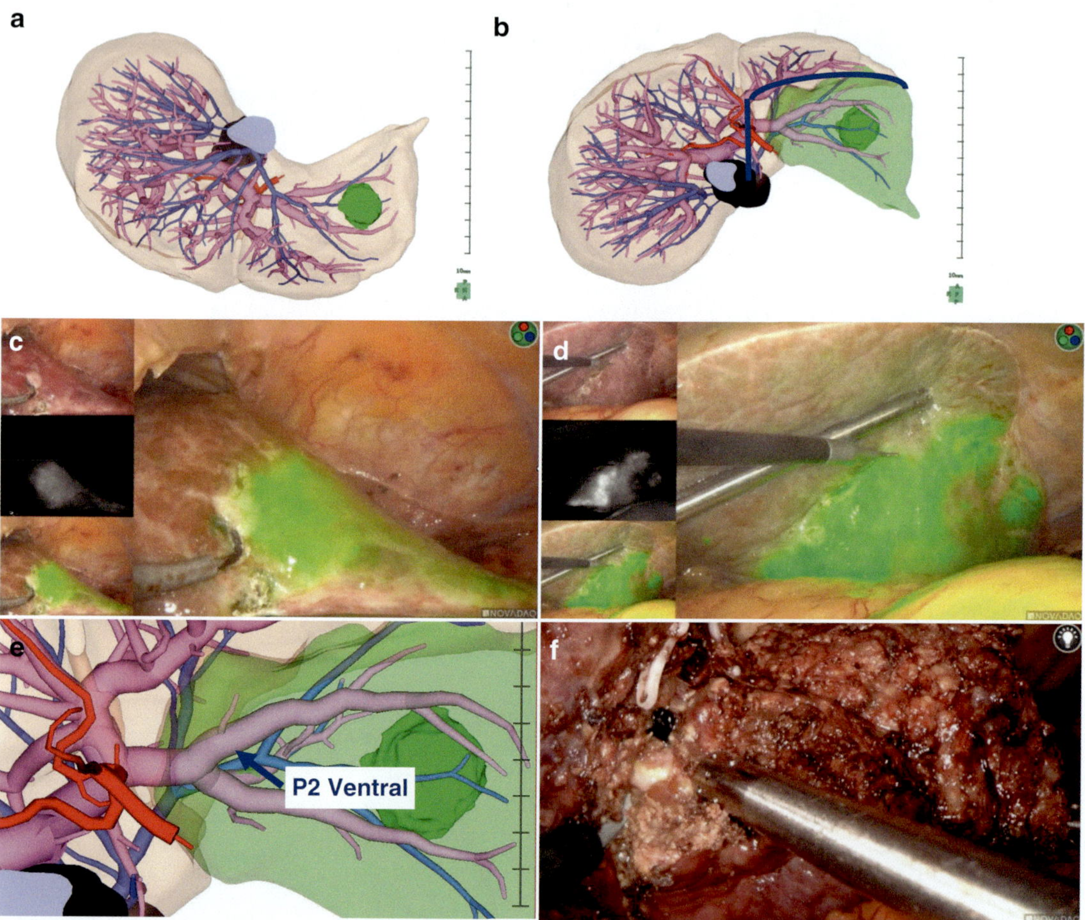

Fig. 13.4 Laparoscopic S2 subsegmentectomy guided by ICG fluorescence method (positive staining). Laparoscopic S2 subsegmentectomy performed in an 85-year-old man with S2 hepatocellular carcinoma. (**a**) Confirmation of tumor location in S2 in the preoperative simulation. (**b**) ICG staining area for cancer-bearing Glissonian vessel (P2). (**c**) S2 fluorescence observed on the ventral surface of the liver following injection of 0.025 mg/ml of ICG into P2. (**d**) S2 fluorescence observed on the dorsal surface of the liver and its marking by cautery. (**e**) P2 ventral branch identified in the preoperative simulation. (**f**) Appearance of the identified P2 ventral branch in the liver transection plane, its encirclement, and dissection. (**g**) Observation of ICG fluorescence on one side of the transection plane. According to this picture, adjustment of the transection plane is required. (**h**) P2 dorsal branch and hepatic vein (V2) identified in the preoperative simulation. (**i**) Dissection of the P2 dorsal branch and V2 appearing in the liver transection plane using a linear stapler. (**j**) Liver transection plane after the completion of laparoscopic S2 subsegmentectomy (see Video 13.1)

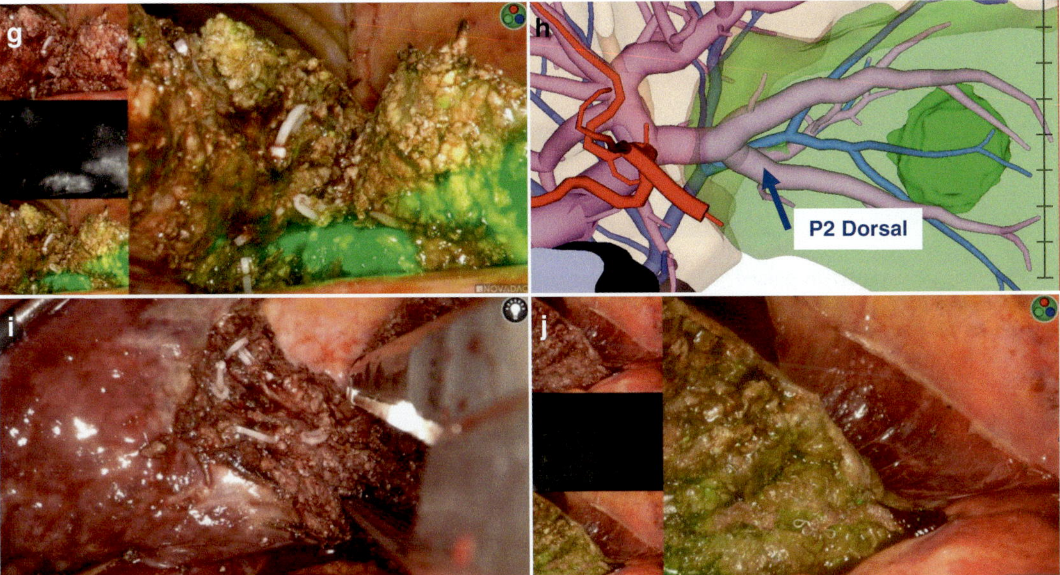

Fig. 13.4 (continued)

Challenges of Laparoscopic ICG Positive Staining Method

The previous section mentioned the technical difficulty of intraoperative dominant portal vein puncture under laparoscopic IOUS guidance and hence the percutaneous technique under transabdominal US guidance was proposed.

However, tertiary portal branch identification with external ultrasonography and their puncture can sometimes be remarkably challenging.

In these cases, IOUS-guided injection remains a viable alternative. Furthermore, the combination of both the percutaneous and the IOUS-guided technique, i.e., we inject the externally accessible branch and then additional ICG is injected under IOUS-guidance into the other portal branches feeding the target area, is possible. The difficulty of laparoscopic IOUS-guided injection can be mitigated by the use of a probe with an injection opening mounted on it (four-way laparoscope, 8666-RF, BK Medical). After identification of the portal radicle by IOUS, the needle is passed via the body surface to pass through the hole in the probe to reach the tip of the vessel. This technique is also effective for additional staining by ICG injection into small portal veins, especially S7 and S8.

Compared to standard ultrasound probes used in conjunction with laparoscopes, this device provides additional assistance with intraoperative laparoscopic vessel puncture (Fig. 13.5). Yet, it would be very helpful to develop them to provide sensory cues facilitating determination of the puncture site and angle on the body surface; thus, the puncture technique is not easy.

In the future, to enhance feasibility of positive staining under IOUS guidance in laparoscopic liver segmentectomy, the development and refinement of a specialized laparoscopic ultrasound probe adapted to the intraoperative penetration method is needed.

Liver Subregional Staining Methods Using ICG Fluorescence

Right Lobe

S7 identification method S7 is frequently fed by a single portal vein which is punctured and injected.

S6 and S8 identification method In 76% of cases, S6 is fed by a single tertiary branch, and in

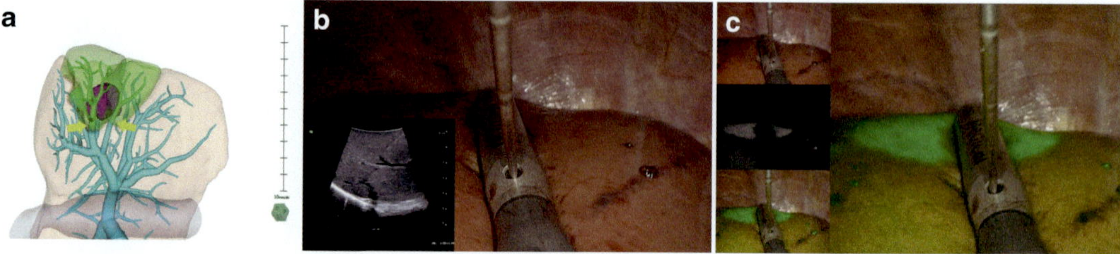

Fig. 13.5 Laparoscopic IOUS-guided puncture of the target portal vein in laparoscopic S7 subsegmentectomy (positive staining). A 68-year-old woman with S7 hepatic segment metastatic liver cancer disease. (**a**) Confirmation of tumor location in S7, identification of the 2 feeding vessels (marked by yellow arrows) and estimation of the staining volume. (**b**) Identification of the designated portal vein on IOUS, its puncture by a needle tip passed through the hole in the IOUS probe. (**c**) Injection of 0.025 mg/ml of ICG into the portal vein and completion of segment staining

24% of cases, it is fed by two branches. In most cases, S8 has a dorsal and a ventral branch.

The portal branch number is confirmed with preoperative diagnostic imaging and either the positive or negative staining method performed.

S5 identification method Since S5 commonly has multiple small feeding vessels, the counterstaining method is selected [3]. The portal vein to the adjacent S8 area is punctured and the plane between S5 and S8 is marked. The right and the middle hepatic veins serve as landmarks for the S5/6 and the S4/5 interface, respectively.

Left Lobe

S2 or S3 identification method The S2/S3 interface is visualized by either direct positive staining or the counterstaining technique by injecting the portal branch to the reciprocal segment.

Cone Unit Resection

In cases of metastatic liver cancer where anatomical resections are not of additional oncological value, ICG fluorescence technique offers the possibility of a cone unit resection [19, 20]. This is valuable as part of the parenchyma sparing principle in lesions where a limited resection would leave behind ischemic liver tissue. Also, in case of HCC on top of a compromised liver, this may prove a useful procedure.

Case Report: Laparoscopic Hepatectomy Using Cone Unit Resection

A laparoscopic segment S4b cone unit resection was performed in a case of CRLM. The root of the Glissonian vessel P4b was identified and clipped along the plane of the falciform ligament. Intravenous injection of 2.5 mg/ml of ICG led to the appearance of a negatively staining volume rendering cone unit resection along the parenchymal interface possible (Fig. 13.6).

Conclusions

ICG fluorescence staining of liver segments clearly outlines segment boundaries on the liver surface. The fluorescence staining is maintained throughout the procedure and drives the transection plane between the fluorescent and the nonfluorescent parenchyma. Therefore, ICG fluorescence serves as a real-time intraoperative navigation tool contributing to the accurate and safe performance of laparoscopic ALR.

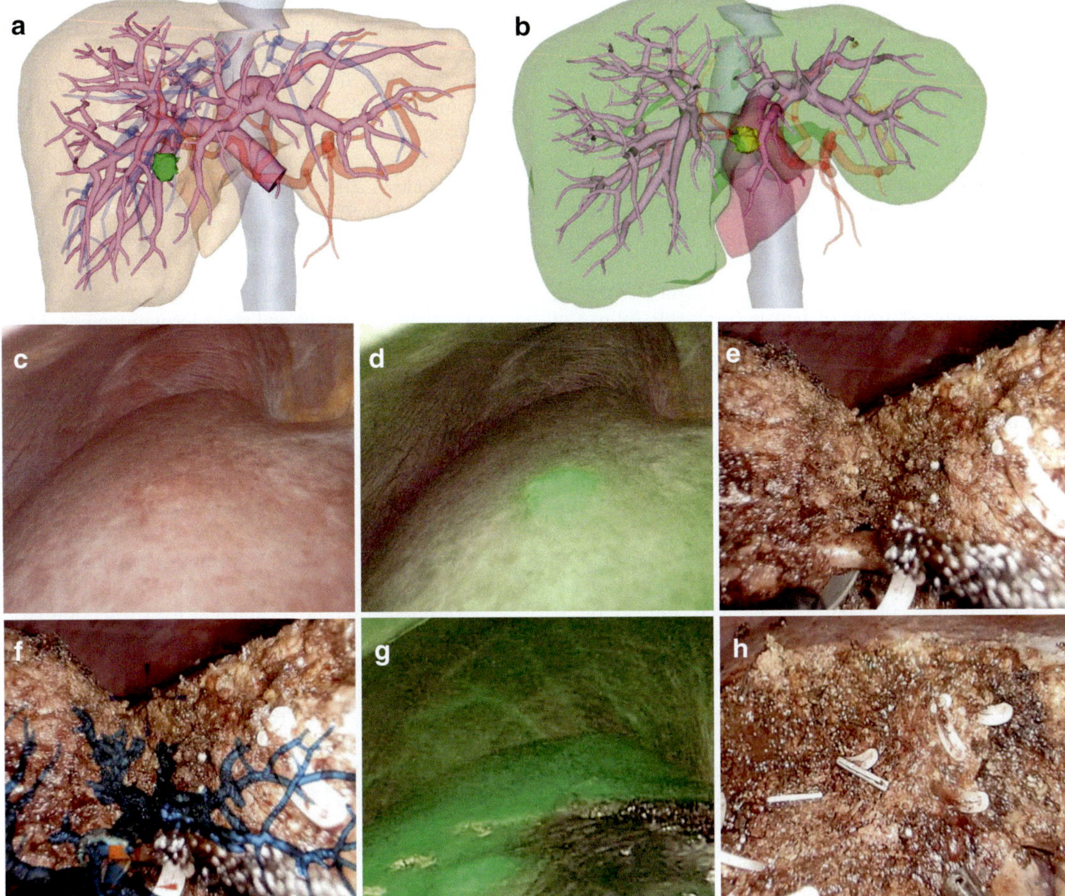

Fig. 13.6 Laparoscopic cone unit resection with ICG fluorescence imaging (negative staining). Laparoscopic S4b cone unit resection performed on a 66-year-old woman with metastatic liver cancer. (**a**) Tertiary branches of the Glissonian vessel identified in the preoperative simulation. (**b**) Simulation of the absence of ICG fluorescence when blood flow to the feeding portal vein was occluded. (**c**) Intraoperative view of ill-defined S4 segment tumor (white light). (**d**) S4 segment tumor localization confirmed by NIR function of the laparoscopic camera (in this patient the tumor has retained the ICG used during the preoperative ICG retention test to determine hepatic functional reserve). (**e**) Appearance of the Glissonian vessel (P4b) in the transection plane and its dissection just before intravenous injection. (**f**) Fusion of the laparoscopic view and the preoperative simulation to show the correlation regarding the Glissonian branch appearing in the liver transection plane. (**g**) ICG fluorescence deficiency in the area fed by P4b on the liver surface and marking of ICG fluorescence-deficient area. (**h**) Liver transection plane after completion of laparoscopic cone unit resection

References

1. Couinaud C. Les enveloppes vasculobiliaries du foie ou capsule de Glisson:leur interet dans la chirurgie vesicularie, les resections hepatiques et l'abord du bile du foie. Lyon Chir. 1954;49:589.
2. Makuuchi M, Hasegawa H, Yamazaki S. Ultrasonically guided subsegmentectomy. Surg Gynecol Obset. 1985;126:346–50.
3. Takayama T, Makuuchi M, Watanabe K, Kosuge T, Takayasu K, Yamazaki S, et al. A new method for mapping hepatic subsegment: counterstaining indetification technique. Surgery. 1991;110:903–4.
4. Ishizawa T, Fukushima N, Shibahara J, Masuda K, Tamura S, Aoki T, et al. Real-time identification of liver cancers by using Indocyanine green fluorescent imaging. Cancer. 2009;115:2491–504. https://doi.org/10.1002/cncr.24291.

5. Ishizawa T, Tamura S, Masuda K, Aoki T, Hasegawa K, Imamura H, et al. Intraoperative fluorescent cholangiography using indocyanine green: a biliary road map for safe surgery. J Am Coll Surg. 2009;208:e1–4. https://doi.org/10.1016/j.jamcollsurg.2008.09.024.

6. Aoki T, Yasuda D, Shimizu Y, Odaira M, Niiya T, Kusano T, et al. Image-guided liver mapping using fluorescence navigation system with indo- cyanine green for anatomical hepatic resecion. World J Surg. 2008;32:1763–7. https://doi.org/10.1007/s00268–008–9620-y.

7. Ishizawa T, Zuker NB, Kokudo N, Gayet B. Positive and negative staining of hepatic segments by use of fluorescent imaging techniques during laparoscopic hepatectomy. Arch Surg. 2012;147:393–4. https://doi.org/10.1001/archsurg.2012.59.

8. Aoki T, Murakami M, Koizumi T, Fujimori A, Gareer H, Enami Y, et al. Three-dimensional virtual endoscopy for laparoscopic and thoracoscopic liver resection. J Am Coll Surg. 2015;221:e21–6. https://doi.org/10.1016/j.jamcollsurg.2015.04.012.

9. Uchiyama K, Ueno M, Ozawa S, Kiriyama S, Shigekawa Y, Hirono S, et al. Combined intraoperative use of contrast-enhanced ultrasonography imaging using a sonazoid and fluorescence navigation system with indocyanine green during anatomical hepatectomy. Langenbeck's Arch Surg. 2011;396:1101–7. https://doi.org/10.1007/s00423–011–0778–7.

10. Sakoda M, Ueno S, Iino S, Minami K, Ando K, Kawasaki Y, et al. Pure laparoscopic subsegmentectomy of the liver using a puncture method for the target portal branch under percutaneous ultrasound with artificial ascites. Surg Laparosc Endosc Percutan Tech. 2013;23:e45–8. https://doi.org/10.1097/SLE.0b013e31826f9598.

11. Inoue Y, Arita J, Sakamoto T, Ono Y, Takahashi M, Takahashi Y, et al. Anatomical liver resections guided by 3-dimensional parenchymal staining using fusion indocyanine green fluorescence imaging. Ann Surg. 2015;262:105–11. https://doi.org/10.1097/SLA.0000000000000775.

12. Miyata A, Ishizawa T, Tani K, Shimizu A, Kaneko J, Aoki T, et al. Reappraisal of a dye staining technique for anatomic hepatectomy by the concomitant use of indocyanine green fluorescence imaging. J Am Coll Surg. 2015;221:e27–36. https://doi.org/10.1016/j.jamcollsurg.2015.05.005.

13. Mizuno T, Sheth R, Yamamoto M, Kang HS, Yamashita S, Aloia TA, et al. Laparoscopic Glissonean pedicle transection (Takasaki) for negative fluorescent counterstaining of segment 6. Ann Surg Oncol. 2017;24:1046–7. https://doi.org/10.1245/s10434–016–5721–2.

14. Kobayashi Y, Kawaguchi Y, Kobayashi K, Mori K, Arita J, Sakamoto Y, et al. Portal vein territory identification using indocyanine green fluorescence imaging: technical details and short-term outcomes. J Surg Oncol. 2017;116:921–31. https://doi.org/10.1002/js0.24752.

15. Terasawa M, Ishizawa T, Mise Y, Inoue Y, Ito H, Takahashi Y, et al. Applications of fusion-fluorescence imaging using indocyanine green in laparoscopic hepatectomy. Surg Endosc. 2017;31:5111–8. https://doi.org/10.1007/s00464–017–5576-z.

16. Ueno M, Hayami S, Sonomura T, Tanaka R, Kawai M, Hirono S, et al. Indocyanine green fluorescence imaging techniques and interventional radiology during laparoscopic anatomical liver resection (with video). Surg Endosc. 2018;32:1051–5. https://doi.org/10.1007/s00464–017–5997–8.

17. Peyrat P, Blanc E, Guillermet S, Chen Y, Ferlay C, Perol D, et al. HEPATOFLUO: a prospective monocentric study assessing the benefits of indocyanine green (ICG) fluorescence for hepatic surgery. J Surg Oncol. 2018;117:922–7. https://doi.org/10.1002/js0.25011.

18. Nishino H, Hatano E, Seo S, Nitta T, Saito T, Nakamura M, et al. Real-time navigation for liver surgery using projection mapping with indocyanine green fluorescence: development of the novel medical imaging projection system. Ann Surg. 2018;267:1134–40. https://doi.org/10.1097/SLA.0000000000002172.

19. Takasaki K. Glissonean pedicle transection method for hepatic resection: a new concept of liver segmentation. J Hepato-Biliary-Pancreat Surg. 1998;5:286–91.

20. Yamamoto M, Katagiri S, Ariizumi S, Kotera Y, Takahashi Y. Glissonean pedicle transection method for liver surgery (with video). J Hepatobiliary Pancreat Sci. 2012;19:3–8.

Takeaki Ishizawa, Daisuke Ito,
and Kiyoshi Hasegawa

Indications

Anatomical (sub)segmentectomy of the liver, which was first reported by Makuuchi and colleagues in 1985 [1], has been widely applied as a standard surgical procedure balancing curability and hepatic parenchymal preservation. Anatomical hepatectomy has oncologic advantages—particularly in the treatment of hepatocellular carcinoma (HCC)—by eradicating possible cancer spread along the portal system, leading to favorable long-term outcomes compared with limited non-anatomical resection [2, 3]. Anatomical hepatectomy can also be indicated for patients with metastatic liver cancers with invasion to the proximal portal pedicle and/or intrasegmental tumor spread. Accurate transection of the liver along its intersegmental planes has the potential advantage of decreasing the risk of postoperative bile leakage because this technique can minimize the need for division of the portal pedicles.

Electronic Supplementary Material The online version of this chapter (https://doi.org/10.1007/978-3-030-38092-2_14) contains supplementary material, which is available to authorized users.

T. Ishizawa · D. Ito · K. Hasegawa (✉)
Hepato-Biliary-Pancreatic Surgery Division,
Department of Surgery, Graduate School of
Medicine, The University of Tokyo, Tokyo, Japan
e-mail: kihase-tky@umin.ac.jp

Techniques

Hepatic segmental boundaries can be delineated by intraoperative indocyanine green (ICG) fluorescence imaging using a positive staining technique or a negative staining technique [4].

Positive Staining Technique

The tumor-bearing portal vein is punctured with a 21–23-G needle under ultrasound guidance, and ICG solution (0.25 mg/5 mL) is injected into the portal vein. The extent of the corresponding hepatic segment can then be visualized on the hepatic surfaces with the use of near-infrared camera systems [4–6]. Even when direct puncture of the portal vein supplying the tumor-bearing hepatic segment is technically difficult, the boundaries of that region can be identified as non-fluorescing regions by identifying the adjacent hepatic segments using the same method (counterstaining technique) [6, 7]. With the positive staining technique, the intrahepatic segmental boundaries can also be identified using intraoperative ultrasonography by mixing ultrasound contrast material with the ICG solution [5]. In contrast to the conventional staining technique with indigo carmine, ICG fluorescence imaging enables continued identification of hepatic segments throughout hepatectomy procedures, as the fluorescence persists for 5 hours and longer [6] (Fig. 14.1 and Video 14.1).

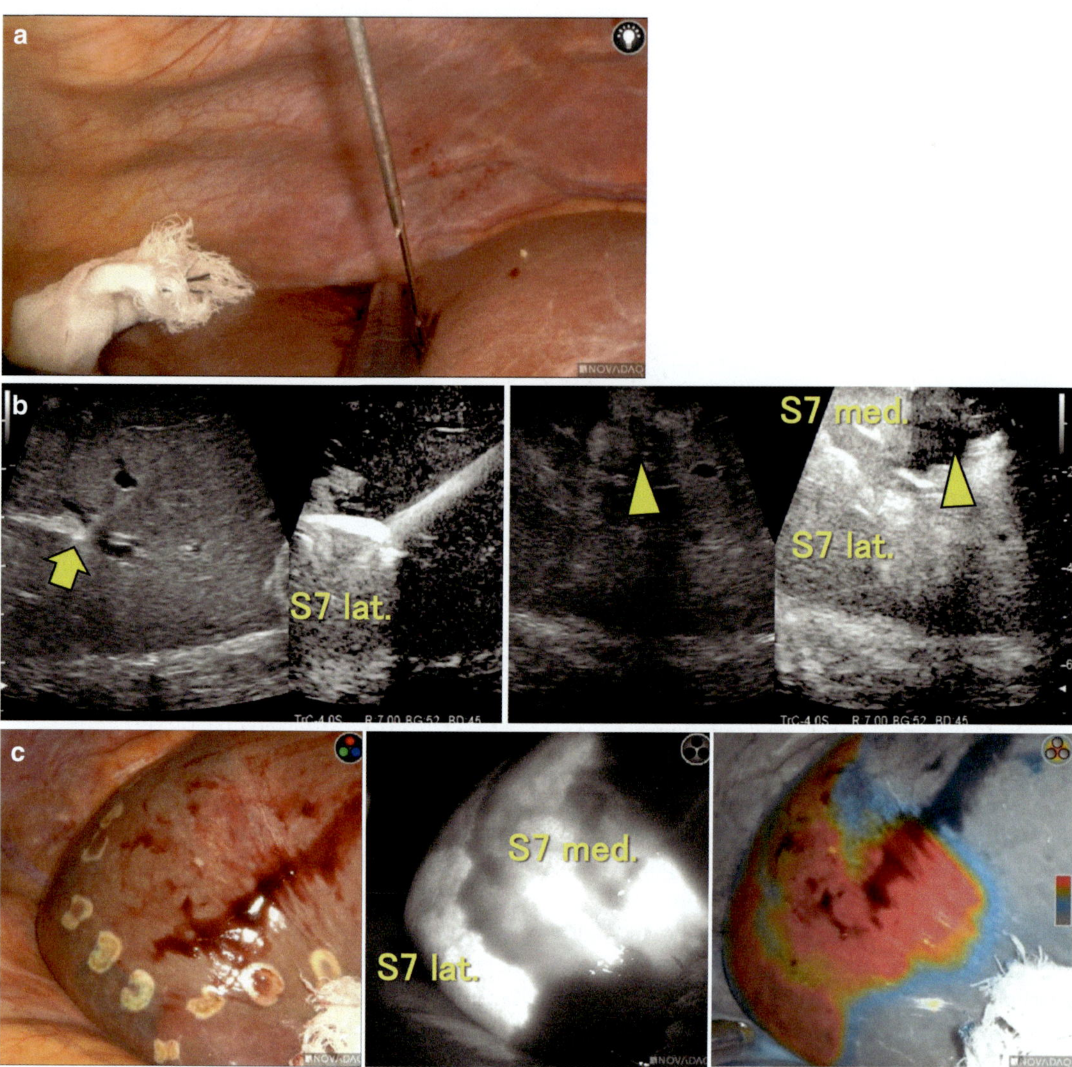

Fig. 14.1 Positive staining technique for the identification of hepatic segment 7. (**a**) The portal branch supplying hepatic segment 7 is punctured with a 21-G needle under ultrasound guidance and indigo carmine solution (5 mL) with ICG (0.25 mg) and ultrasound contrast material is injected into the portal vein. (**b**) Contrast-enhanced ultrasonography demonstrates hyperechoic signals in the lateral region of segment 7 (S7 lat.) and slightly increased echoic signals in the medial region of this segment (S7 med.). The arrow and arrowhead shows a tumor (colorectal liver metastasis) and the tip of the needle in the portal vein, respectively. (**c**) Gray-scale fluorescence imaging (middle) enables clearer demarcation between S7 lat., S7. med., and the non-fluorescing surrounding hepatic parenchyma compared with blue staining observed with white-light color imaging (left). Fusion fluorescence imaging (right) also enables clear identification of S7, although the boundary between S7 med. and S7 lat. is unclear. (**d**) The boundaries of S7 lat. on the visceral surfaces of the liver. (**e**) Because the tumor is located in the medial aspect of S7, the hepatic transection lines are extended to non-fluorescing regions to remove the hepatic parenchyma of S7 med. and part of segment 8 (S8). (**f**) The hepatic parenchyma is transected using the clamp-crushing method, with the occasional use of fluorescence imaging to confirm the intersegmental planes between the fluorescing region of S7 and the non-fluorescing region of S8 (dotted line). (**g**) The portal pedicle of S7 med. (arrowhead) is ligated and divided, preserving the portal pedicle supplying S7 lat. (arrow). (**h**) The operative site after completion of the hepatectomy. Fluorescence imaging clearly shows the boundaries of S7 lat. and the surrounding hepatic regions on the hepatic raw surfaces. The PINPOINT™ Endoscopic Fluorescence Imaging System (Stryker, Kalamazoo, Michigan, USA) was used in this case. Please see also Video 14.1

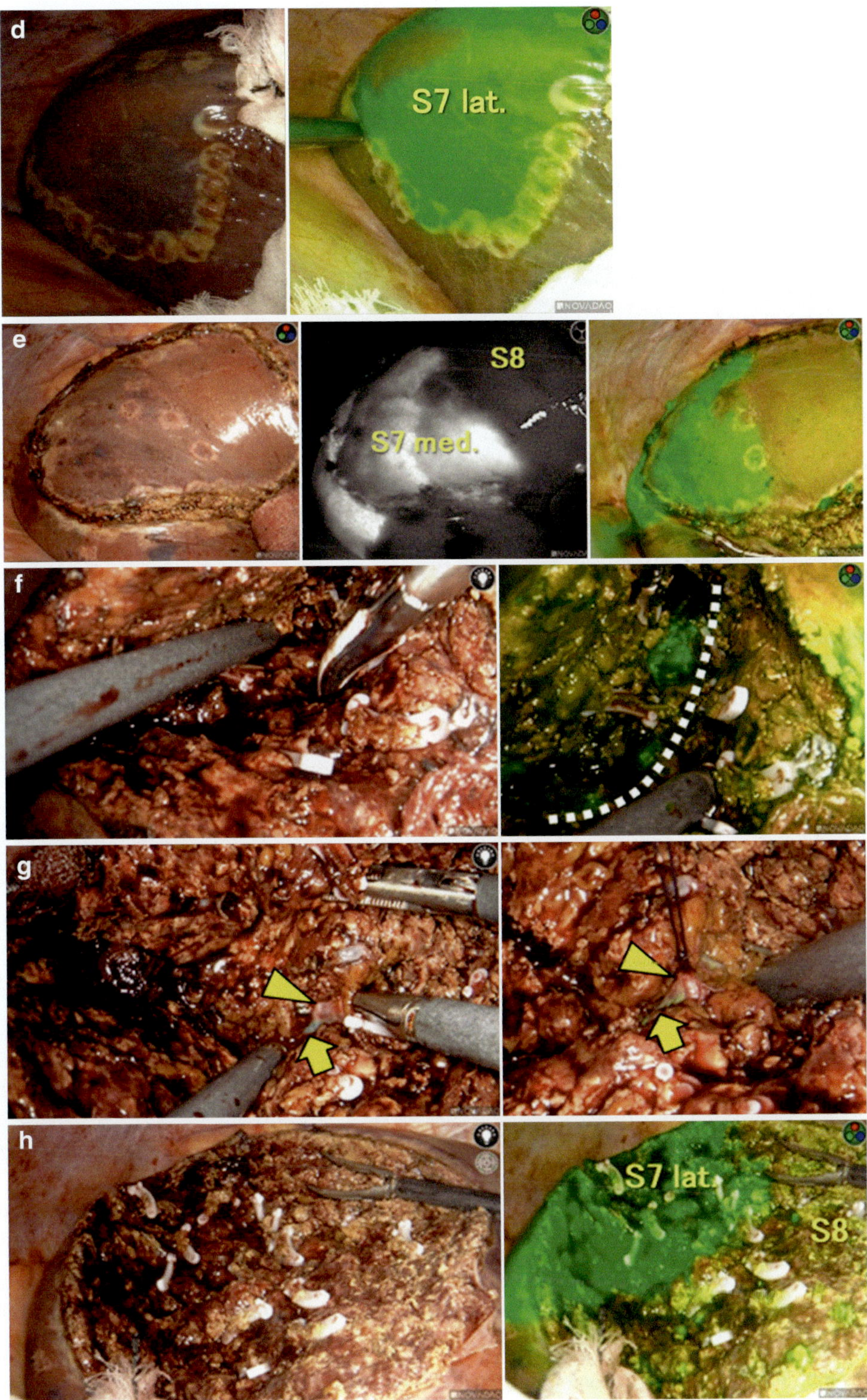

Fig. 14.1 (continued)

Negative Staining Technique

Indocyanine green (2.5 mg) is injected intravenously following closure or division of the tumor-bearing

portal pedicle. Fluorescence imaging can then be used to identify corresponding hepatic segments as non-fluorescing ischemic regions of the liver throughout subsequent surgical procedures (Fig. 14.2

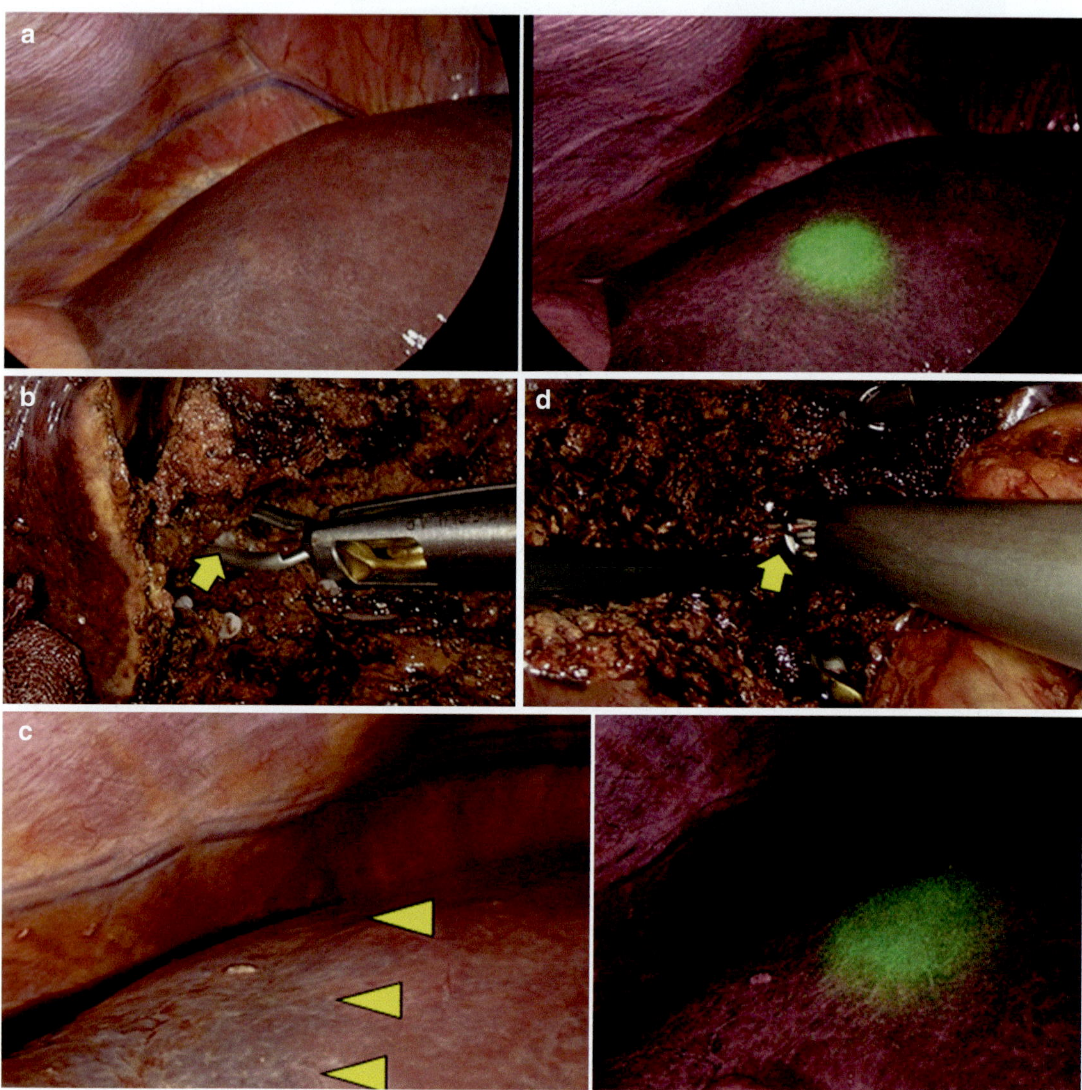

Fig. 14.2 Negative staining technique for the identification of hepatic segment 6. (**a**) The tumor (hepatocellular carcinoma [HCC]), located in the subcapsular region of segment 6 (S6), is identified by fluorescence imaging because of accumulation of the indocyanine green that was injected intravenously prior to surgery. (**b**) The main portal pedicle of segment 6 (arrow) is closed with a vascular clamp at its root. (**c**) Fluorescence imaging (right) indicates that the tumor is located on the intersegmental boundary (arrowheads) between the ischemic region (S6) and the nonischemic hepatic parenchyma (S5), as demonstrated in the white-light color image (left). (**d**) Hepatic parenchymal transection is added to identify and close portal branch of the lateral region of S5 (arrow). (**e**) Indocyanine green (2.5 mg) is then injected intravenously, enabling clear visualization of the boundaries around the ischemic regions of S5 and S6, which include the tumor (arrowhead), by fluorescence imaging. (**f**) The hepatic parenchyma is further transected, with occasional use of fluorescence imaging to confirm accurate intersegmental planes (dotted line). (**g**) The operative site after completion of the hepatectomy. The arrow indicates the stump of the S6 portal pedicle. The residual hepatic parenchyma of S7 still shows ICG fluorescence signals. (**h**) On the cut surface of the resected specimen, the tumor (well-differentiated HCC) shows cancerous fluorescence signals because of accumulation of the ICG that was administered before surgery [11]. The VISERA ELITE II infrared imaging system (OLYMPUS MEDICAL SYSTEMS CORP., Tokyo, Japan) was used in this case. Please see also Video 14.2

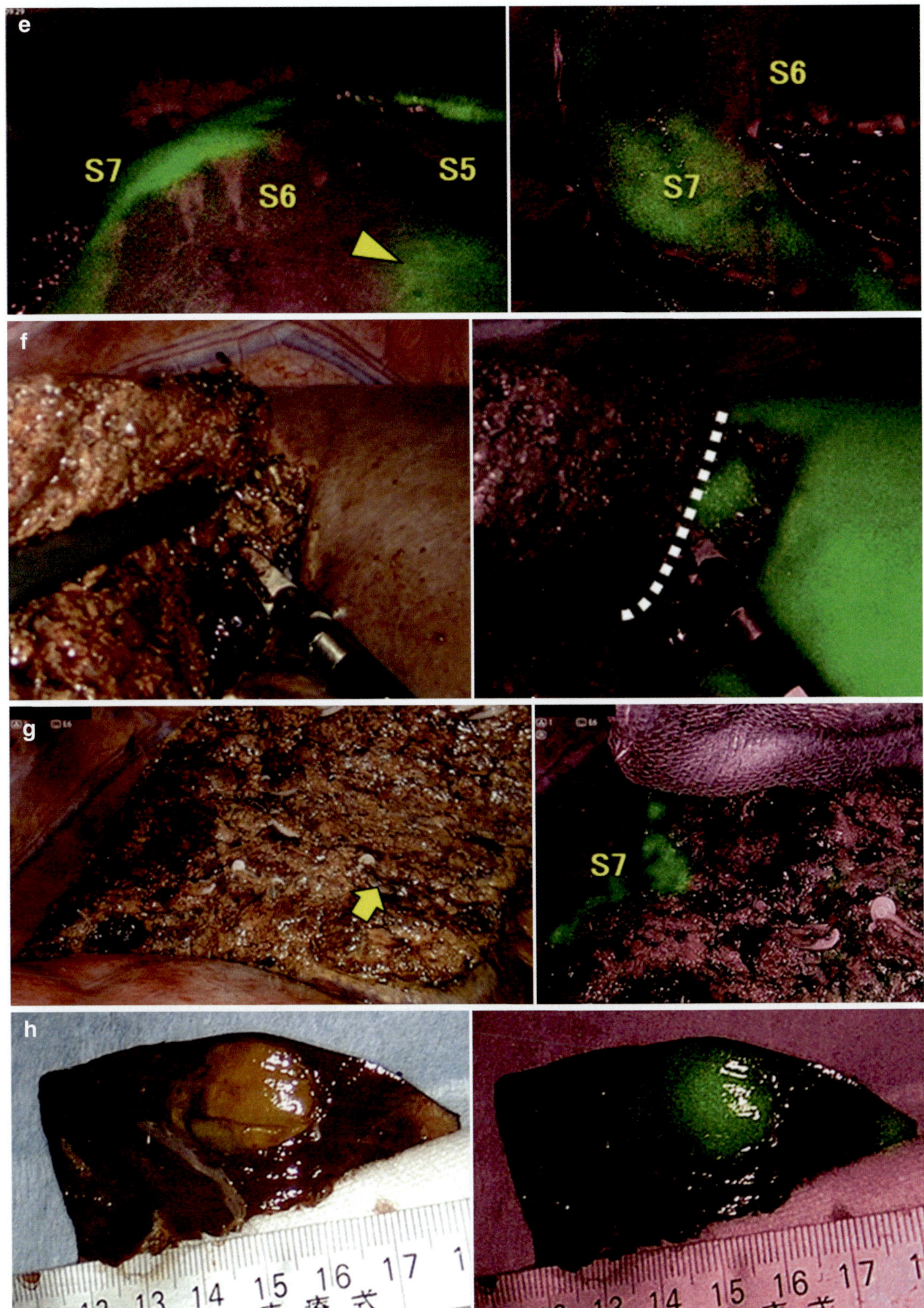

Fig. 14.2 (continued)

and Video 14.2). The negative staining technique has been used frequently in laparoscopic hepatectomy [4, 8] because puncture of a thin portal branch followed by injection of ICG solution is technically demanding in this setting. This technique can also be used for intraoperative estimation of portal uptake function in veno-occlusive hepatic regions [9].

Interpretation

Makuuchi's original technique for the identification of hepatic segments involves the injection of blue dye (indigo carmine) instead of ICG into the portal branch, staining the hepatic surfaces of the corresponding segments in blue [1]. While this conventional dye-staining technique has been used by liver surgeons for more than 20 years, the short duration of hepatic staining (2–3 minutes) makes it difficult to accurately identify segmental boundaries throughout hepatectomy procedures. In 2008, Aoki and colleagues [10] first reported the fluorescence imaging technique using ICG for the delineation of hepatic segments. Their protocol specifies the injection of 5 mg ICG into the portal veins, resulting in a 94% success rate of hepatic segment identification. Based on our preliminary experience, however, 5 mg of ICG seemed to be excessive, resulting in overflow from the liver into the systemic circulation and a massive increase in background fluorescence of the rest of the liver.

To maintain a high enough signal-to-background ratio to identify segmental boundaries by fluorescence imaging throughout hepatectomy, it is important to administer a dose of ICG that can be completely taken up by hepatocytes occupying the corresponding hepatic segments. In 2012, Ishizawa and Gayet [4] reported that hepatic segments could be identified by fluorescence imaging following the injection of diluted ICG solution (0.025 mg/mL) into the portal branch during laparoscopic hepatectomy. Inoue and colleagues [5] injected 2.5 mg of ICG into the portal branches, achieving a 100% success rate of hepatic segment identification compared with 42% using the conventional dye-staining technique. The authors have used

0.25 mg of ICG diluted in 5 mL of indigo carmine solution for the portal vein injection, enabling identification of hepatic segments both by gross examination of blue-stained regions and by fluorescence imaging [6]. In our previous series, concomitant use of fluorescence imaging enhanced the detection of hepatic segments during anatomic resection, especially in the cirrhotic liver or when the liver is covered with connective tissues from a previous surgery. Another advantage of fluorescence imaging is that it enables long-lasting (5 hours and longer [6]) identification of segmental boundaries not only from the hepatic surfaces but also from the raw surfaces during hepatic dissection.

As demonstrated in this chapter, the above positive staining technique can be reproduced even in laparoscopic hepatectomy by surgeons with excellent puncture skills and spatial ability [4]. In general, however, positive staining is technically demanding; the negative staining technique, i.e., enhancement of ischemic hepatic segments by fluorescence imaging, is more feasible in the setting of laparoscopic surgery [8, 12]. Even when using the negative staining technique, surgeons can accurately identify intersegmental planes during hepatic dissection because fluorescence signals in the nonischemic hepatic parenchyma last for several hours following the intravenous injection of ICG (at a dose of 2.5 mg).

Pitfalls

The major limitation of hepatic fluorescence imaging is that, once ICG is administered, it is almost impossible to "delete" the fluorescence signals emitted from the hepatic parenchyma retaining ICG, in contrast to the conventional dye-staining technique. Thus, the anatomic relationships between the tumor and the portal pedicles should be fully considered prior to intraportal or intravenous injection of ICG. To obtain clear images of segmental boundaries, it is important to adjust the intensity of illumination, the distance between the camera and the hepatic surfaces, and the mode of fluorescence imaging. With the positive staining technique in particular, fluorescence imaging using appropriate camera settings (a sufficient imaging distance and use of black and white mode) may enable the visualization of hepatic subsegment boundaries based on minute difference in the amount of ICG in each region, which may be useful for determining hepatic transection lines (Fig. 14.1 and Video 14.1). During open surgery, operation lamps should be turned off to avoid nonspecific fluorescence signals from the background structures.

Summary

Hepatic segmental boundaries can be identified by intraoperative fluorescence imaging using positive staining technique (injection of ICG into the portal veins under ultrasound guidance) or negative staining technique (intravenous administration of ICG following closure of the portal pedicle). These techniques enable clear and long-lasting identification of segmental boundaries, enhancing safety, and accuracy of anatomic hepatectomy.

References

1. Makuuchi M, Hasegawa H, Yamazaki S. Ultrasonically guided subsegmentectomy. Surg Gynecol Obstet. 1985;161:346–50.
2. Hasegawa K, Kokudo N, Imamura H, et al. Prognostic impact of anatomic resection for hepatocellular carcinoma. Ann Surg. 2005;242:252–9.
3. Shindoh J, Makuuchi M, Matsuyama Y, Mise Y, Arita J, Sakamoto Y, et al. Complete removal of the tumor-bearing portal territory decreases local tumor recurrence and improves disease-specific survival of patients with hepatocellular carcinoma. J Hepatol. 2016;64:594–600.
4. Ishizawa T, Zuker NB, Kokudo N, Gayet B. Positive and negative staining of hepatic segments by use of fluorescent imaging techniques during laparoscopic hepatectomy. Arch Surg. 2012;147:393–4.
5. Inoue Y, Arita J, Sakamoto T, et al. Anatomical liver resections guided by 3-dimensional parenchymal staining using fusion indocyanine green fluorescence imaging. Ann Surg. 2015;262:105–11.
6. Miyata A, Ishizawa T, Tani K, Shimizu A, Kaneko J, Aoki T, et al. Reappraisal of a dye-staining technique for anatomic hepatectomy by the concomitant use of indocyanine green-fluorescence imaging. J Am Coll Surg. 2015;221:e27–36.
7. Takayama T, Makuuchi M, Watanabe K, et al. A new method for mapping hepatic subsegment: counterstaining identification technique. Surgery. 1991;109:226–9.
8. Terasawa M, Ishizawa T, Saiura A, et al. Applications of fusion fluorescence imaging using indocyanine green in laparoscopic hepatectomy. Surg Endosc. 2017;31:5111–8.
9. Kawaguchi Y, Ishizawa T, Miyata Y, et al. Portal uptake function in veno-occlusive regions evaluated by real-time fluorescent imaging using indocyanine green. J Hepatol. 2013;58:247–53.
10. Aoki T, Yasuda D, Shimizu Y, et al. Image-guided liver mapping using fluorescence navigation system with indocyanine green for anatomical hepatic resection. World J Surg. 2008;32:1763–7.
11. Ishizawa T, Fukushima N, Shibahara J, et al. Real-time identification of liver cancers by using indocyanine green fluorescent imaging. Cancer. 2009;115:2491–504.
12. Ito D, Ishizawa T, Kokudo T, et al. Laparoscopic positive staining of hepatic segments using ICG-fluorescence imaging. J Hepatobiliary Pancreat Sci. 2020 (in press).

Identification of Hepatocellular Carcinoma Recurrence after Resection

Yoshikuni Kawaguchi, Kosuke Kobayashi, and Kiyoshi Hasegawa

Introduction

Intraoperative navigation using fluorescence imaging was reported in the 1990s. Indocyanine green (ICG) was used as a fluorophore to assess the patency of coronary artery bypass graft [1, 2]. This technique was then applied for visualizing lymphatic vessels [3] and for identifying sentinel lymph nodes during breast cancer surgery [4] and gastric cancer surgery [5, 6]. The principle of ICG-fluorescent imaging is that protein-bound ICG emits light with a peak wavelength of around 840 nm when illuminated with near-infrared light (750–810 nm). Because ICG is taken into the hepatocyte and then exclusively excreted into the bile, the technique is used for various purposes during hepatobiliary surgery. ICG-fluorescence imaging visualizes the flow of hepatic artery and portal vein [7, 8], primary and metastatic liver tumors [9, 10], the

bile duct [11, 12], and portal venous territory [13–15]. The technique was used for evaluating hepatic perfusion of regions with outflow obstruction [16–18]. The technique was originally used for open liver resection and has been increasingly applied for laparoscopic liver resection [19–23]. This chapter focuses on intraoperative navigation using ICG-fluorescence imaging for identifying recurrence of hepatocellular carcinoma (HCC) after resection.

Technical Description of the Procedure

Mechanism of Fluorescence Imaging for Hepatocellular Carcinoma

Mechanism of ICG-fluorescence imaging of HCC was studied using the analyses of immunohistochemical staining and gene expression [24–27]. The mechanism of HCC fluorescence is different between well/moderately differentiated type and poorly differentiated type. For well/moderately differentiated type, ICG is taken into HCC tissues through transporters (organic anion-transporting polypeptide 8 and Na⁺/taurocholate cotransporting polypeptide). ICG is retained in cancerous tissues longer than non-cancerous tissues because functional

Electronic Supplementary Material The online version of this chapter (https://doi.org/10.1007/978-3-030-38092-2_15) contains supplementary material, which is available to authorized users.

Y. Kawaguchi · K. Kobayashi · K. Hasegawa (✉)
Hepato-Biliary-Pancreatic Surgery Division,
Department of Surgery, Graduate School of
Medicine, The University of Tokyo, Tokyo, Japan
e-mail: kihase-tky@umin.ac.jp

or morphological biliary excretion is impaired. In contrast, for poorly differentiated type, the transporters of ICG are downregulated in cancerous tissues, and ICG is generally not taken into cancerous tissues. Biliary excretion function in non-cancerous tissues surrounding cancerous tissues is also impaired. As a result, surrounding non-cancerous tissue retains ICG longer than other liver parenchyma and can provide fluorescence of peripheral areas of liver tumors.

Administration of ICG for Visualizing Liver Tumors

The most common method for administering a fluorophore is to intravenously inject ICG at a dose of 0.5 mg/kg as a routine liver function test within 14 days before surgery [9, 10, 20, 28–31]. Another method was rarely reported for visualizing HCC as fluorescence except intravenous injection of ICG (10 mg) 24 hours before surgery [32]. Figure 15.1 and Video 15.1 show typical fluorescence imaging of HCC.

Interpretation

Usefulness of Fluorescence Imaging of HCC Recurrence

Liver resection is the optimal treatment for HCC and provides overall survival rates which range from 40% to 80% at 3 years and from 20% to 70% at 5 years after resection [33–35]. However, cumulative recurrence rates remain high (50–60% at 3 years and 70–100% at 5 years) [33–37]. Repeat hepatectomy was reported to lead better cumulative long-term survival from initial resection [38–40]. The challenge in performing repeat hepatectomy is due to the technical complexity caused by adhesions of and changes in liver anatomy after the previous operation. These changes may create a challenge in identifying liver tumors during surgery. Figure 15.2 and Video 15.2 show typical fluorescence imaging for HCC recurrence after initial hepatectomy. Fluorescence of HCC was clearly visualized on the thick connective tissues around the liver surface. Previous reports also showed that fluorescence imaging was helpful for visualizing HCC recurrence on the thick connective tissues [8, 10, 41] and viable areas of

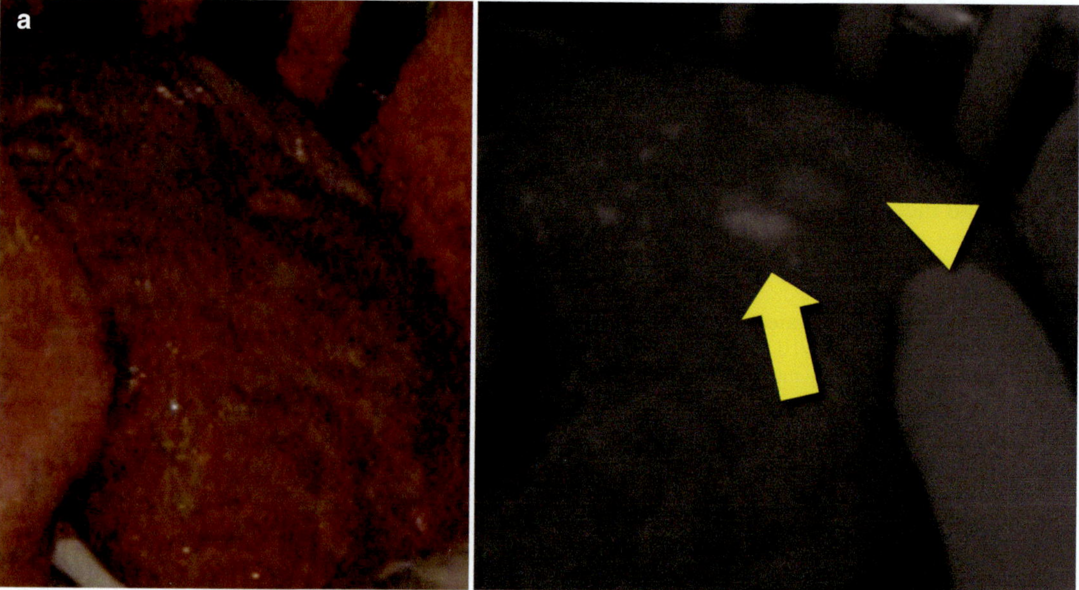

Fig. 15.1 Fluorescence imaging of hepatocellular carcinoma. (**a**) Fluorescence imaging visualized 2 HCCs on the surface of cirrhotic liver. (**b**) ICG fluorescence is confirmed in the HCC tissues (yellow arrow and arrowhead)

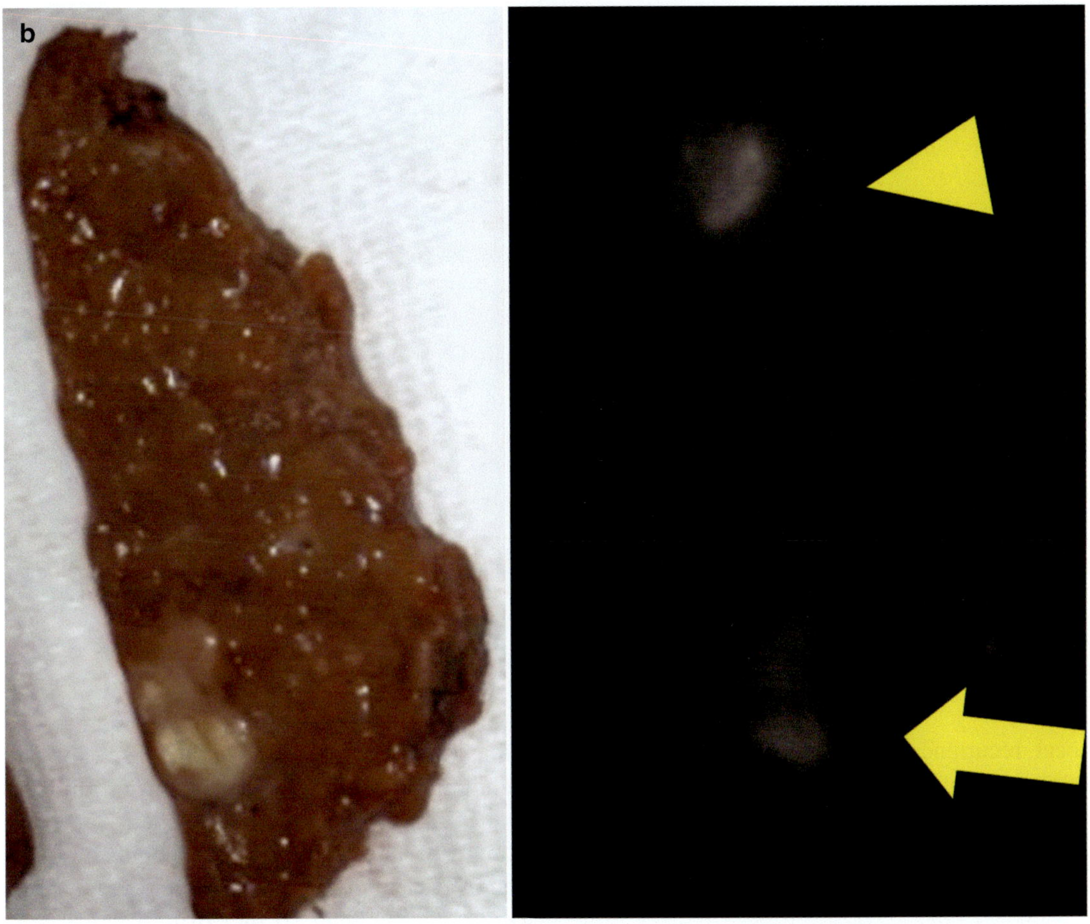

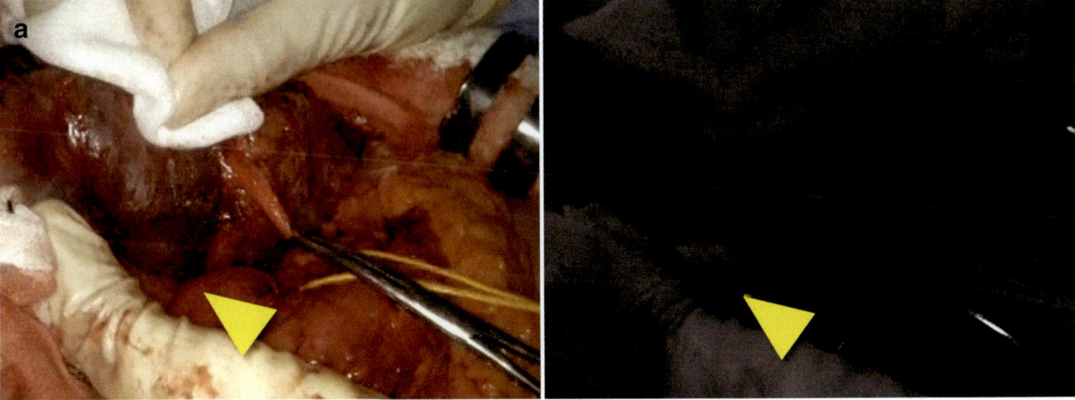

Fig. 15.1 (continued)

Fig. 15.2 Fluorescence imaging of recurrence of hepatocellular carcinoma. (**a**) Fluorescence imaging clearly visualized HCC on the liver surface with connective tissue caused by previous surgery (arrowhead). (**b**) ICG fluorescence is confirmed in HCC tissue

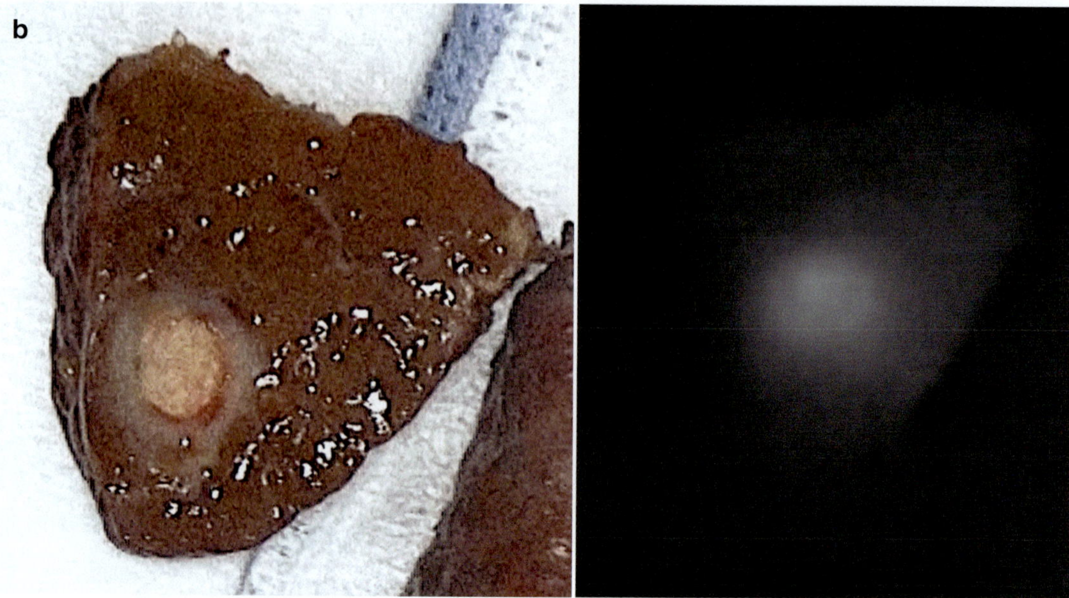

Fig. 15.2 (continued)

local recurrence of HCC, which was initially treated by ablation [20].

Pitfalls

One of the drawbacks of ICG-fluorescence imaging for visualizing liver tumors as fluorescence is a relatively high false-positive rate, ranging from 5% to 40% [26, 30, 42]. It is an issue whether false-positive lesions (i.e., fluorescing lesions but no malignancy) should be resected or not. This false-positive rate may increase in patients who previously underwent resection or ablation. Previous intervention causes focal bile stasis around the area of treatment. Such focal areas with bile stasis are likely to retain ICG longer than the other areas and result in providing fluorescence. We hypothesized that false-positive rate can be reduced by altering the timing and dose of ICG administration. Currently, we are conducting a clinical research trial to determine the timing and dose of ICG administration, which are associated with high sensitivity and high positive predictive value for identifying liver malignancies with fluorescence. Another drawback of the technique is that the tissue penetration ability of near-infrared light is limited to about 8–10 mm from the liver surface. This is a technical limitation of ICG-fluorescence imaging. Liver lesions located deeper than 10 mm from the liver surface cannot be visualized as fluorescence using the current imaging systems. Nonetheless, ICG-fluorescence imaging is helpful for visualizing vanishing tumors after chemotherapy, and for identifying viable areas of local recurrence after ablation, although these tumors are hard to visualize using intraoperative ultrasonography [20].

Summary

ICG-fluorescence imaging can be used for visualizing recurrent HCC in patients undergoing repeat liver resection as in patients undergoing initial liver resection. It clearly visualizes HCC as fluorescence on the thick connective tissue because of adhesions after initial liver resection. The technique may be useful for complementing visual inspection, palpation, and intraoperative ultrasonography.

References

1. Rubens FD, Ruel M, Fremes SE. A new and simplified method for coronary and graft imaging during CABG. Heart Surg Forum. 2002;5:141–4.
2. Taggart DP, Choudhary B, Anastasiadis K, Abu-Omar Y, Balacumaraswami L, Pigott DW. Preliminary experience with a novel intraoperative fluorescence imaging technique to evaluate the patency of bypass grafts in total arterial revascularization. Ann Thorac Surg. 2003;75:870–3.
3. Ogata F, Narushima M, Mihara M, Azuma R, Morimoto Y, Koshima I. Intraoperative lymphography using indocyanine green dye for near-infrared fluorescence labeling in lymphedema. Ann Plast Surg. 2007;59:180–4.
4. Kitai T, Inomoto T, Miwa M, Shikayama T. Fluorescence navigation with indocyanine green for detecting sentinel lymph nodes in breast cancer. Breast Cancer. 2005;12:211–5.
5. Kusano M, Tajima Y, Yamazaki K, Kato M, Watanabe M, Miwa M. Sentinel node mapping guided by indocyanine green fluorescence imaging: a new method for sentinel node navigation surgery in gastrointestinal cancer. Dig Surg. 2008;25:103–8.
6. Miyashiro I, Miyoshi N, Hiratsuka M, Kishi K, Yamada T, Ohue M, et al. Detection of sentinel node in gastric cancer surgery by indocyanine green fluorescence imaging: comparison with infrared imaging. Ann Surg Oncol. 2008;15:1640–3.
7. Kubota K, Kita J, Shimoda M, Rokkaku K, Kato M, Iso Y, et al. Intraoperative assessment of reconstructed vessels in living-donor liver transplantation, using a novel fluorescence imaging technique. J Hepato-Biliary-Pancreat Surg. 2006;13:100–4.
8. Kawaguchi Y, Ishizawa T, Masuda K, Sato S, Kaneko J, Aoki T, et al. Hepatobiliary surgery guided by a novel fluorescent imaging technique for visualizing hepatic arteries, bile ducts, and liver cancers on color images. J Am Coll Surg. 2011;212:e33–9.
9. Gotoh K, Yamada T, Ishikawa O, Takahashi H, Eguchi H, Yano M, et al. A novel image-guided surgery of hepatocellular carcinoma by indocyanine green fluorescence imaging navigation. J Surg Oncol. 2009;100:75–9.
10. Ishizawa T, Fukushima N, Shibahara J, Masuda K, Tamura S, Aoki T, et al. Real-time identification of liver cancers by using indocyanine green fluorescent imaging. Cancer. 2009;115:2491–504.
11. Mitsuhashi N, Kimura F, Shimizu H, Imamaki M, Yoshidome H, Ohtsuka M, et al. Usefulness of intraoperative fluorescence imaging to evaluate local anatomy in hepatobiliary surgery. J Hepato-Biliary-Pancreat Surg. 2008;15:508–14.
12. Ishizawa T, Bandai Y, Ijichi M, Kaneko J, Hasegawa K, Kokudo N. Fluorescent cholangiography illuminating the biliary tree during laparoscopic cholecystectomy. Br J Surg. 2010;97:1369–77.
13. Aoki T, Murakami M, Yasuda D, Shimizu Y, Kusano T, Matsuda K, et al. Intraoperative fluorescent imaging using indocyanine green for liver mapping and cholangiography. J Hepatobiliary Pancreat Sci. 2010;17:590–4.
14. Miyata A, Ishizawa T, Tani K, Shimizu A, Kaneko J, Aoki T, et al. Reappraisal of a dye-staining technique for anatomic hepatectomy by the concomitant use of indocyanine green fluorescence imaging. J Am Coll Surg. 2015;221:e27–36.
15. Kobayashi Y, Kawaguchi Y, Kobayashi K, Mori K, Arita J, Sakamoto Y, et al. Portal vein territory identification using indocyanine green fluorescence imaging: technical details and short-term outcomes. J Surg Oncol. 2017;116:921.
16. Kawaguchi Y, Ishizawa T, Miyata Y, Yamashita S, Masuda K, Satou S, et al. Portal uptake function in veno-occlusive regions evaluated by real-time fluorescent imaging using indocyanine green. J Hepatol. 2013;58:247–53.
17. Kawaguchi Y, Sugawara Y, Ishizawa T, Satou S, Kaneko J, Tamura S, et al. Identification of veno-occlusive regions in a right liver graft after reconstruction of vein segments 5 and 8: application of indocyanine green fluorescence imaging. Liver Transpl. 2013;19:778–9.
18. Kawaguchi Y, Nomura Y, Nagai M, Koike D, Sakuraoka Y, Ishida T, et al. Liver transection using indocyanine green fluorescence imaging and hepatic vein clamping. Br J Surg. 2017;104:898–906.
19. Kudo H, Ishizawa T, Tani K, Harada N, Ichida A, Shimizu A, et al. Visualization of subcapsular hepatic malignancy by indocyanine-green fluorescence imaging during laparoscopic hepatectomy. Surg Endosc. 2014;28:2504–8.
20. Kawaguchi Y, Nagai M, Nomura Y, Kokudo N, Tanaka N. Usefulness of indocyanine green-fluorescence imaging during laparoscopic hepatectomy to visualize subcapsular hard-to-identify hepatic malignancy. J Surg Oncol. 2015;112:514.
21. Kawaguchi Y, Velayutham V, Fuks D, Christidis C, Kokudo N, Gayet B. Usefulness of indocyanine green-fluorescence imaging for visualization of the bile duct during laparoscopic liver resection. J Am Coll Surg. 2015;221:e113–7.
22. Terasawa M, Ishizawa T, Mise Y, Inoue Y, Ito H, Takahashi Y, et al. Applications of fusion-fluorescence imaging using indocyanine green in laparoscopic hepatectomy. Surg Endosc. 2017;31:5111.
23. Aoki T, Murakami M, Koizumi T, Matsuda K, Fujimori A, Kusano T, et al. Determination of the surgical margin in laparoscopic liver resections using infrared indocyanine green fluorescence. Langenbeck's Arch Surg. 2018;403:671.
24. Kitao A, Zen Y, Matsui O, Gabata T, Kobayashi S, Koda W, et al. Hepatocellular carcinoma: signal intensity at gadoxetic acid-enhanced MR imaging--correlation with molecular transporters and histopathologic features. Radiology. 2010;256:817–26.

25. de Graaf W, Hausler S, Heger M, van Ginhoven TM, van Cappellen G, Bennink RJ, et al. Transporters involved in the hepatic uptake of (99m)Tc-mebrofenin and indocyanine green. J Hepatol. 2011;54:738–45.

26. Ishizawa T, Masuda K, Urano Y, Kawaguchi Y, Satou S, Kaneko J, et al. Mechanistic background and clinical applications of indocyanine green fluorescence imaging of hepatocellular carcinoma. Ann Surg Oncol. 2014;21:440–8.

27. Shibasaki Y, Sakaguchi T, Hiraide T, Morita Y, Suzuki A, Baba S, et al. Expression of indocyanine green-related transporters in hepatocellular carcinoma. J Surg Res. 2015;193:567–76.

28. Uchiyama K, Ueno M, Ozawa S, Kiriyama S, Shigekawa Y, Yamaue H. Combined use of contrast-enhanced intraoperative ultrasonography and a fluorescence navigation system for identifying hepatic metastases. World J Surg. 2010;34:2953–9.

29. Tanaka T, Takatsuki M, Hidaka M, Hara T, Muraoka I, Soyama A, et al. Is a fluorescence navigation system with indocyanine green effective enough to detect liver malignancies? J Hepatobiliary Pancreat Sci. 2014;21(3):199–204.

30. Morita Y, Sakaguchi T, Unno N, Shibasaki Y, Suzuki A, Fukumoto K, et al. Detection of hepatocellular carcinomas with near-infrared fluorescence imaging using indocyanine green: its usefulness and limitation. Int J Clin Oncol. 2013;18:232–41.

31. Zhang YM, Shi R, Hou JC, Liu ZR, Cui ZL, Li Y, et al. Liver tumor boundaries identified intraoperatively using real-time indocyanine green fluorescence imaging. J Cancer Res Clin Oncol. 2017;143:51–8.

32. Boogerd LS, Handgraaf HJ, Lam HD, Huurman VA, Farina-Sarasqueta A, Frangioni JV, et al. Laparoscopic detection and resection of occult liver tumors of multiple cancer types using real-time near-infrared fluorescence guidance. Surg Endosc. 2017;31:952–61.

33. Belghiti J, Panis Y, Farges O, Benhamou JP, Fekete F. Intrahepatic recurrence after resection of hepatocellular carcinoma complicating cirrhosis. Ann Surg. 1991;214:114–7.

34. Grazi GL, Ercolani G, Pierangeli F, Del Gaudio M, Cescon M, Cavallari A, et al. Improved results of liver resection for hepatocellular carcinoma on cirrhosis give the procedure added value. Ann Surg. 2001;234:71–8.

35. Poon RT, Fan ST, Lo CM, Liu CL, Wong J. Long-term survival and pattern of recurrence after resection of small hepatocellular carcinoma in patients with preserved liver function: implications for a strategy of salvage transplantation. Ann Surg. 2002;235:373–82.

36. Imamura H, Matsuyama Y, Miyagawa Y, Ishida K, Shimada R, Miyagawa S, et al. Prognostic significance of anatomical resection and des-gamma-carboxy prothrombin in patients with hepatocellular carcinoma. Br J Surg. 1999;86:1032–8.

37. Nakajima Y, Ko S, Kanamura T, Nagao M, Kanehiro H, Hisanaga M, et al. Repeat liver resection for hepatocellular carcinoma. J Am Coll Surg. 2001;192:339–44.

38. Adam R, Bhangui P, Vibert E, Azoulay D, Pelletier G, Duclos-Vallee JC, et al. Resection or transplantation for early hepatocellular carcinoma in a cirrhotic liver: does size define the best oncological strategy? Ann Surg. 2012;256:883–91.

39. Zheng Z, Liang W, Milgrom DP, Schroder PM, Kong NS, Yang C, et al. Liver transplantation versus liver resection in the treatment of hepatocellular carcinoma: a meta-analysis of observational studies. Transplantation. 2014;97:227–34.

40. Mise Y, Hasegawa K, Shindoh J, Ishizawa T, Aoki T, Sakamoto Y, et al. The feasibility of third or more repeat hepatectomy for recurrent hepatocellular carcinoma. Ann Surg. 2015;262:347–57.

41. Kawaguchi Y, Aoki T, Ishizawa T, Arita J, Satou S, Kaneko J, et al. Education and imaging: hepatobiliary and pancreatic: identification of recurrent hepatocellular carcinoma by intraoperative fluorescent imaging. J Gastroenterol Hepatol. 2013;28:587.

42. Abo T, Nanashima A, Tobinaga S, Hidaka S, Taura N, Takagi K, et al. Usefulness of intraoperative diagnosis of hepatic tumors located at the liver surface and hepatic segmental visualization using indocyanine green-photodynamic eye imaging. Eur J Surg Oncol. 2015;41:257–64.

Tomotake Koizumi, Takeshi Aoki,
and Masahiko Murakami

Indications

Intraoperative fluorescence imaging, particularly near-infrared (NIR) fluorescence imaging, techniques using indocyanine green (ICG) have been widely applied in various fields of surgery [1–10]. In the field of liver surgery, NIR imaging has been adopted to intraoperatively identify tumors on the basis of the characteristic accumulation of ICG in the cancerous tissues of hepatocellular carcinoma and in noncancerous hepatic parenchyma around the adenocarcinoma foci [11, 12]. The mechanism of ICG fluorescence signal retention following preoperative intravenous injection has reportedly been caused by the decreased bile excretion ability of immature hepatocytes that surround the tumor [13]. This technique has been applied not only during open surgery but also during laparoscopic hepatectomy [14] because the limited visual inspection and palpation during laparoscopic surgery can be complemented by NIR imaging.

For the treatment of liver metastasis (LM), liver resection has played a leading role in modern multimodality therapy, which includes systemic chemotherapy and radiation therapy [15]. Despite recent advances in imaging modalities, 3–17% of LM from colorectal carcinoma can be detected only by microscopic examination [16–19]. In addition, the administration of chemotherapy can make it more difficult to detect LM by preoperative and intraoperative ultrasound. Furthermore, the intraoperative detection and diagnosis of small tumors remain insufficient.

NIR imaging technique is reportedly an excellent method to identify LM during surgery [11–14] and is useful in determining the surgical margins along the transection plane of the liver [20]. This review reports the techniques, present applications, and future perspectives on NIR imaging for LM.

Technical Description of the Procedures

The technique for NIR imaging for LM is safe and simple. As a fluorescent source, ICG (Diagnogreen, Daiichi Sankyo, Tokyo, Japan) is used and commonly administered to the patient intravenously at a dose of 0.5 mg/kg body weight; this is part of the routine preoperative liver function tests to determine

---

Electronic Supplementary Material The online version of this chapter (https://doi.org/10.1007/978-3-030-38092-2_16) contains supplementary material, which is available to authorized users.

T. Koizumi (✉) · T. Aoki · M. Murakami
Division of Gastroenterological and General Surgery,
Department of Surgery, Showa University,
Tokyo, Japan
e-mail: t-koiz@med.showa-u.ac.jp

the operative indications and procedures. The interval between the ICG injection and surgery ranges from 2 to 14 days.

During surgery, the liver surface is observed, and the location of subcapsular hepatic tumor is identified using a commercially available NIR fluorescence imaging system, followed by preoperative intravenous injection of ICG. NIR fluorescence imaging has the ability to identify newly detected lesions that cannot be preoperatively detected by ultrasound, contrast-enhanced computed tomography (CT), and gadolinium ethoxybenzyl diethylenetriamine pentaacetic acid-enhanced magnetic resonance imaging (EOB-MRI). Furthermore, the information provided by fluorescence imaging helps the surgeon set a dissection line for parenchymal transection during surgery.

Various commercial NIR fluorescence imagers exist for open and laparoscopic surgery, and they have the capability to image ICG fluorescence signals with different levels of sensitivity and features [21]. The only contraindication to ICG administration and application of NIR imaging is the presence of allergy to ICG.

Interpretation

NIR Fluorescence Imaging

NIR fluorescence imaging has the characteristics of tissue penetration, which allows effective rejection of excitation light and detection of deep tissues within the organs. The NIR imaging system irradiated the ICG combined with serum protein with infrared light at wavelengths of 700–850 nm, which is the range that has the advantage of preventing light absorption by hemoglobin in the visible light spectrum (<600 nm) and by the other molecules in the infrared spectrum (>900 nm). Therefore, a wavelength of 845 nm after illumination by an NIR ray offers a better contrast of the NIR fluorescence signal emitted from the ICG, enabling real-time intraoperative visualization of the LM location [22–24].

Timing and Dose of ICG Administration

ICG has been generally applied as a fluorescence source for NIR fluorescence imaging. The majority of studies that adopted an ICG dose of 0.5 mg/kg body weight and a timing of ICG administration of 1–14 days before surgery reported NIR fluorescence imaging accuracy rates of 68.8–100% for the detection of LM [11, 14, 20, 23, 25–30] (Table 16.1). Alfano et al. reported that the administration of ICG at a dose of 0.2 mL/kg, given 24–48 h prior to the scheduled surgery, was the best for patients who underwent the ICG test at ≥7 days before the scheduled surgery [24]. Some studies have reported that ICG administration in doses of 7.5, 10, and 20 mg at 24 or 48 h before surgery yielded NIR fluorescence imaging accuracy rates of 61.4–69.2% for the detection of LM (Table 16.1) [31, 32]. Takahashi et al. reported that the best contrast distinction between the tumors and the normal parenchyma was obtained by ICG administration at 24 h preoperatively than by ICG administration at 48 h preoperatively or intraoperatively [31]. Several studies have reported that the intraoperative administration of ICG at different doses of 0.25 mg/kg body weight, 5 mg per injection, and 25 mg per injection enable the identification of a tumor as a deflected area of fluorescence signal by infrared light irradiation [31, 33, 34].

Mechanism of ICG Accumulation in the Tumor

The preferential accumulation of ICG in malignant or benign nodules relative to normal liver tissue has been attributed to biliary excretion disorders in the surrounding noncancerous liver tissue that has been compressed by the tumor [11, 25]. Van der Vorst et al. reported that on microscopic examination, ICG fluorescence was noted to be located both intracellularly and extracellularly, in the liver tissue directly surrounding the tumor, implying entrapment around the CK7-positive hepatocytes compressed by the tumor. Moreover, the area of liver tissue near the tumor

Table 16.1 Identification of liver metastasis via near-infrared fluorescence imaging

Study	Number of LM patients	Preoperative diagnosis	Surgical approach	Imaging system	Fluorescence agent dosage	Injection timing (before surgery)	Accuracy (%)	References
Ishizawa 2009	12	CRLM	Open	PDE	ICG 0.5 mg/kgBW	1–14 days	100	[11]
Uchiyama 2010	32	CRLM	Open	PDE	ICG 0.5 mg/kgBW	1–14 days	94.4	[25]
Yokoyama 2012	49	Pancreatic cancer	Open	PDE	ICG 25 mg	Intraoperative	42.9	[33]
Ishizuka 2012	7	CRLM	Open	–	ICG 0.1 mg/kg	1–14 days	97.9	[26]
van der Vorst 2013	40	CRLM	Open	Mini-FLARE	ICG 10 or 20 mg	24 or 48 h	76.8	[13]
Peloso 2013	25	CRLM	Open	FDE	ICG 0.5 mg/kgBW	24 h	–	[27]
Kudo 2014	7	CRLM/uterine cancer	Lap	Ollympus medical system	ICG 0.5 mg/kgBW	1–14 days	68.8	[14]
Tummers 2015	3	Uveal melanoma	Lap	Karl Storz	ICG 10 mg	24 h	–	[35]
Shimada 2015	7	CRLM	Open	PDE	ICG 0.5 mg/kgBW	2–14 days	–	[28]
Abo 2015	12	CRLM	Open	PDE	ICG 0.5 mg/kgBW	4–7 days	86.1	[22]
Kawaguchi 2015	1	CRLM	Lap	Ollympus medical system	ICG 0.5 mg/kgBW	1–14 days	100	[29]
Kaibori 2016	13	CRLM	Open	PDE	ICG 0.5 mg/kgBW	ICG 1–14 days	ICG 94[a]	[30]
				SBI Pharmaceuticals	5-ALA 750 mg	5-ALA 3 h	5-ALA 58[a]	
Takahashi 2016	15	CRLM/benign lesion	Open/lap	Fluorescence firefly imaging/SPY	ICG 5–7.5 mg	Intraoperative or 1–2 days	54	[31]
Handgraaf 2017	86	CRLM	Open/lap	FLARE/Artemis/Karl Storz	ICG 10 or 20 mg	1–2 days	–	[38]
Terasawa 2017	41	CRLM/GIST	Lap	SPY	ICG 0.5 mg/kgBW	1–3 days	84.9[a]	[37]
Boogerd 2017	14	CRLM/uveal melanoma/breast cancer	Lap	Karl Storz	ICG 10 mg	24 h	78.3[a]	[32]
Zhang 2017	9	CRLM/other/ benign lesion	Open	SPY	ICG 0.25 mg/ kgBW	Intraoperqative	–	[34]
Lieto 2018	6	CRLM	–	–	ICG 0.5 mg/kgBW	24 h	–	[23]
Aoki 2018	12	CRLM	Lap	SPY	ICG 0.5 mg/kgBW	2–14 days	100	[20]
Alfano 2018	5	CRLM	Open	Karl Stortz/SPY	ICG 0.5 mg/kgBW	1–2 days	–	[24]
Benedicenti 2018	1	CRLM	Open	–	ICG 0.5 mg/kgBW	10days	–	[36]

CRLM colorectal liver metastasis, *PDE* photo dynamic eye, *ICG* indocyanine green, *SPY* fluorescence imaging system of Stryker
[a]Included other malignancy (HCC, ICC)

was observed to have compressed hepatocytes and increased ductular transformation, periportal fibrosis, and Kupffer cells. Immunohistochemical analysis showed a close relationship between fluorescence and staining for CK7, which was expressed by the immature hepatocytes in the areas of ductular transformation. Notably, fluorescence was observed to have no relationship with the presence of Kupffer cells (CD68) and blood vessels (CD31) [13].

Tumor Detection

LM from colorectal cancer has been commonly delineated as rim-fluorescing lesions (Fig. 16.1) [11, 13, 22, 27, 28, 35, 36]. Using fluorescent microscopy, several studies have confirmed that rim fluorescence originates in the noncancerous liver parenchyma surrounding the LM [11, 28]. Conversely, some cases of LM have been delineated as completely (Fig. 16.2) or partially

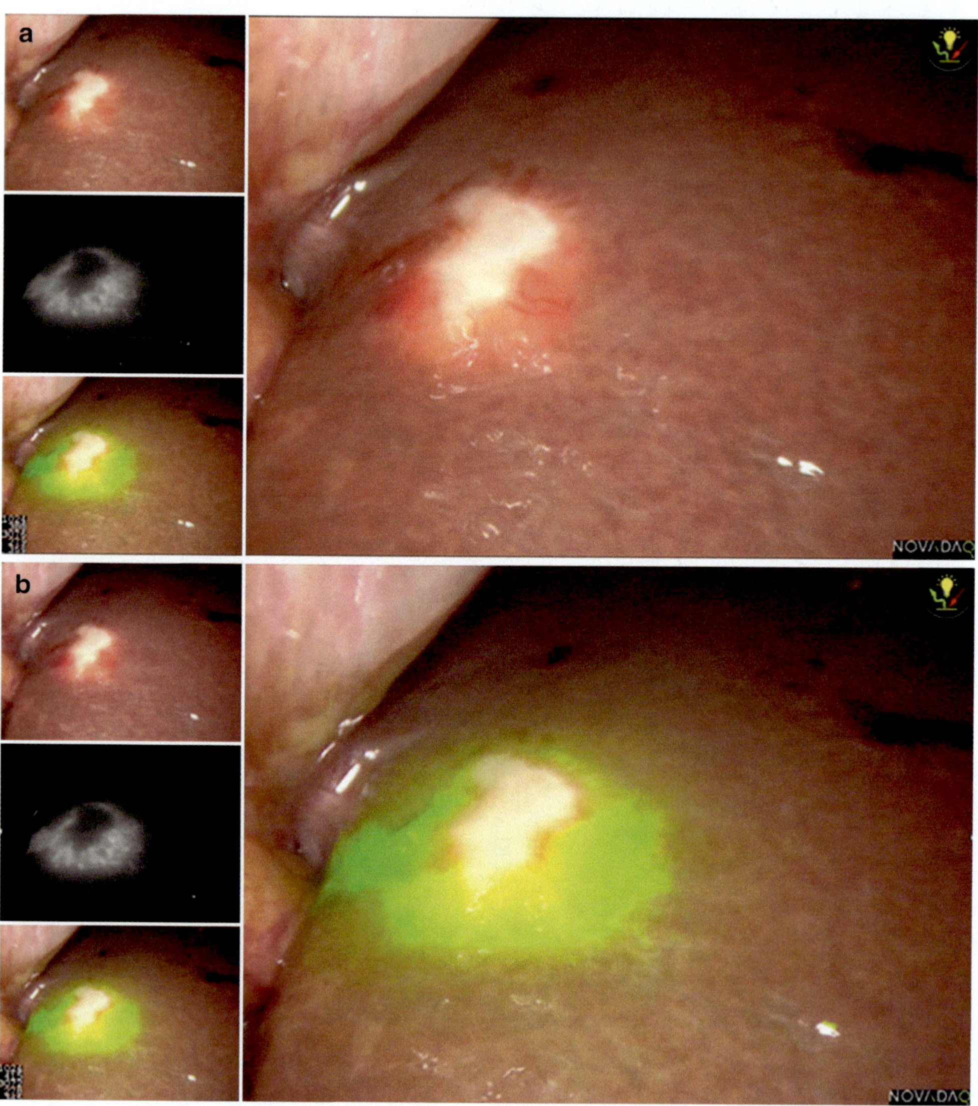

Fig. 16.1 Clinical application of intraoperative NIR fluorescence imaging. (**a**) A 58-year-old female with colorectal liver metastasis in segment 3. Normal laparoscopic color image (right). (**b**) NIR fluorescence superimposed in a pseudo-color (green) on a white-light image. NIR fluorescence was detected in the noncancerous liver parenchyma around the tumor (right). NIR imaging was used to visualize the planned point of the tumor lesion. (**c**) Black and white NIR fluorescent image (right)

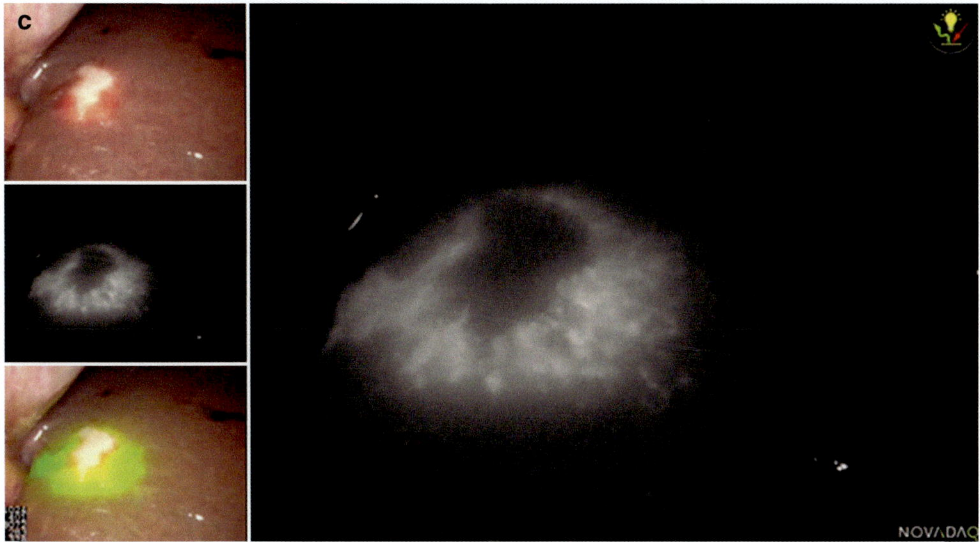

Fig. 16.1 (continued)

enhanced fluorescing lesions [24, 25]. Uchiyama et al. reported that the average diameters of the completely and partially enhanced types of LM lesions were smaller compared with those of the rim-enhanced type [25], and that there was no relationship between fluorescence imaging type and histological differentiation of metastases [22, 25].

LM from pancreatic cancer, uterine cancer, uveal melanoma, breast cancer, and colorectal squamous cell carcinoma have been shown to exhibit NIR fluorescence signal in accordance with the tumor location. In cases of LM from pancreatic cancer with abnormal hepatic fluorescence of at least 1.5 mm in greatest dimension but without any apparent liver tumor, histologic examination confirmed the presence of micrometastases in 16% of patients [33]. Among cases of partial or complete response to preoperative chemotherapy, NIR fluorescence imaging was found to be superior to visual inspection and contrast-enhanced ultrasound in detecting LM [37]. Moreover, the use of neoadjuvant chemotherapy did not significantly influence the contrast between the fluorescent rim around the LM and normal liver tissue [13].

Several studies have reported that the detection of LM significantly improved with the concomitant use of NIR imaging and intraoperative ultrasound (IOUS), with or without Perflubutane, than with preoperative diagnostic imaging [14, 25, 27, 32]. The propensity of metastatic tumor detection has been reported to be significantly smaller with the use of NIR fluorescent imaging alone than with the combined use of inspection, palpation, and IOUS [38]. In addition, the stratification of nodules by size showed that the combined use of IOUS and NIR fluorescent imaging has a significant advantage in the detection of nodules ≤3 mm [27].

Newly Detected Lesions by NIR Fluorescence Imaging

NIR fluorescence imaging technique can be used to achieve enhanced detection of LM that is undetectable by conventional preoperative imaging, including US, CT, EOB-MRI, IOUS, palpation, and visual inspection (Fig. 16.3). Previously published studies have reported that during hepatic resection in patients with LM, observation by NIR fluorescence imaging is useful for detecting fine residual tumors that could not be revealed under visible light (Table 16.2) [13, 14, 23, 26, 29, 30, 32, 34, 37, 38]. These new lesions

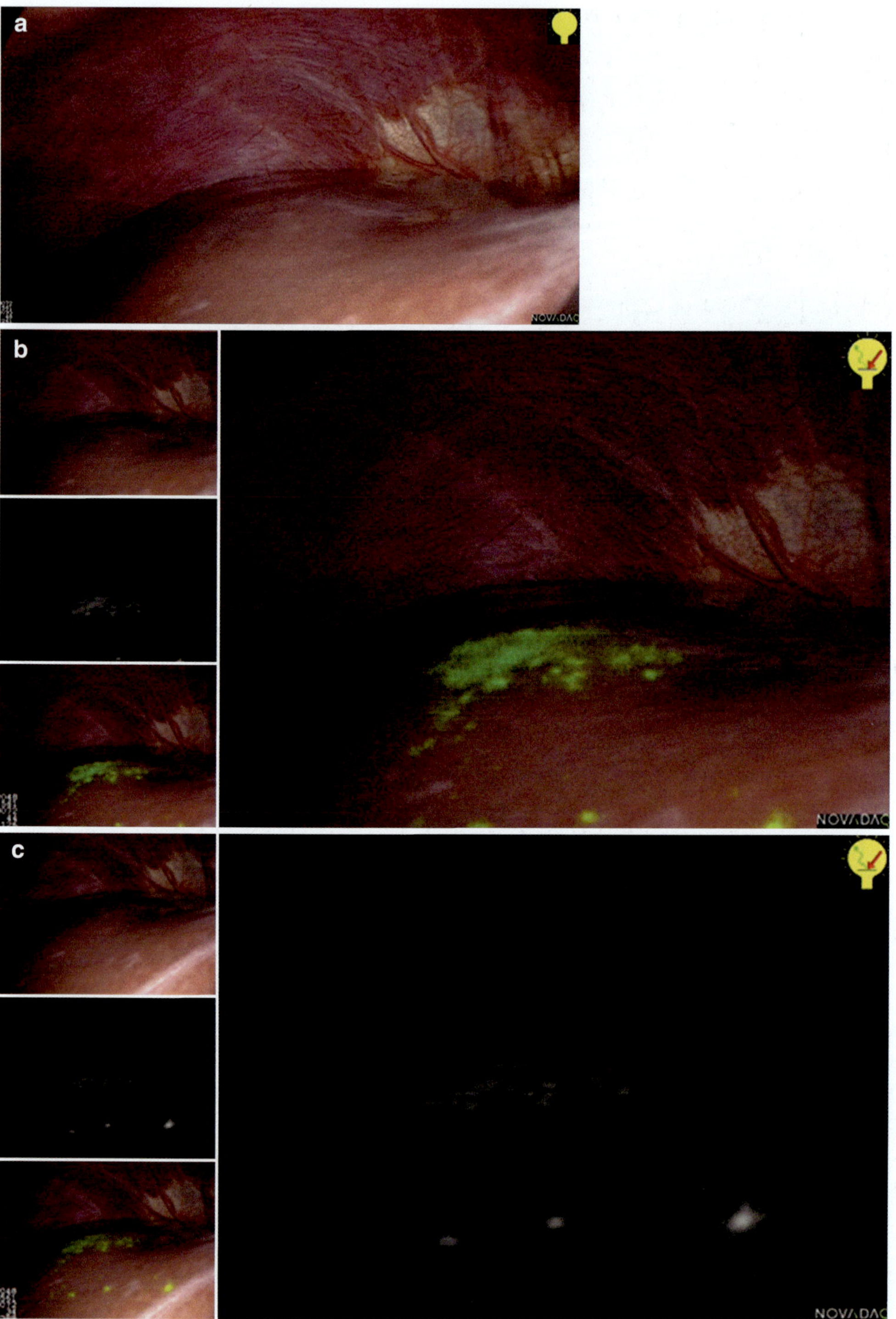

Fig. 16.2 A colorectal liver metastasis in segment 8 of a 71-year-old male. (**a**) Normal laparoscopic color image. (**b**) NIR fluorescence superimposed in a pseudo-color (green) on a white-light image. NIR fluorescence was detected in the liver tumor (right). (**c**) Black and white NIR fluorescent image (right). (**d**) Observation of the liver surface after the transection. No remaining fluorescent dye is seen in the residual liver

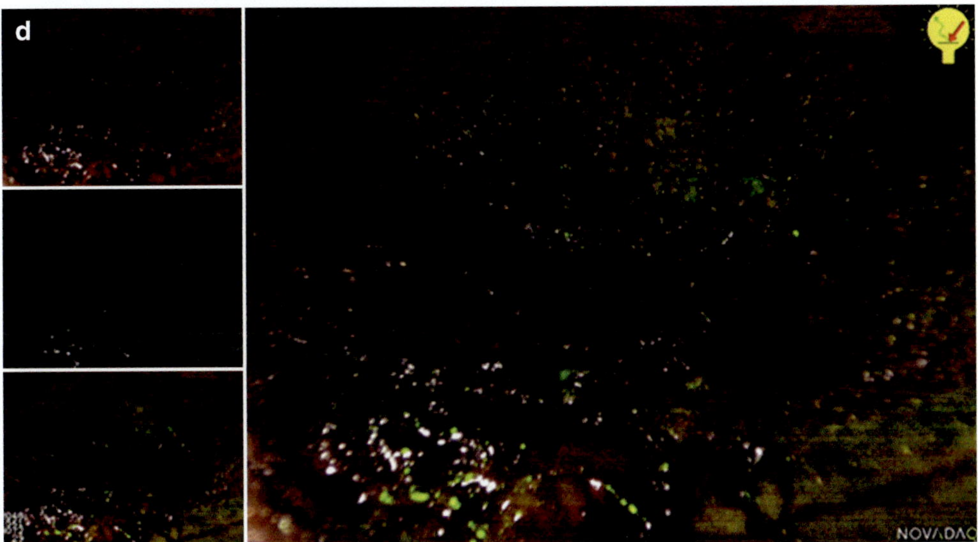

Fig. 16.2 (continued)

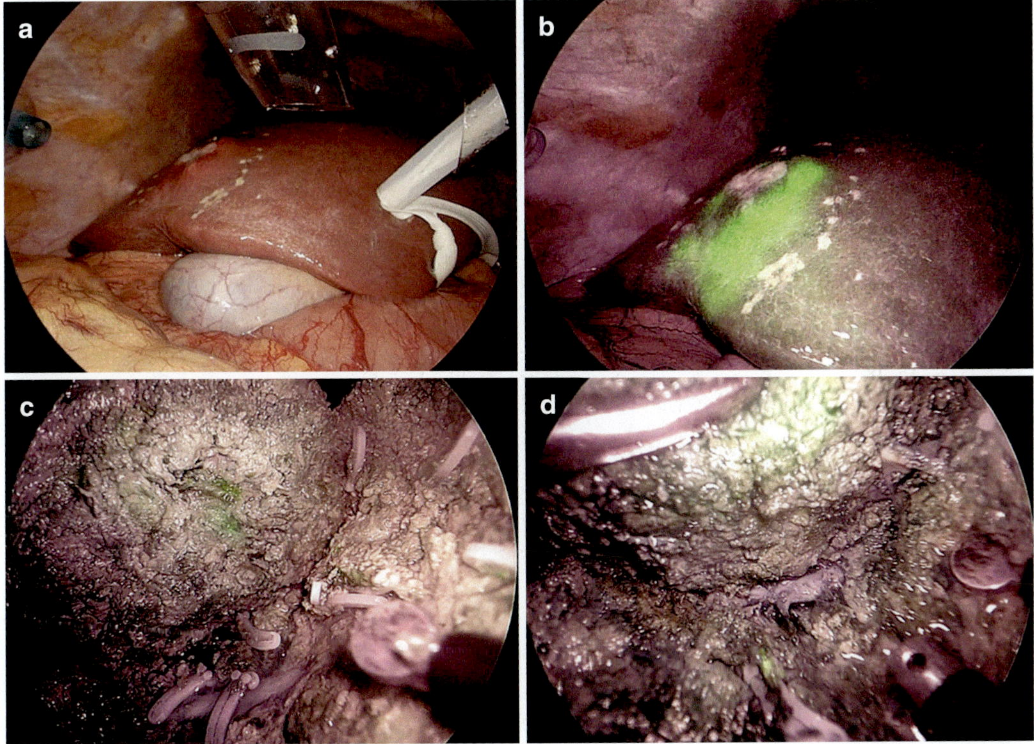

Fig. 16.3 A colorectal liver metastasis in segment 5 of a 42-year-old female. (**a**) Normal laparoscopic color image. (**b**) NIR fluorescence superimposed in a pseudo-color (green) on a white-light image. NIR fluorescence was detected in the noncancerous liver parenchyma around the tumor. (**c**, **d**) Observation of the liver surface during the transection. The appropriate transection plane should be identified to avoid the exposure of NIR fluorescence from the tumor

Table 16.2 Identification of liver metastasis via near-infrared fluorescence imaging. Sensitivity/Positive predictive value

Study	Number of LM patients	Preoperative diagnosis	Surgical approach	Imaging system	Number of LM	Sensitivity (%)	New lesion cancer/ other	Positive predictive value (%)	References
Ishizawa 2009	12	CRLM	Open	PDE	28	100	0/0	100	[11]
Uchiyama 2010	32	CRLM	Open	PDE	52	98.1	4/0	96.3	[25]
Ishizuka 2012	7	CRLM	Open	–	46	100	0/1	97.9	[26]
van der Vorst 2013	40	CRLM	Open	Mini-FLARE	97	73.2	5/0	100	[13]
Peloso 2013	25	CRLM	Open	PDE	77	100	32/1	98.7	[27]
Kudo 2014	7	CRLM/uterine cancer	Lap	Olympus medical system	16	68.8	0/0	100	[14]
Shimada 2015	7	CRLM	Open	PDE	9	100	0/0	100	[28]
Abo 2015	12	CRLM	Open	PDE	36	86.1	0/0	100	[22]
Kaibori 2016	13	CRLM	Open	PDE	N/A	95.7[a]	5/4	97.8[a]	[30]
				SBI pharmaceuticals	N/A	56.5[a]	5/0	100[a]	
Takahashi 2016	15	CRLM/benign lesion	Open/lap	Fluorescence firefly imaging/SPY	61	61.4	12/–	–	[31]
Terasawa 2017	41	CRLM/GIST	Lap	SPY	46	84.9[a]	4/0	100[a]	[37]
Boogerd 2017	14	CRLM/uveal melanoma/ breast cancer	Lap	Karl Storz	21	90.5	3/1	71.1	[32]
Lieto 2018	6	CRLM	–	–	9	100	2/0	100	[23]
Aoki 2018	12	CRLM	Lap	SPY	17	100	5/0	100	[20]

CRLM Colorectal liver metastasis, *PDE* Photo Dynamic Eye, *ICG* indocyanine green, *SPY* fluorescence imaging system of Styker
[a]Included other maligmnancy (HCC, ICC)

that can be detected by NIR fluorescence only and not by preoperative CT, IOUS, visual inspection, and palpation tend to be small and superficially located [11, 13, 38]. Moreover, NIR fluorescence imaging has been shown to be superior in detecting lesions treated using chemotherapy or radiofrequency ablation (RFA) [29, 37].

One of the limitations of IOUS is the inaccurate detection of superficial tumors, which can be detected by NIR fluorescence imaging. Although intraoperative NIR fluorescence imaging can detect false-positive lesions and may be limited to detecting lesions that are located deep inside the liver, it can be expected as a powerful complementary modality to conventional imaging techniques for the intraoperative detection of LM. Furthermore, additional resection of newly detected LM by NIR fluorescence imaging may prevent recurrence in a subset of patients with LM from colorectal cancer [38].

Determination of the Surgical Margin

Surgical resection of LM typically involves either anatomical resection or parenchymal-sparing hepatectomy [39]. The latter approach has mostly been performed for nonanatomical liver resection under IOUS guidance. The basic principles of oncological resection of LM include achievement of tumor-free surgical margins and avoidance of possible iatrogenic spread.

In cases of laparoscopic liver resection, one of the challenges faced by surgeons is missing lesions in uncertain anatomical areas because of the limited visualization through a laparoscope, inability to palpate, and the difficulty in interpreting the IOUS images. Several studies, including ours, reported the utility of NIR fluorescence imaging in determining the surgical margin in the transection plane of the liver [14, 20, 23, 31]. As described above, the accumulation of ICG in or around a tumor enables NIR fluorescence imaging to provide valuable visualization of tumors and to guide the setting of the transection plane (Figs. 16.4 and 16.5, Video 16.1).

Here, we described the technical details for the determination of surgical margin by NIR fluorescence imaging [20]. First, 0.5 mg/kg of ICG was intravenously administered at 2–14 days prior to the surgery. During surgery, NIR fluorescence images on the liver surface were obtained before and after the completion of hepatic mobilization. The surgical margin and the planned point of tumor resection were assessed by NIR fluorescence imaging immediately before, during, and after completion of the resection. Using the NIR fluorescence images for guidance, the transection plane is set and changed accordingly, so as not to expose the fluorescence signal from the tumor lesion [20]. The absence of fluorescent

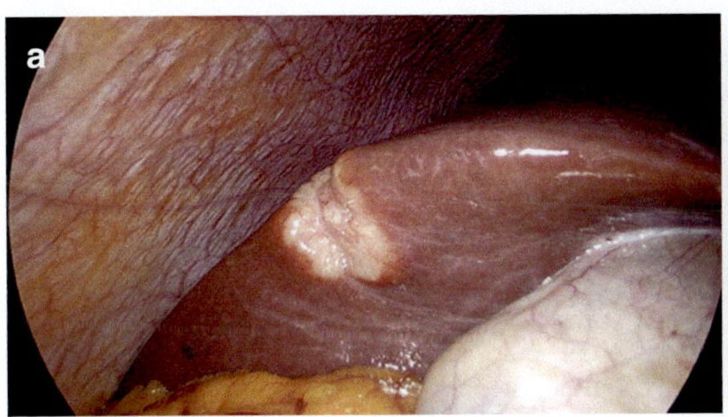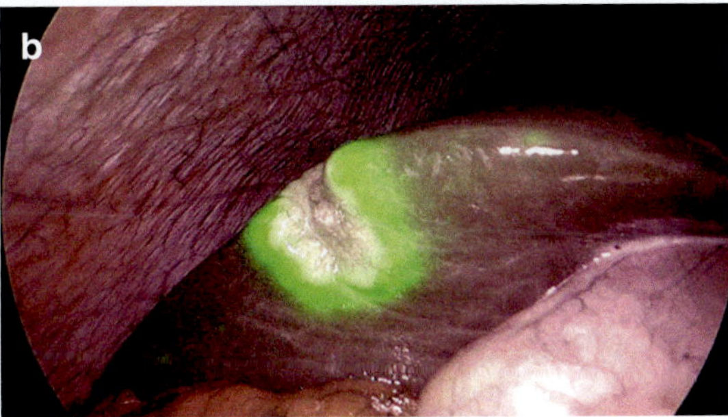

Fig. 16.4 A colorectal liver metastasis in segment 5 of a 61-year-old female. (**a**) Normal laparoscopic color image. (**b**) NIR fluorescence superimposed in a pseudo-color (green) on a white-light image. NIR fluorescence was detected in the noncancerous liver parenchyma around the tumor. (**c**) Black and white NIR fluorescent image. (**d, e**) Observation of the liver surface during the transection. The appropriate transection plane should be identified to avoid the exposure of NIR fluorescence from the tumor. (**f**) Observation of the liver surface after the transection

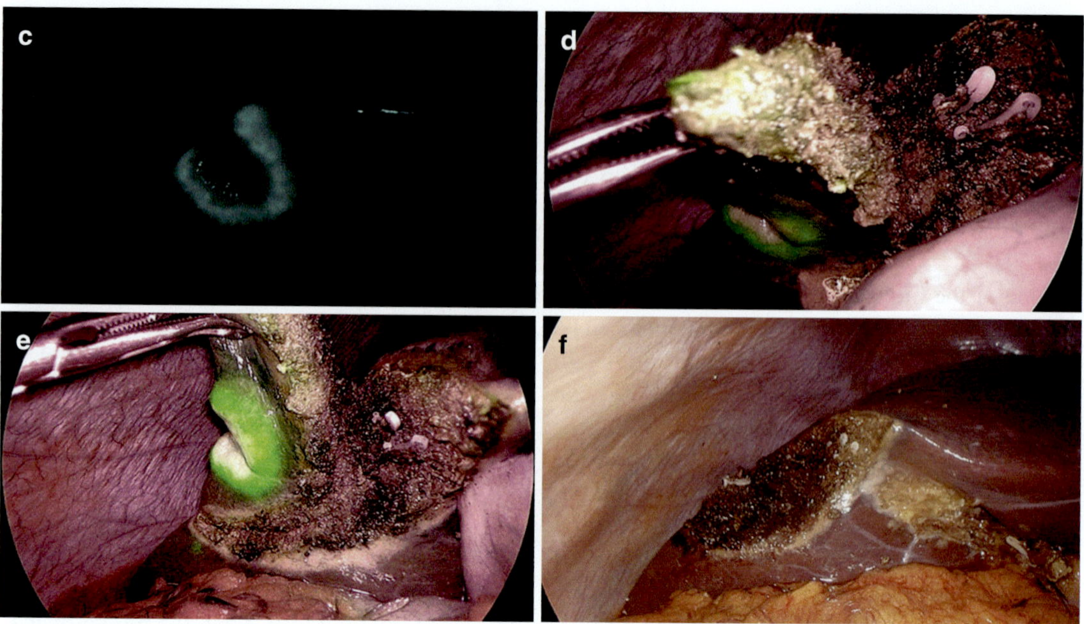

Fig. 16.4 (continued)

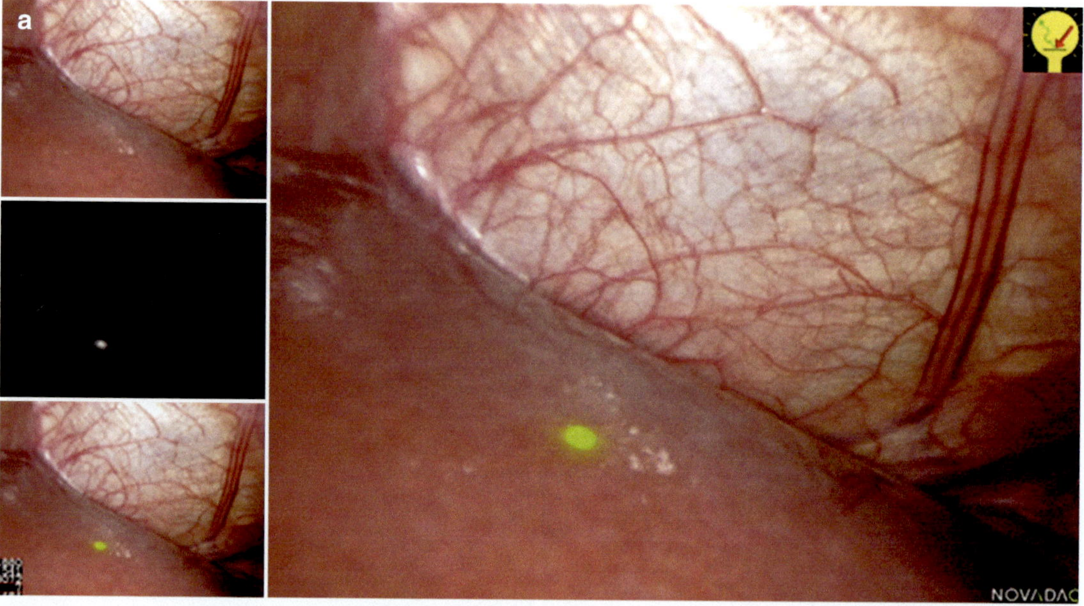

Fig. 16.5 Newly detected fluorescing lesions without preoperative diagnosis. (**a**) A 75-year-old male with colorectal liver metastasis. The main tumor was located in the right lobe, and the tumor in the left lateral segment could not be identified by visual inspection of the normal laparoscopic color image and not diagnosed preoperatively. NIR fluorescence imaging enabled the identification of the new lesion (right). (**b**) Observation of the liver surface after the transection. Pathological diagnosis of the newly detected tumor was also colorectal liver metastasis

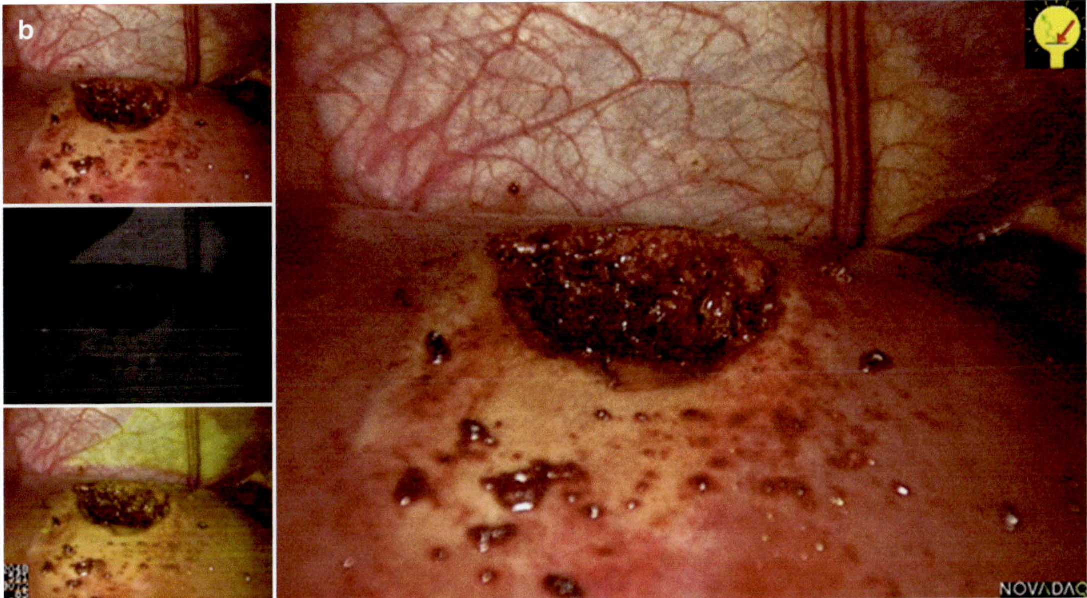

Fig. 16.5 (continued)

dye in the residual liver is considered to indicate a decreased risk for a positive tumor margin. Therefore, the surgeon should frequently verify the presence of any tissue with a fluorescent area in the transection plane and ensure removal of this tissue. Our data suggested that in cases of LM, the presence of fluorescence in the transection plane may indicate that the tumor is exposed, because the fluorescence area around the tumor should be <5 mm. The visualization of fluorescence dye on the side of the resected area would indicate a risk for positive tumor margins.

Pitfalls

False-Positive Lesions

Previous studies demonstrated the possibility of ICG accumulation and NIR fluorescence imaging detection of nonmalignant lesions (Fig. 16.6), such as regenerative nodules, dysplastic nodules, bile duct proliferation, biliary cysts, angiomyoli-poma, biliary adenoma, bile duct hamartoma, biliary adenofibroma, hemangioma, focal nodular hyperplasia, hepatic steatosis, and normal liver parenchyma (Table 16.3) [11, 22, 24, 32–34, 37]. Intraoperative NIR fluorescence imaging reportedly has a relatively high false-positive rate of approximately 40% [11] and positive predictive value for LM of 71.1–100% (Table 16.2). Because ICG is not a cancer-specific dye, distinguishing LM from benign lesions using only NIR fluorescence imaging may be difficult.

Sensitivity

The sensitivity of NIR fluorescence imaging for main tumor detection was reported to range from 61.4% to 100% (Table 16.2). Moreover, the inability to visualize deeply located tumors is a major limitation of NIR fluorescence imaging. In fact, LM identified by conventional imaging could not be detected using NIR fluorescence imaging when the tumor was located deeper than 8–10 mm

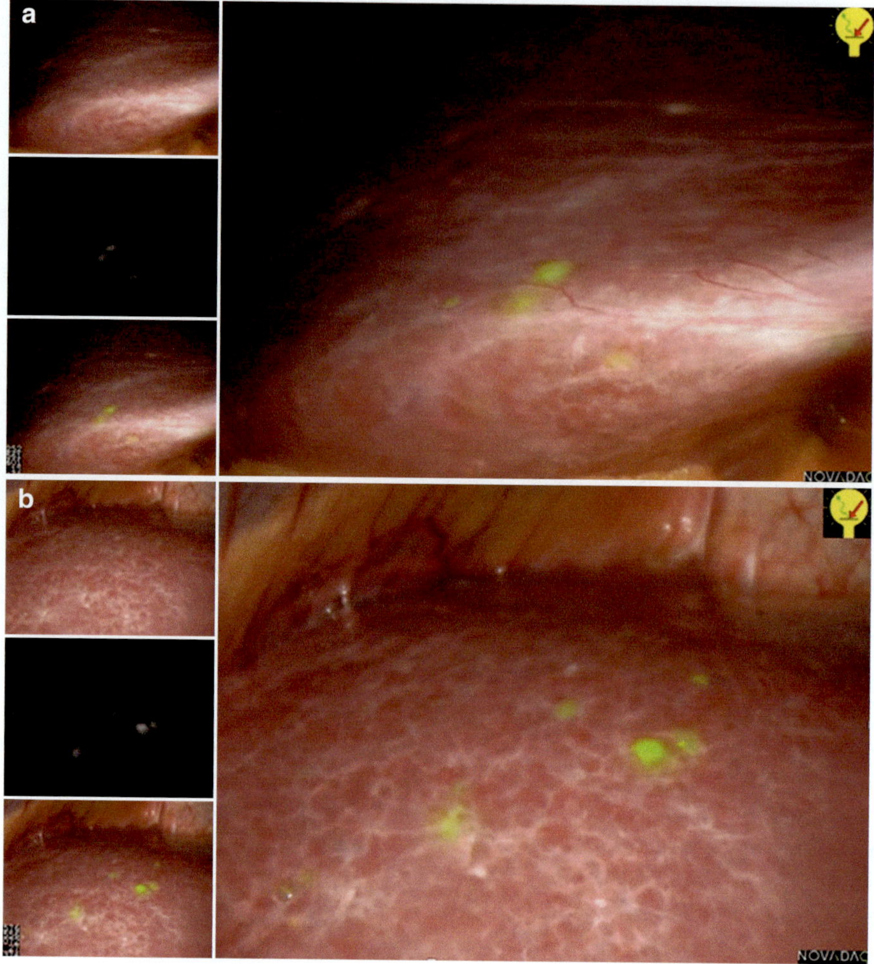

Fig. 16.6 Fluorescence image findings in benign tumor. Liver cyst. (**a, b**) NIR fluorescence superimposed in a pseudo-color (green) on a white-light image. NIR fluorescence was detected in the multiple cysts in the right lobe of the liver (right). (**b**) NIR fluorescence was also detected in the multiple cysts in the left lobe (right). (**c**) CT images show multiple liver cysts preoperatively

from the liver surface [11, 27, 32, 37]. Conversely, IOUS has been considered to be a mandatory diagnostic tool during laparoscopic and open hepatectomy [14], and the use of contrast-enhanced IOUS with NIR fluorescence imaging is reported to improve the diagnostic sensitivity [25].

Future Perspectives

It is expected that fluorescence tagging of cancer specific elements e.g. antibodies will realistically facilitate tumor detection in the future [38]. Several clinical investigators [40–42] have reported their experience using this principle. Identification of liver metastases originating from carcinoma of the pancreas or colorectum by a CEA-specific monoclonal antibody conjugated with BM104 fluorochrome (absorbing around 700 nm), has been demonstrated [43, 44]. The advantages of these target specific fluorescent antibodies, just like ICG, are their safety, availability and cost effectiveness. They are clinically relevant fluorescent tracers of both diagnostic and therapeutic value.

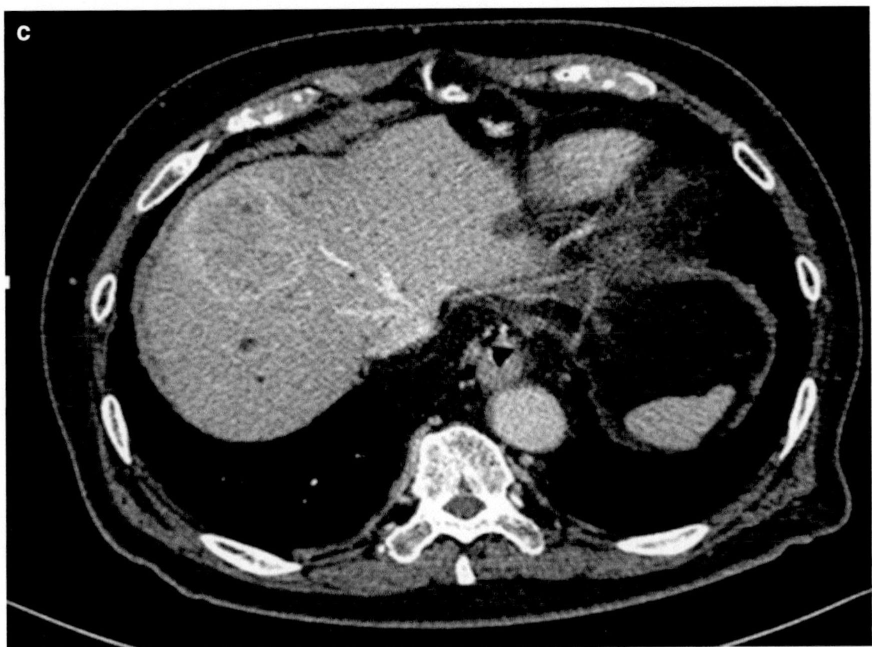

Fig. 16.6 (continued)

Table 16.3 Indentification of liver metastasis via near-infrared fluorescence imaging. False positive lesions

Study	Number of LM patients	Preoperative diagnosis	Number of tumor	New lesion cancer/ other	False positive lesion	References
Ishizawa 2009	12	CRLM	28	0/0	4 large regenerative nodules, 1 bile duct proliferation	[11]
Yokoyama 2012	49	Pancreatic cancer	N/A	N/A	Bile- secreting foci, biliary cysts (number not provided)	[33]
Abo 2015	12	CRLM	36	0/–	Angiomyolipoma 1, biliary adenoma 1, cavernous hemangioma 1, Local fibrosis 1, organizing 1, hematoma 1, simple cyst 7, small hemangioma 4, cirrhotic small nodule 6, ablated lesion 1(rim stain)	[22]
Takahashi 2016	15	CRLM/ benign lesion	61	12/–	Focal nodular hyperplasia (number not provided)	[31]
Terasawa 2017	41	CRLM/GIST	46	4/0	5 hemangiomas and 1 nodule of lymphoid cell hyperplasia were *negative* for NIR fluorescence	[37]
Boogerd 2017	14	CRLM/uveal melanoma/ breast cancer	21	3/1	Bile duct hamartoma, steatotic liver tissue, necrosis (3 times), cholestatic and inflamed liver tissue, FNH, and a biliary adenofibroma	[32]
Zhang 2017	9	CRLM/other/ benign lesion	N/A	5(HCC)/7	Recurrent nodular cirrhosis (2 patients), liver macrovesicular steatosis (1 patient), hemangioma (2 patients), and hepatic focal hyperplasia (2 patients) were detected as a *shadow with a PDE (lack of fluorescent signal)*	[34]
Alfano 2018	5	CRLM	N/A	N/A	Biliary cyst	[24]

CRLM colorectal liver metastasis, *N/A* not available

Conclusions

The clinical value of NIR fluorescence in the detection of liver metastases has been repeatedly demonstrated. With further advancements in imaging technology and target specific tracers, this technique may well become an integral part of diagnosis and therapy of liver metastases.

References

1. Guyer DR, Puliafito CA, Monés JM, Friedman E, Chang W, Verdooner SR. Digital indocyanine-green angiography in chorioretinal disorders. Ophthalmology. 1992;99:287–91.
2. Ogata F, Azuma R, Kikuchi M, Koshima I, Morimoto Y. Novel lymphography using indocyanine green dye for near-infrared fluorescence labeling. Ann Plast Surg. 2007;58:652–5.
3. Kitai T, Inomoto T, Miwa M, Shikayama T. Fluorescence navigation with indocyanine green for detecting sentinel lymph nodes in breast cancer. Breast Cancer. 2005;12:211–5.
4. Kusano M, Tajima Y, Yamazaki K, Kato M, Watanabe M, Miwa M. Sentinel node mapping guided by indocyanine green fluorescence imaging: a new method for sentinel node navigation surgery in gastrointestinal cancer. Dig Surg. 2008;25:103–8. https://doi.org/10.1159/000121905.
5. Rubens FD, Ruel M, Fremes SE. A new and simplified method for coronary and graft imaging during CABG. Heart Surg Forum. 2002;5:141–4.
6. Raabe A, Nakaji P, Beck J, Kim LJ, Hsu FP, Kamerman JD, et al. Prospective evaluation of surgical microscope-integrated intraoperative near-infrared indocyanine green videoangiography during aneurysm surgery. J Neurosurg. 2005;103:982–9.
7. Kubota K, Kita J, Shimoda M, Rokkaku K, Kato M, Iso Y, et al. Intraoperative assessment of reconstructed vessels in living-donor liver transplantation, using a novel fluorescence imaging technique. J Hepato-Biliary-Pancreat Surg. 2006;13:100–4.
8. Mitsuhashi N, Kimura F, Shimizu H, Imamaki M, Yoshidome H, Ohtsuka M, et al. Usefulness of intraoperative fluorescence imaging to evaluate local anatomy in hepatobiliary surgery. J Hepato-Biliary-Pancreat Surg. 2008;15:508–14. https://doi.org/10.1007/s00534–007–1307–5.
9. Aoki T, Yasuda D, Shimizu Y, Odaira M, Niiya T, Kusano T, et al. Image-guided liver mapping using fluorescence navigation system with indocyanine green for anatomical hepatic resection. World J Surg. 2008;32:1763–7. https://doi.org/10.1007/s00268–008–9620-y.
10. Ishizawa T, Tamura S, Masuda K, Aoki T, Hasegawa K, Imamura H, et al. Intraoperative fluorescent cholangiography using indocyanine green: a biliary road map for safe surgery. J Am Coll Surg. 2009;208:e1–4. https://doi.org/10.1016/j.jamcollsurg.2008.09.024.
11. Ishizawa T, Fukushima N, Shibahara J, Masuda K, Tamura S, Aoki T, et al. Real-time identification of liver cancers by using indocyanine green fluorescent imaging. Cancer. 2009;115:2491–504. https://doi.org/10.1002/cncr.24291.
12. Ishizawa T, Masuda K, Urano Y, Kawaguchi Y, Satou S, Kaneko J, et al. Mechanistic background and clinical applications of indocyanine green fluorescence imaging of hepatocellular carcinoma. Ann Surg Oncol. 2014;21:440–8. https://doi.org/10.1245/s10434–013–3360–4.
13. van der Vorst JR, Schaafsma BE, Hutteman M, Verbeek FP, Liefers GJ, Hartgrink HH, et al. Near-infrared fluorescence-guided resection of colorectal liver metastases. Cancer. 2013;119:3411–8. https://doi.org/10.1002/cncr.28203.
14. Kudo H, Ishizawa T, Tani K, Harada N, Ichida A, Shimizu A, et al. Visualization of subcapsular hepatic malignancy by indocyanine-green fluorescence imaging during laparoscopic hepatectomy. Surg Endosc. 2014;28:2504–8. https://doi.org/10.1007/s00464–014–3468-z.
15. Xu F, Tang B, Jin TQ, Dai CL. Current status of surgical treatment of colorectal liver metastases. World J Clin Cases. 2018;26(6):716–34. https://doi.org/10.12998/wjcc.v6.i14.716.
16. Sahani DV, Kalva SP, Tanabe KK, Hayat SM, O'Neill MJ, Halpern EF, et al. Intraoperative US in patients undergoing surgery for liver neoplasms: comparison with MR imaging. Radiology. 2004;232:810–4.
17. Zhang K, Kokudo N, Hasegawa K, Arita J, Tang W, Aoki T, et al. Detection of new tumors by intraoperative ultrasonography during repeated hepatic resections for hepatocellular carcinoma. Arch Surg. 2007;142:1170–5.
18. Machi J, Isomoto H, Kurohiji T, Yamashita Y, Shirouzu K, Kakegawa T, et al. Accuracy of intraoperative ultrasonography in diagnosing liver metastasis from colorectal cancer: evaluation with postoperative follow-up results. World J Surg. 1991;15:551–6.
19. Nomura K, Kadoya M, Ueda K, Fujinaga Y, Miwa S, Miyagawa S. Detection of hepatic metastases from colorectal carcinoma: comparison of histopathologic features of anatomically resected liver with results of preoperative imaging. J Clin Gastroenterol. 2007;41:789–95.
20. Aoki T, Murakami M, Koizumi T, Matsuda K, Fujimori A, Kusano T, et al. Determination of the surgical margin in laparoscopic liver resections using infrared indocyanine green fluorescence. Langenbeck's Arch Surg. 2018;403:671–80. https://doi.org/10.1007/s00423–018–1685-y.
21. DSouza AV, Lin H, Henderson ER, Samkoe KS, Pogue BW. Review of fluorescence guided surgery systems: identification of key performance capabilities beyond indocyanine green imaging. J Biomed

Opt. 2016;21:80901. https://doi.org/10.1117/1.JBO.21.8.080901.

22. Abo T, Nanashima A, Tobinaga S, Hidaka S, Taura N, Takagi K, et al. Usefulness of intraoperative diagnosis of hepatic tumors located at the liver surface and hepatic segmental visualization using indocyanine green-photodynamic eye imaging. Eur J Surg Oncol. 2015;41:257–64. https://doi.org/10.1016/j.ejs0.2014.09.008.

23. Lieto E, Galizia G, Cardella F, Mabilia A, Basile N, Castellano P, et al. Indocyanine green fluorescence imaging-guided surgery in primary and metastatic liver tumors. Surg Innov. 2018;25(1):62–8. https://doi.org/10.1177/1553350617751451.

24. Alfano MS, Molfino S, Benedicenti S, Molteni B, Porsio P, Arici E, et al. Intraoperative ICG-based imaging of liver neoplasms: a simple yet powerful tool. Preliminary results. Surg Endosc. 2019;33(1):126–34. https://doi.org/10.1007/s00464-018-6282-1.

25. Uchiyama K, Ueno M, Ozawa S, Kiriyama S, Shigekawa Y, Yamaue H. Combined use of contrast-enhanced intraoperative ultrasonography and a fluorescence navigation system for identifying hepatic metastases. World J Surg. 2010;34:2953–9. https://doi.org/10.1007/s00268-010-0764-1.

26. Ishizuka M, Kubota K, Kita J, Shimoda M, Kato M, Sawada T. Intraoperative observation using a fluorescence imaging instrument during hepatic resection for liver metastasis from colorectal cancer. Hepato-Gastroenterology. 2012;59:90–2. https://doi.org/10.5754/hge11223.

27. Peloso A, Franchi E, Canepa MC, Barbieri L, Briani L, Ferrario J, et al. Combined use of intraoperative ultrasound and indocyanine green fluorescence imaging to detect liver metastases from colorectal cancer. HPB (Oxford). 2013;15:928–34. https://doi.org/10.1111/hpb.12057.

28. Shimada S, Ohtsubo S, Ogasawara K, Kusano M. Macro- and microscopic findings of ICG fluorescence in liver tumors. World J Surg Oncol. 2015;13:198. https://doi.org/10.1186/s12957-015-0615-5.

29. Kawaguchi Y, Nagai M, Nomura Y, Kokudo N, Tanaka N. Usefulness of indocyanine green-fluorescence imaging during laparoscopic hepatectomy to visualize subcapsular hard-to-identify hepatic malignancy. J Surg Oncol. 2015;112:514–6. https://doi.org/10.1002/js0.24021.

30. Kaibori M, Matsui K, Ishizaki M, Iida H, Okumura T, Sakaguchi T, et al. Intraoperative detection of superficial liver tumors by fluorescence imaging using indocyanine green and 5-aminolevulinic acid. Anticancer Res. 2016;36:1841–9.

31. Takahashi H, Zaidi N, Berber E. An initial report on the intraoperative use of indocyanine green fluorescence imaging in the surgical management of liver tumorss. J Surg Oncol. 2016;114:625–9. https://doi.org/10.1002/js0.24363.

32. Boogerd LS, Handgraaf HJ, Lam HD, Huurman VA, Farina-Sarasqueta A, Frangioni JV, et al. Laparoscopic detection and resection of occult liver tumors of multiple cancer types using real-time near-infrared fluorescence guidance. Surg Endosc. 2017;31:952–61. https://doi.org/10.1007/s00464-016-5007-6.

33. Yokoyama N, Otani T, Hashidate H, Maeda C, Katada T, Sudo N, et al. Real-time detection of hepatic micrometastases from pancreatic cancer by intraoperative fluorescence imaging: preliminary results of a prospective study. Cancer. 2012;118:2813–9. https://doi.org/10.1002/cncr.26594.

34. Zhang YM, Shi R, Hou JC, Liu ZR, Cui ZL, Li Y, et al. Liver tumor boundaries identified intraoperatively using real-time indocyanine green fluorescence imaging. J Cancer Res Clin Oncol. 2017;143:51–8. https://doi.org/10.1007/s00432-016-2267-4.

35. Tummers QR, Verbeek FP, Prevoo HA, Braat AE, Baeten CI, Frangioni JV, et al. First experience on laparoscopic near-infrared fluorescence imaging of hepatic uveal melanoma metastases using indocyanine green. Surg Innov. 2015;22:20–5. https://doi.org/10.1177/1553350614535857.

36. Benedicenti S, Molfino S, Alfano MS, Molteni B, Porsio P, Portolani N, et al. Indocyanine-green fluorescence-GUIDED liver resection of metastasis from squamous cell carcinoma invading the biliary tree. Case Rep Gastrointest Med. 2018;2018:5849816. https://doi.org/10.1155/2018/5849816.

37. Terasawa M, Ishizawa T, Mise Y, Inoue Y, Ito H, Takahashi Y, et al. Applications of fusion-fluorescence imaging using indocyanine green in laparoscopic hepatectomy. Surg Endosc. 2017;31:5111–8. https://doi.org/10.1007/s00464-017-5576-z.

38. Handgraaf HJM, Boogerd LSF, Höppener DJ, Peloso A, Sibinga Mulder BG, Hoogstins CES, et al. Long-term follow-up after near-infrared fluorescence-guided resection of colorectal liver metastases: a retrospective multicenter analysis. Eur J Surg Oncol. 2017;43:1463–71. https://doi.org/10.1016/j.ejs0.2017.04.016.

39. Moris D, Ronnekleiv-Kelly S, Rahnemai-Azar AA, Felekouras E, Dillhoff M, Schmidt C, et al. Parenchymal-sparing versus anatomic liver resection for colorectal liver metastases: a systematic review. J Gastrointest Surg. 2017;21:1076–85. https://doi.org/10.1007/s11605-017-3397-y.

40. Hoogstins CE, Tummers QR, Gaarenstroom KN, de Kroon CD, Trimbos JB, Bosse T, et al. A novel tumor-specific agent for intraoperative near-infrared fluorescence imaging: a translational study in healthy volunteers and patients with ovarian cancer. Clin Cancer Res. 2016;22:2929–38. https://doi.org/10.1158/1078-0432.CCR-15-2640.

41. Rosenthal EL, Warram JM, de Boer E, Chung TK, Korb ML, Brandwein-Gensler M, et al. Safety and tumor specificity of Cetuximab-IRDye800 for surgical navigation in head and neck cancer. Clin Cancer Res. 2015;21:3658–66. https://doi.org/10.1158/1078-0432.CCR-14-3284.

42. Lamberts LE, Koch M, de Jong JS, Adams ALL, Glatz J, Kranendonk MEG, et al. Tumor-specific

uptake of fluorescent bevacizumab-IRDye800CW microdosing in patients with primary breast cancer: a phase I feasibility study. Clin Cancer Res. 2017;23:2730–41. https://doi.org/10.1158/1078-0432.CCR-16-0437.

43. Boogerd LSF, Hoogstins CES, Schaap DP, Kusters M, Handgraaf HJM, van der Valk MJM, et al. Safety and effectiveness of SGM-101, a fluorescent antibody targeting carcinoembryonic antigen, for intraoperative detection of colorectal cancer: a dose-escalation pilot study. Lancet Gastroenterol Hepatol. 2018;3:181–91. https://doi.org/10.1016/S2468-1253(17)30395-3.

44. Hoogstins CES, Boogerd LSF, Sibinga Mulder BG, Mieog JSD, Swijnenburg RJ, van de Velde CJH, et al. Image-guided surgery in patients with pancreatic cancer: first results of a clinical trial using SGM-101, a novel carcinoembryonic antigen-targeting, near-infrared fluorescent agent. Ann Surg Oncol. 2018;25:3350–7. https://doi.org/10.1245/s10434-018-6655-7.

Minimally Invasive Hepatectomy

Jesse K. Sulzer, Patrick N. Salibi, John B. Martinie, and David A. Iannitti

Indications

Minimally invasive hepatectomy remains an evolving field. The first laparoscopic liver resections were reported in the early 1990s, but widespread adoption of minimally invasive liver surgery has been a slow process [1]. Initial operations were limited to peripherally located lesions and non-anatomic resections. Increasing experience and improved instrumentation has allowed surgeons to expand to larger resections including anatomic hemi-hepatectomy and even more complex procedures. Over time, concerns such as oncologic equivalence, risk of CO_2 embolization, and ability to control bleeding with limited options for manual compression were invalidated [2]. Today, indications for minimally invasive or laparoscopic hepatectomy should mirror those of traditional open hepatectomy in experienced hands. Indeed, a large review by Nguyen et al. encompassing 2804 patients confirmed the safety and feasibility of laparoscopic liver surgery [3]. Increasingly complex procedures are now being reported including associated liver partition and portal vein ligation for staged hepatectomy and living liver donor hepatectomy [4–6].

The learning curve for minimally invasive hepatectomy is reported as 45–60, comparable to other complex laparoscopic and open hepatobiliary procedures [7]. The above noted concerns and steep learning curve for minimally invasive liver resection have contributed to an increase in recent interest and reports of robotic-assisted hepatectomy [8]. Robotic-assisted hepatectomy has been shown to be comparable to other minimally invasive approaches as well as open procedures in estimated blood loss, operative time, conversion rates, R0 resection rates, and complications [9, 10].

The increasing utilization of the minimally invasive approach to liver resection has resulted in expansion of the available instruments and technologies to aid in safe and effective surgery. Near-infrared fluorescence imaging has been identified as a promising technology with several applications in minimally invasive hepatectomy. Prior reports have shown successful utilization of indocyanine green (ICG) and near-infrared fluorescence cameras to improve identification of occult lesions [11], assist in identifying anatomic landmarks, and delineate pathologic margins as

Electronic Supplementary Material The online version of this chapter (https://doi.org/10.1007/978-3-030-38092-2_17) contains supplementary material, which is available to authorized users.

J. K. Sulzer · P. N. Salibi · J. B. Martinie
D. A. Iannitti (✉)
Department of Hepatopancreaticobiliary Surgery, Carolinas Medical Center, Atrium Health, Charlotte, NC, USA
e-mail: David.iannitti@atriumhealth.org

E. M. Aleassa, K. M. El-Hayek (eds.), *Video Atlas of Intraoperative Applications of Near Infrared Fluorescence Imaging*, https://doi.org/10.1007/978-3-030-38092-2_17

well as reveal more precisely lines of transection for resection [12].

We currently utilize ICG fluorescence imaging in two distinct methods as dictated by the needs of the case. ICG cholangiography can be performed following either an intrabiliary or intravenous injection of ICG. Intravenous injection of 2.5–5 mg of ICG can be administered intraoperatively to guide parenchymal transection. Two methodologies for fluorescence-guided transection exist. The positive-staining technique utilizes a similar approach as the previously reported blue dye approach [13]. In this approach the portal branch of the segment of interest is isolated or identified by intraoperative ultrasound and then punctured with a fine needle. ICG is administered and fluorescence used to identify the borders of the area to be resected. While the positive staining approach has been reported with good success, it can be cumbersome to perform in minimally invasive cases. The negative staining approach has thus been suggested as an easier technique in minimally invasive hepatectomy. In the negative staining approach ICG is administered intravenously following clamping or ligation of the pedicle to the area to be resected. The resection margin can then be identified by lack of fluorescence. This approach can be particularly useful in assisting with identifying intersegmental planes during transection, albeit not with the same clarity as the line of demarcation on the liver surface [12].

Alternatively, biliary cholangiography has received much attention recently as a potential tool to limit bile duct injuries in cases with unclear anatomy. ICG cholangiography involves intravenous administration of ICG preoperatively. When administered intravenously 30–60 minutes preoperatively ICG concentrates in the biliary tree and can be distinguished from the hepatic parenchymal background [14]. The safety and efficacy of ICG cholangiography has been well established in laparoscopic and robotic cholecystectomy. Preoperative injection of ICG can provide fluorescence of the bile ducts for several hours depending on the dose administered and underlying hepatic function [15]. Advantages of ICG cholangiography for hilar dissection include removing the need for catheterization of the biliary tree, ease of repeated use by switching between white light and fluorescence cameras, and the ability to overlay fluorescence images [16]. The safety and sensitivity of this method is evidenced by its use for identification of biliary anatomy in living donor hepatectomies [17].

Technical Description

Laparoscopic Setup

ICG is administered preoperatively for cases in which fluorescence cholangiography is planned. Standard perioperative antibiotics and prophylactic anticoagulation are administered and re-dosed as appropriate per typical surgical guidelines. Sequential compression devices are applied prior to anesthesia. A urinary catheter, arterial line, and nasogastric tube are placed following induction. Fluid management is guided throughout the procedure by monitoring stroke volume variation using the Vigileo® device (Edwards Lifesciences). The patient is secured to the table ensuring appropriate padding and placed in slight reverse Trendelenburg. Flexing the bed to widen the angle of the torso often provides additional space on the anterior abdominal wall for ergonomic port placement. The patient is prepped and draped in standard surgical fashion. Trauma drapes with integrated pouches or dedicated laparoscopic drapes aid in control of cables and tubing for the laparoscopic equipment and desired energy devices.

Left hepatectomy and left lateral sectionectomy are performed in the supine position. For these resections entry into the abdomen is typically achieved at the infraumbilical position unless this is unsafe due to prior operations or other concerns. Our preferred method of entry is direct cut down and 10 mm Hasson trocar placement at this site. For left-sided hepatic resections this location is typically in line for transection and stapler use. We then place 5 mm ports in the left and right flanks. Additional ports are placed based on the intended transection line and need for additional access such as for lysis of adhesions.

Right hepatectomy and right posterior resection patients are placed in a modified right side up position at about 30–45° left lateral decubitus. Entry is achieved with cut down and Hasson trocar placement in the anterior axillary line. An additional two 5 mm ports are placed near the midline and in the posterior axillary line. Additional assistant or stapler ports are placed as dictated by anatomy or body habitus.

Robot Setup

For cases in which IGC cholangiography is planned patients receive ICG in the preoperative care unit to assist with identification of the biliary tree utilizing the Firefly technology available on the da Vinci robotic system. Preoperative antibiotics and prophylactic anticoagulation are administered and re-dosed as appropriate per typical surgical guidelines. Sequential compression devices are applied prior to anesthesia. Following induction of anesthesia, a urinary catheter, arterial line, and nasogastric tube are placed. Fluid management is guided throughout the procedure by monitoring stroke volume variation using the Vigileo® device (Edwards Lifesciences). We now perform the majority of our liver resections on the da Vinci Xi® system allowing for more freedom in patient position and room arrangement. Patients are placed supine on the operating room table with arms extended for all resections with the exception of a right posterior sectionectomy for which the patient is placed in the left lateral position. The bed is oriented at a 30–45° angle from anesthesia. Ample clearance for the robot and ergonomic working space for the bedside assistant are provided by the side-docking ability of the da Vinci Xi® and this room layout. Additionally, this setup allows anesthesia continued access to the airway and both arms.

After ensuring appropriate padding and securing of the patient to the operating room table, the patient is placed in slight reverse Trendelenburg. This usually ranges from 8° to 12° depending on the body habitus of the patient. The patient is prepped and draped in standard surgical fashion. We have found the use of trauma drapes with attached pouches to be of benefit in organizing the necessary cables and tubing.

Entry method can be by Veress needle, open Hasson, or optical entry at the discretion of the operating surgeon and taking into consideration the patient's body habitus and prior operations. For all but right posterior sectionectomy we typically initiate insufflation and entry into the abdomen at the infraumbilical position with a Veress needle followed by a 12 mm port. For a right posterior sectionectomy entry is typically made in the right anterior axillary line. The robotic ports are then placed ideally in symmetrical spacing along a horizontal line above the umbilicus. General locations for the ports include the right anterior axillary line, the right midclavicular line, left midclavicular line, and left anterior axillary line. The four robotic ports may need to be adjusted based on body habitus.

Our standard technique places the camera in the right midclavicular line with two robotic instruments controlled by the right side. Additional modifications to spacing may be required depending on preference for having two arms to the right or left of the camera. Placement of assistant ports will be dictated by the final location of robotic ports and body habitus. In our common layout, the 12 mm infraumbilical port placed at the time of entry is utilized as the assistant port as well as the extraction site. Should this site not be ergonomic for the assistant or impeded by body habitus, an additional 5 mm port can be placed away from the remaining ports. The robot is then docked from the patient's right side. The camera is attached and targeting performed with the resection area as the primary target.

Hilar Dissection

Left Hepatectomy

Both laparoscopic and robotic left liver resections are performed in the standard American supine position as opposed to the French position in which patients are placed in modified lithotomy.

The patient is placed in slight reverse Trendelenburg position. Entry is typically achieved at the infra-umbilical location and insufflation begun. Additional ports are placed as detailed above. The falciform ligament is divided up toward the insertion of the coronary ligament where the liver is attached to the diaphragm and mobilization of the left lateral sector of the liver performed. Attention is then turned to the porta hepatis. The peritoneum overlying the portal structures is opened using monopolar cautery to expose the common hepatic artery and its bifurcation. The left hepatic artery branches are dissected out and ligated with silk ties and divided sharply. Once the artery is transected the portal vein is exposed and the left and right branches clearly identified. The left portal vein is ligated between silk ties or clips; alternatively a stapler can be utilized. ICG cholangiography can then be utilized to positively identify the left hepatic duct prior to ligation and transection. Outflow control can be obtained at this point or the hepatic vein controlled intraparenchymally with clips, ties, or a stapler depending on caliber (see Video 17.1). Parenchymal transection is performed as detailed below.

Right Hepatectomy

ICG is administered preoperatively in preparation of fluorescence cholangiography during the hilar dissection. The patient is placed in the supine position. For robotic cases, the patient is placed supine and entry and insufflation is typically achieved at the infraumbilical position and trocars placed in a linear fashion angled slightly toward the right upper quadrant with an assistant port at an ergonomic location. For laparoscopic cases, the patient is placed in the modified left lateral decubitus position and entry achieved in the anterior axillary line. The gallbladder is dissected off the liver bed in a dome down fashion and left attached to the common hepatic duct to act as a retractor. The location of the common hepatic duct can be confirmed at this time by fluorescence imaging. The cystic artery is divided between clips or using a bipolar sealing device. The lateral aspect of the hepatoduodenal ligament is opened with monopolar scissors and the

bile duct elevated exposing the right hepatic artery and portal vein. The hepatic artery is divided between clips or ties and the bifurcation of the portal vein dissected out. The right portal vein branch is then ligated between clips or ties or alternatively can be stapled. Confirmation of the location of the common hepatic duct can be confirmed as needed during the dissection by switching between white light and fluorescence imaging. Once the vascular supply has been divided, attention is turned to dissection of the right hepatic duct which is facilitated by ICG cholangiography. The right hepatic duct is then ligated between ties and divided sharply (see Video 17.2). Parenchymal transection then proceeds as detailed below.

Right Posterior Sectionectomy

ICG is administered preoperatively if fluorescence cholangiography is planned. The patient is placed in the left lateral decubitus position for right posterior sectionectomy. Insufflation is achieved and trocars placed in a linear fashion with an assistant port at an ergonomic location. The gallbladder is dissected off the liver bed in a dome down fashion and left attached to the common hepatic duct to act as a retractor. The lateral aspect of the hepatoduodenal ligament is opened with monopolar scissors and the bile duct elevated anteriorly off the portal vein. The dissection is continued cephalad until the trifurcation of the portal vein can be identified. The right posterior portal vein branch is ligated and divided opening the posterior pedicle window. The right posterior hepatic artery can then be identified and ligated. If ICG has been administered preoperatively, fluorescence cholangiography can be performed at this time and the bile duct divided once clearly identified. If not, ICG can now be administered to assist with identification of the dissection plane between the right anterior and posterior segments and the bile duct divided intraparenchymally (see Video 17.3).

Left Lateral Sectionectomy

If planning on utilizing fluorescence cholangiography ICG is administered preoperatively. The patient is placed in the supine position. Entry and trocar placement are performed as detailed above. The falciform is dissected off the abdominal wall but the round ligament is typically left in place which assists in retracting the medial sector and can be used as a vascularized pedicle to cover the resection margin. The pedicles to segments 2 and 3 are identified to the left of the umbilical fissure to preserve perfusion and biliary drainage to the medial sector. Once the branches to the left lateral sector are dissected and identified, they are ligated between silk ties and clips and then divided. Following inflow control, ICG can be administered to help delineate the transection plane. The parenchyma is then divided along this line using a bipolar vessel sealing device toward the diaphragm. The bile duct is identified intraparenchymally after transection has begun. It is then ligated between silk ties and clips with subsequent division. Transection is continued superiorly until the left hepatic vein is identified. This is ligated between clips or stapled depending on caliber. The remaining parenchyma is divided with the bipolar vessel sealing device and the coronary attachments divided.

Parenchymal Transection

Laparoscopic Parenchymal Transection with Negative Fluorescence Guidance

The second indication for near-field infrared fluorescence with ICG is to guide parenchymal transection for anatomic resections. Inflow to the segment or lobe to be transected is controlled temporarily or divided as detailed above, and ICG is administered intravenously at this time. The resection line is marked using monopolar electrocautery using the negative fluorescence technique. Parenchymal transection is then begun using a bipolar energy device in a pre-coagulation crush-clamp technique. Larger hepatic venous tributaries and pedicles are controlled with locking plastic clips prior to transection or with staplers. The transection plane can be reaffirmed repeatedly by switching back to fluorescence imaging to ensure that the dissection is continu-

ing in the proper line. The draining hepatic vein is typically taken intraparenchymally with a stapler, or if it is of smaller caliber it can be controlled with locking plastic clips (see Video 17.4).

Robot Parenchymal Transection with Negative Fluorescence Guidance

Following appropriate inflow control as detailed above, ICG is administered intraoperatively. Fluorescence imaging is then utilized to confirm the transection plane using negative fluorescence guidance. In addition to identifying the line of transection, the observed fluorescence may identify areas still perfused by crossing vessels or aberrant anatomy which may contribute to increased bleeding during parenchymal division. The line of transection is marked with a monopolar energy device using fluorescence imaging. Parenchymal transection is then performed using the bipolar vessel sealing device with larger vessels and pedicles controlled with locking clips. We have largely moved to a no stapler hepatectomy when using the robotic platform. Fluorescence can be rechecked at any point to ensure that the line of transection is continuing along the intended plane. If not divided extrahepatically prior to initiation of parenchymal transection, the hepatic vein for the segment of interest is divided intraparenchymally with locking plastic clips or a stapler depending on the caliber of the vessel. Mobilization is often performed after completion of the hepatectomy (see Video 17.5).

Interpretation

Accurate identification of the biliary tree requires proper timing of ICG administration. As demonstrated in the videos included with this chapter, preoperative administration allows for clear delineation of the bile duct of interest from the surrounding background parenchymal signal assuming sufficient dissection has been performed. Studies on cholecystectomy have demonstrated improved accuracy in identification of extrahepatic biliary structures [18]. As would be expected given the limited tissue penetration of near-field fluorescence, these results are altered in patients with higher body mass indexes [19]. Likewise, identification of the proper location for intrahepatic bile duct division has been demonstrated sensitive enough for use in complex cases such as living donor hepatectomy [17].

Fluorescence guided parenchymal transection utilizing the negative technique requires that proper inflow control be achieved prior to ICG administration. Accurate identification of the transection plane has been reported as high as 100% in some studies [20]. Importantly, negative counterstaining can reveal patient-specific variations which are often not linear and can be difficult to identify laparoscopically [21].

Pitfalls

While fluorescence cholangiography and ICG-guided transection have been demonstrated to be safe and efficacious, there are several potential pitfalls. A major drawback to ICG fluorescence is the limited penetration of 5–10 mm. As reported in studies examining ICG cholangiography, there can be a failure to identify structures in the setting of obesity or severe inflammation [18]. Importantly when using fluorescence imaging to aid in identifying biliary anatomy, studies on cholecystectomy demonstrate that repeated imaging and continued meticulous dissection ultimately allow for satisfactory identification. Another potential pitfall is limited efficacy following spillage of bile. This has been reported following perforation of the gallbladder when using ICG cholangiography during cholecystectomy [18].

Proper timing of the ICG administration is key for cases in which cholangiography is planned. This can represent a logistical concern for some settings, although the range of administration times has been reported to be quite wide [22]. Likewise, there may be delayed excretion and concentration of the dye in the biliary tree in patients with compromised liver function [23].

A final concern is for the potential of allergic reaction. ICG use is contraindicated in patients with iodine allergy. While rare, anaphylactic reaction to ICG has been reported with an incidence of 3/1000 [24].

Summary

Use of near-field infrared fluorescence during hepatic resections has several benefits and will continue to provide novel techniques to improve the accuracy and safety of minimally invasive hepatic resections. It can be used to aid in identification of biliary structures and anatomy to guide portal and hilar dissection. This allows for more confident identification of key structures during this tedious dissection. Secondly, it greatly assists in detailing the transection planes during anatomic parenchymal transections after appropriate inflow control has been achieved. This allows for a precise and visual confirmation of viable parenchyma that will be left behind after transection.

References

1. Yohanathan L, Cleary SP. Minimally invasive management of secondary liver cancer. Surg Oncol Clin N Am. 2019;28(2):229–41. Epub 2019/01/07. https://doi.org/10.1016/j.soc.2018.11.003. PubMed PMID: 30851825.
2. Swaid F, Geller DA. Minimally invasive primary liver cancer surgery. Surg Oncol Clin N Am. 2019;28(2):215–27. Epub 2019/02/02. https://doi.org/10.1016/j.soc.2018.11.002. PubMed PMID: 30851824.
3. Nguyen KT, Gamblin TC, Geller DA. World review of laparoscopic liver resection-2,804 patients. Ann Surg. 2009;250(5):831–41. https://doi.org/10.1097/SLA.0b013e3181b0c4df. PubMed PMID: 19801936.
4. Melandro F, Giovanardi F, Hassan R, Larghi Laureiro Z, Ferri F, Rossi M, et al. Minimally invasive approach in the setting of ALPPS procedure: a systematic review of the literature. J Gastrointest Surg. 2019. Epub 2019/06/13. https://doi.org/10.1007/s11605-018-04092-x. PubMed PMID: 31197682.
5. Lee B, Choi Y, Han HS, Yoon YS, Cho JY, Kim S, et al. Comparison of pure laparoscopic and open living donor right hepatectomy after a learning curve. Clin Transplant. 2019. Epub 2019/08/01. https://doi.org/10.1111/ctr.13683. PubMed PMID: 31368582.
6. Park J, Kwon DCH, Choi GS, Kim SJ, Lee SK, Kim JM, et al. Safety and risk factors of pure laparoscopic living donor right hepatectomy: comparison to open

technique in propensity score-matched analysis. Transplantation. 2019. Epub 2019/06/24. https://doi.org/10.1097/TP.0000000000002834. PubMed PMID: 31283680.

7. Brown KM, Geller DA. What is the learning curve for laparoscopic major hepatectomy? J Gastrointest Surg. 2016;20(5):1065–71. Epub 2016/03/08. https://doi.org/10.1007/s11605-016-3100-8. PubMed PMID: 26956007.

8. Hu L, Yao L, Li X, Jin P, Yang K, Guo T. Effectiveness and safety of robotic-assisted versus laparoscopic hepatectomy for liver neoplasms: a meta-analysis of retrospective studies. Asian J Surg. 2018;41(5):401–16. Epub 2017/09/12. https://doi.org/10.1016/j.asjsur.2017.07.001. PubMed PMID: 28912048.

9. Tsung A, Geller DA, Sukato DC, Sabbaghian S, Tohme S, Steel J, et al. Robotic versus laparoscopic hepatectomy: a matched comparison. Ann Surg. 2014;259(3):549–55. https://doi.org/10.1097/SLA.0000000000000250. PubMed PMID: 24045442.

10. Kingham TP, Leung U, Kuk D, Gönen M, D'Angelica MI, Allen PJ, et al. Robotic liver resection: a case-matched comparison. World J Surg. 2016;40(6):1422–8. https://doi.org/10.1007/s00268-016-3446-9. PubMed PMID: 26913732; PubMed Central PMCID: PMCPMC4870111.

11. Kudo H, Ishizawa T, Tani K, Harada N, Ichida A, Shimizu A, et al. Visualization of subcapsular hepatic malignancy by indocyanine-green fluorescence imaging during laparoscopic hepatectomy. Surg Endosc. 2014;28(8):2504–8. Epub 2014/02/25. https://doi.org/10.1007/s00464-014-3468-z. PubMed PMID: 24566751.

12. Urade T, Sawa H, Iwatani Y, Abe T, Fujinaka R, Murata K, et al. Laparoscopic anatomical liver resection using indocyanine green fluorescence imaging. Asian J Surg. 2019. Epub 2019/04/28. https://doi.org/10.1016/j.asjsur.2019.04.008. PubMed PMID: 31043331

13. Ishizawa T, Gumbs AA, Kokudo N, Gayet B. Laparoscopic segmentectomy of the liver: from segment I to VIII. Ann Surg. 2012;256(6):959–64. https://doi.org/10.1097/SLA.0b013e31825ffed3.

14. Verbeek FP, Schaafsma BE, Tummers QR, van der Vorst JR, van der Made WJ, Baeten CI, et al. Optimization of near-infrared fluorescence cholangiography for open and laparoscopic surgery. Surg Endosc. 2014;28(4):1076–82. https://doi.org/10.1007/s00464-013-3305-9. PubMed PMID: 24232054; PubMed Central PMCID: PMCPMC4021038.

15. Ishizawa T, Bandai Y, Kokudo N. Fluorescent cholangiography using indocyanine green for laparoscopic cholecystectomy: an initial experience. Arch Surg. 2009;144(4):381–2. https://doi.org/10.1001/archsurg.2009.9.

16. Ishizawa T, Saiura A, Kokudo N. Clinical application of indocyanine green-fluorescence imaging during hepatectomy. Hepatobiliary Surg Nutr. 2016;5(4):322–8. https://doi.org/10.21037/hbsn.2015.10.01. PubMed PMID: 27500144; PubMed Central PMCID: PMCPMC4960410.

17. Hong SK, Lee KW, Kim HS, Yoon KC, Ahn SW, Choi JY, et al. Optimal bile duct division using real-time indocyanine green near-infrared fluorescence cholangiography during laparoscopic donor hepatectomy. Liver Transpl. 2017;23(6):847–52. https://doi.org/10.1002/lt.24686.

18. Osayi SN, Wendling MR, Drosdeck JM, Chaudhry UI, Perry KA, Noria SF, et al. Near-infrared fluorescent cholangiography facilitates identification of biliary anatomy during laparoscopic cholecystectomy. Surg Endosc. 2015;29(2):368–75. Epub 2014/07/02. https://doi.org/10.1007/s00464-014-3677-5. PubMed PMID: 24986018; PubMed Central PMCID: PMCPMC4415528.

19. Pesce A, Latteri S, Barchitta M, Portale TR, Di Stefano B, Agodi A, et al. Near-infrared fluorescent cholangiography—real-time visualization of the biliary tree during elective laparoscopic cholecystectomy. HPB (Oxford). 2018;20(6):538–45. Epub 2017/12/29. https://doi.org/10.1016/j.hpb.2017.11.013. PubMed PMID: 29292071.

20. Nomi T, Hokuto D, Yoshikawa T, Matsuo Y, Sho M. A novel navigation for laparoscopic anatomic liver resection using indocyanine green fluorescence. Ann Surg Oncol. 2018;25(13):3982. Epub 2018/09/14. https://doi.org/10.1245/s10434-018-6768-z. PubMed PMID: 30218249.

21. Mizuno T, Sheth R, Yamamoto M, Kang HS, Yamashita S, Aloia TA, et al. Laparoscopic glissonean pedicle transection (Takasaki) for negative fluorescent counterstaining of segment 6. Ann Surg Oncol. 2017;24(4):1046–7. Epub 2016/12/19. https://doi.org/10.1245/s10434-016-5721-2. PubMed PMID: 27995453.

22. Schols RM, Bouvy ND, Masclee AA, van Dam RM, Dejong CH, Stassen LP. Fluorescence cholangiography during laparoscopic cholecystectomy: a feasibility study on early biliary tract delineation. Surg Endosc. 2013;27(5):1530–6. Epub 2012/10/18. https://doi.org/10.1007/s00464-012-2635-3. PubMed PMID: 23076461.

23. Mitsuhashi N, Kimura F, Shimizu H, Imamaki M, Yoshidome H, Ohtsuka M, et al. Usefulness of intraoperative fluorescence imaging to evaluate local anatomy in hepatobiliary surgery. J Hepatobiliary Pancreat Surg. 2008;15(5):508–14. Epub 2008/10/04. https://doi.org/10.1007/s00534-007-1307-5. PubMed PMID. 18836805.

24. Speich R, Saesseli B, Hoffmann U, Neftel KA, Reichen J. Anaphylactoid reactions after indocyanine-green administration. Ann Intern Med. 1988;109(4):345–6. https://doi.org/10.7326/0003-4819-109-4-345_2. PubMed PMID: 3395048.

Shiksha Joshi, Emanuele Lo Menzo, Fernando Dip,
Samuel Szomstein, and Raul J. Rosenthal

Introduction

Laparoscopic cholecystectomy (LC) has become the gold standard surgical treatment for benign diseases of the gallbladder. The superiority of the minimally invasive technique over the open one results from the shorter postoperative hospital stay, less postoperative pain, and the cosmetic superiority. However, the rate of iatrogenic vascular injuries and bile duct injuries remains double than the open. In fact, the reported rate of common bile duct injury is estimated to be 0.4% with LC [1]. The clinical and economic consequences of such injuries are very significant, with need for prolonged rehospitalization, multiple procedures, and long-term strictures.

The intrinsic property of indocyanine green (ICG) to bind to serum proteins and be com-

pletely excreted by the liver in the bile has been increasingly utilized as a method of intraoperative identification of the biliary anatomy. This technique has been found to be simple, cost-effective, and reproducible. In addition, it also seems to be superior to other traditional techniques of intraoperative bile duct identification such as the intraoperative cholangiogram (IOC). In fact, the need for incision of the biliary tract, expensive equipment, radiation, and learning curve makes the use of IOC less practical. On the contrary, FC does not require an incision, avoids potential injury to the biliary tree, is cheap, can be repeated many times by simply switching the light wavelength, and gives a real-time visualization of the anatomy.

Indications

Fluorescent cholangiography can be used during any benign condition that requires removal of the gallbladder like cholelithiasis, acute cholecystitis, and polyps. The use of FC is particularly beneficial in the following conditions.

Anatomical Variations

Misidentification of the biliary anatomy can be due to the presence of anatomical variation and aberrancies. Confirming the anatomy is an inte-

Electronic Supplementary Material The online version of this chapter (https://doi.org/10.1007/978-3-030-38092-2_18) contains supplementary material, which is available to authorized users.

S. Joshi · E. Lo Menzo · S. Szomstein
R. J. Rosenthal (✉)
Department of General Surgery, The Bariatric and Metabolic Institute, Cleveland Clinic Florida, Weston, FL, USA
e-mail: ROSENTR@CCF.ORG

F. Dip
Hospital de Clinicas Jose de San Martin,
Buenos Aires, Argentina

gral part of the surgery with use of CT scan. Magnetic resonance cholangiopancreatography (MRCP) to study these anatomical variations is limited by the two-dimensional type of imaging, radiation exposure, and inability to be performed intraoperatively. ICG use makes the ducts fluorescent, thereby simplifying the identification of these structures intraoperatively [1]. Similarly, aberrancy of cystic ducts and gallbladder can also be successfully visualized. A recently reported case of cholelithiasis in retrohepatic gallbladder used FC to identify the biliary structure and successfully avoided any iatrogenic damage [2].

Acute Cholecystitis

The severe inflammation surrounding the gallbladder, cystic duct, and bile duct causes difficulty in recognition of these structures. In fact, the rate of bile duct injuries significantly increases in the cases of severe inflammation. The use of ICG fluorescence in this scenario can help the surgeon identify the ducts and reduce the risk of bile duct injury. In a recent study on the use of ICG in delayed LC after percutaneous transhepatic gallbladder drainage (PTGBD) in 130 patients with acute cholecystitis, the authors found a statistically significant reduction in operative time (129 ± 46 vs. 150 ± 56 min), low conversion rate to laparotomy (2.6% vs. 22%), and lower proportion of subtotal cholecystectomy (0% vs. 6.6%), when compared with the group without the use of ICG fluorescence [3]. The rate of post-surgical complication in both the groups remained same at 10%. LC without ICG in the setting of PTGBD has been described as an independent risk factor for conversion to laparotomy [3].

Obesity

Gallbladder diseases are very common in patients with obesity. The presence of obesity can significantly affect exposure and visualization of the biliary tree. The use of fluorescence cholangiography was explored in a study that compared ICG use in LC in patients who were obese versus non-obese. A total of 70% of the hepatic duct and 87% of the common bile duct were visualized with no significant differences in identification of hepatic duct, common bile duct, and accessory duct in the groups with obesity versus groups without obesity. The authors found that obesity did not affect the visualization of bile ducts with ICG, making this technique suitable in this patient population [4].

Technique and Description

The U.S. Food and Drug Administration (FDA) approved the use of ICG for clinical studies in 1956. Since then, it has been intensively studied and used in many fields such as in cardiology for evaluation of the cardiac output, patency of coronary bypass grafts, assessment of hepatic function and perfusion in bowel anastomosis post-resection, and in plastic surgery to assess the circulation in free flaps for reconstruction.

The ability of ICG to show this fluorescence lies in its inherent property to absorb the light at a wavelength of 750–800 nm and to then radiate at a wavelength of 800 nm and above, which comes under infrared region of the light spectra. Cameras can capture this emission with specific filters to collect multiple images.

The ICG forms covalent bonds with plasma proteins, and this property results in a restricted bioavailability and keeps the molecule intravascularly. The half-life of ICG is 4–5 min, and it is completely eliminated by the liver and excreted into the bile without any metabolism. The toxicity profile of ICG is minimal. The cost-effectiveness of this dye along with its safety profile makes it a superior choice for imaging the vascular structures [5, 6].

After gaining the peripheral venous access, a single bolus dose of 0.05 mg/kg of ICG is administered intravenously 1 h prior to surgery. The ICG is then circulated through the system and excreted by liver into bile. The flow of bile with ICG can be recorded intraoperatively, in form of images through cameras with filters for immediate analysis. The light of the laparoscope can be toggled between with light and infrared light by simply depressing a pedal. This results in a repeatable and real-time picture of the fluorescence (Figs. 18.1 and 18.2). In addition to the biliary tree, the vascular anatomy can be visualized by an additional peripheral intravenous injection of ICG with nearly immediate visualization through the camera [7] (Fig. 18.3). Refer to Video 18.1 for the stepwise approach to laparoscopic cholecystectomy with use of ICG.

Discussion

The unarguable advantages of LC have been well demonstrated. Unfortunately, the rate of bile duct injury (BDI) remains higher than in open surgery (0.2–0.7% vs. 0.16–0.2%). One of the main reasons for such difference between open and LC is the misidentification of the biliary structures. Several techniques to attempt to reduce such injuries have been described. Among these, the "critical view of safety," first described by Strasberg in 1995, is the most commonly utilized

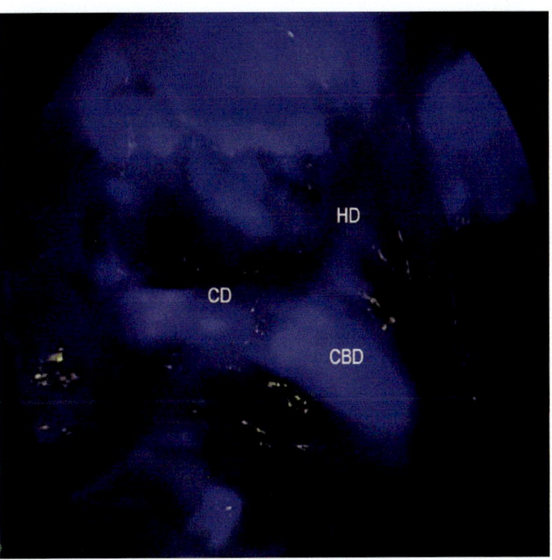

Fig. 18.2 Imaging with indocyanine green shows common bile duct (CBD) and hepatic duct (HD)

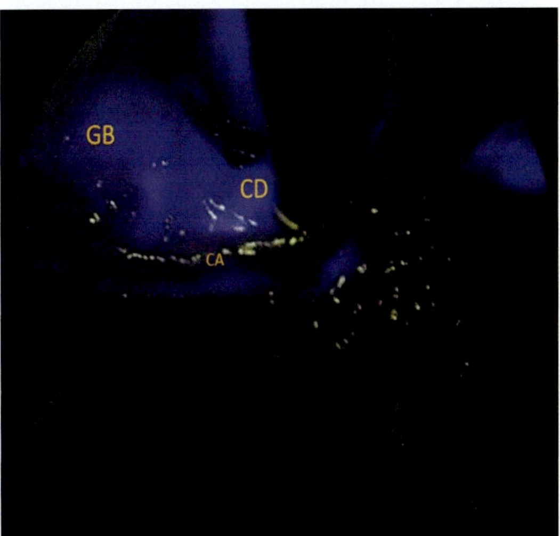

Fig. 18.3 Imaging with indocyanine green shows relationship between cystic duct (CD), cystic artery (CA), and gall bladder (GB)

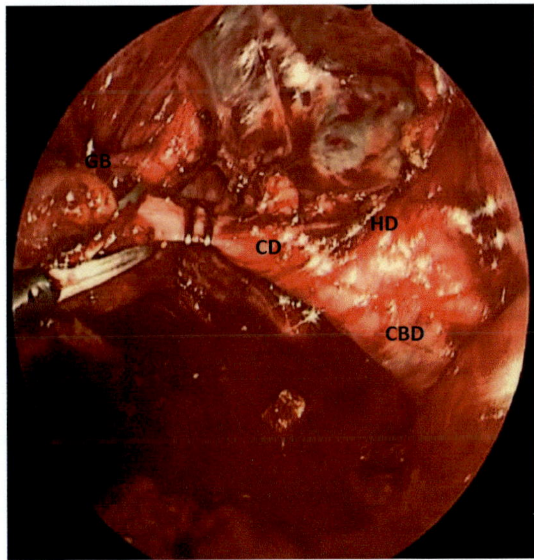

Fig. 18.1 Image with white light showing gall bladder (GB), common bile duct (CBD), and hepatic duct (HD). Cystic duct (CD) is clipped

technique intraoperatively. Additionally, intraoperative cholangiogram (IOC) has been extensively reported to provide adequate visualization of the extrahepatic bile ducts and to successfully identify common bile duct stones. However, IOC has not been demonstrated to reduce the incidence of BDI, but only to provide earlier diagnosis of them. Part of the reason for this finding has to do with the intrinsic technique, which requires an incision of the biliary tree in order to gain access into it. Also, IOC presents other disadvantages, such as radiation exposure, need for specialized equipment, significant additional time to perform and coordinate, and higher costs.

Fluorescent cholangiography has shown promising results regarding identification of the anatomic structures. As previously described, ICG is injected intravenously, 1 h before the planned surgery, or alternatively directly into the gallbladder [8]. A systematic review of 27 clinical trials focused its analysis on dose optimization and found that the administration of 5 mg of ICG resulted in highest bile duct-to-liver ratio in 3–7 hours, though most of the studies used 2.5 mg of ICG dose. This study supported the idea of administering 5 mg of ICG in advance of 3 hours for best visualization of bile ducts [9].

Dip et al. compared the process of fluorescent cholangiography (FC) with intraoperative invasive cholangiogram, which is the standard of choice for imaging the biliary structures. The authors found a statistical significance difference in terms of cost-effectiveness and shorter intraoperative time with FC. The use of FC helped in successful identification of the cystic duct in 97% of the cases and common bile duct in 80% of the cases. In general, several reasons have been identified to use ICG. Table 18.1 shows 10 reasons to use cholangiography in LC [7].

A recently published randomized multicenter trial compared the efficiency of FC with white light versus white light alone in laparoscopic cholecystectomy cases. They found that identification of biliary structures like the cystic duct, common bile duct, right hepatic duct, and common hepatic duct was high with FC when compared to white light alone, and the result was statistically significant [10, 11]. Also, the same trial showed a trend toward fewer BDI in the FC group.

A Canadian study on use of FC in LC showed 100% visualization of cystic duct and identification of CBD in 83% of cases. They found consensus in 83% of surgeons in support of the use of FC for efficient visualization of the extrahepatic biliary tree [12].

Robotic cholecystectomy is a latest innovative technique for gallbladder removal, and the use of fluorescence has been studied in this with similar results when compared to LC. At least one biliary structure was identified in 99% of cases with a 3.2% postoperative complication rate [13].

All the above studies show the significant utility of FC in LC. It is an incisionless cost-effective simple technique with a high safety profile, and it

Table 18.1 Ten reasons to use fluorescent cholangiography in laparoscopic cholecystectomy

1	Feasibility	FC 45 (100%) vs. IOC 42 (93%), $p < 0.078$
2	Cost/cheaper	FC—13.97 ± 4.3 vs. IOC—778.43 ± 0.4 U.S. dollars per patient, $p = 0.0001$
3	Time/faster	FC—0.71 ± 0.26 vs. IOC—7.15 ± 3.76 min, $p < 0.0001$
4	Specificity	Identification by FC of cystic duct—44 out of 45 patients (97.77%); the common hepatic duct—27 out of 45 patients (60%); the common bile duct—36 out of 45 (80%) patients
5	Teaching tool/can be used repeatedly	Residents identified the extrahepatic structures in all 45 cases (100%) with FC
6	Safety	No complications reported with the use of FC
7	Lack of learning curve	No statistical difference in the time needed for identification of structures between the first group and the second group (0.77 ± 0.3 vs. 0.65 ± 0.2 min, $p = 0.13$)
8	Lack of X-ray exposure	X-ray leads were only used for IOC
9	Simplicity	FC could be performed by all residents at different levels of training in 100% of the cases
10	*Real-time surgery*	*Dissection, transection, and resection could be safely performed in 45 cases (100%) with FC*

From: Dip et al. [7]; used with permission
FC fluorescent cholangiography, *IOC* intraoperative cholangiogram

can be used intraoperatively. Time required for the imaging is comparatively short, and it does not require extra training to use. It can also be used as a teaching tool for residents to identify the biliary structures.

Pitfalls

FC is an incisionless simple technique to identify Calot's triangle, but it cannot be used to visualize intraduct obstruction such as in the case of common bile duct stones. The sensitivity of FC is affected by the thickness of the tissue being investigated due to the limitation of the penetration of the light. This can be a limiting factor in the cases of acute cholecystitis with severe inflammation of the tissues surrounding the gallbladder and bile duct, limiting the identification of the biliary structures. Fluorescence from ICG has a low penetrance, and the structures may not be visualized with clarity if there is excess abdominal fat or inflammation.

In addition, the inadvertent spillage of bile during the procedure will also cause wide diffusion of the ICG with reduced ability to accurately identify the biliary structures.

References

1. Tsuruda Y, Okumura H, Setoyama T, Hiwatashi K, Minami K, Ando K, Wada M, Maenohara S, Natsugoe S. Laparoscopic cholecystectomy with aberrant bile duct detected by intraoperative fluorescent cholangiography concomitant with angiography: a case report. Int J Surg Case Rep. 2018;51:14–6.
2. Mattone E, Latteri S, Teodoro M, Pesce A, Mannino M, Romano G, Russello D, La Greca G. Dystopic retrohepatic gallbladder and cholecysto-choledocho lithiasis: the rendez-vous and indocyanine green fluorescence. Clin Case Rep. 2018;6:522–6.
3. Yoshiya S, Minagawa R, Kamo K, et al. Usability of intraoperative fluorescence imaging with indocyanine green during laparoscopic cholecystectomy after percutaneous transhepatic gallbladder drainage. World J Surg. 2019;43:127–33.
4. Dip F, Nguyen D, Montorfano L, Szretter Noste ME, Lo Menzo E, Simpfendorfer C, Szomstein S, Rosenthal R. Accuracy of near infrared-guided surgery in morbidly obese subjects undergoing laparoscopic cholecystectomy. Obes Surg. 2016;26:525–30.
5. Menzo EL, Lo Menzo E, Dip FD, Szomstein S, Rosenthal RJ. Economic impact of fluorescent cholangiography. In: Fluorescence imaging for surgeons. Cham: Springer; 2015. p. 99–106.
6. Boni L, David G, Mangano A, Dionigi G, Rausei S, Spampatti S, Cassinotti E, Fingerhut A. Clinical applications of indocyanine green (ICG) enhanced fluorescence in laparoscopic surgery. Surg Endosc. 2015;29:2046–55.
7. Dip F, Roy M, Lo Menzo E, Simpfendorfer C, Szomstein S, Rosenthal RJ. Routine use of fluorescent incisionless cholangiography as a new imaging modality during laparoscopic cholecystectomy. Surg Endosc. 2015;29:1621–6.
8. Graves C, Ely S, Idowu O, Newton C, Kim S. Direct gallbladder indocyanine green injection fluorescence cholangiography during laparoscopic cholecystectomy. J Laparoendosc Adv Surg Tech A. 2017;27:1069–73.
9. Boogerd LSF, Handgraaf HJM, Huurman VAL, Lam H-D, Mieog JSD, van der Made WJ, van de Velde CJH, Vahrmeijer AL. The best approach for laparoscopic fluorescence cholangiography: overview of the literature and optimization of dose and dosing time. Surg Innov. 2017;24:386–96.
10. Dip F, LoMenzo E, Sarotto L, et al. Randomized trial of near-infrared incisionless fluorescent cholangiography. Ann Surg. 2019;270:992. https://doi.org/10.1097/SLA.0000000000003178.
11. Rosenthal RJ, Dip F, Lo Menzo E, Sarotto LL, Schneider SS, Matthew Walsh R, Carus T, Boni L, Ishizawa T, Phillips EH. Multicenter trial evaluating the efficacy of near-infrared incisionless fluorescent cholangiography during laparoscopic cholecystectomy. J Am Coll Surg. 2018;227:e2.
12. Zroback C, Chow G, Meneghetti A, Warnock G, Meloche M, Chiu CJ, Panton ON. Fluorescent cholangiography in laparoscopic cholecystectomy: the initial Canadian experience. Am J Surg. 2016;211:933–7.
13. Daskalaki D, Fernandes E, Wang X, Bianco FM, Elli EF, Ayloo S, Masrur M, Milone L, Giulianotti PC. Indocyanine green (ICG) fluorescent cholangiography during robotic cholecystectomy: results of 184 consecutive cases in a single institution. Surg Innov. 2014;21:615–21.

Part VI

Applications in Colorectal Surgery

Anastomosis Viability Assessment in Colorectal Surgery

Mahmoud Abu Gazala and Steven D. Wexner

Introduction

Anastomotic leak (AL) remains one of the most dreaded complications in colorectal surgery and is responsible for significant morbidity and mortality. In spite of improvements in technique and technology, the AL rate for colorectal anastomosis ranges 20% [1]. The more distal the anastomosis, the higher the risk for AL. The highest AL rates are found in patients undergoing proctectomy with anastomosis lower than 10 cm from the anal verge (AV) and/or patients who received preoperative neoadjuvant chemoradiation. In these high-risk patients, an AL rate of 10–20% is common; thus loop ileostomy is often performed [2]. Table 19.1 presents the reates of reoperation due to AL.

Consequences of AL are devastating and, accordingly, have been extensively studied. In addition to the increased risk for short-term morbidity and mortality associated with AL, there are other consequences including worsened oncologic outcomes, worsened functional outcomes, reduced quality of life, and increased financial burden. Hammond et al. [3] evaluated the Premier Perspective™ database for patients who underwent colorectal procedures and identified 6174 patients (6.18%) with colorectal AL. Patients who had AL were prone to significantly higher postoperative infection rate (X0.8–1.9), higher 30-day re-admission rates (X1.3), and longer duration of hospitalization (7.3 more days) compared with patients who did not have AL. This translated to excess hospitalization cost of $24,129 per patient for patients who suffered an AL.

Anastomotic leak is also strongly linked to significantly worse functional outcomes, reduced quality of life, and increased risk of permanent stoma [4–6]. In patients who underwent restorative proctectomy and developed AL, increased pelvic fibrosis significantly hinders the compliance and distensibility of the "neo-rectum," increasing the urge to defecate and reducing the maximum tolerated volume, resulting in anterior resection syndrome symptoms including urgency, frequency, impaired evacuation, and incontinence [7, 8]. This worsened function also increases the risk for a permanent stoma. Another

Electronic Supplementary Material The online version of this chapter (https://doi.org/10.1007/978-3-030-38092-2_19) contains supplementary material, which is available to authorized users.

M. Abu Gazala
Colorectal Department, Cleveland Clinic Florida, Weston, FL, USA

S. D. Wexner (✉)
Department of Colorectal Surgery, Digestive Disease Center, Cleveland Clinic Florida, Weston, FL, USA
e-mail: WexnerS@CCF.org

E. M. Aleassa, K. M. El-Hayek (eds.), *Video Atlas of Intraoperative Applications of Near Infrared Fluorescence Imaging*, https://doi.org/10.1007/978-3-030-38092-2_19

Table 19.1 Colorectal anastomosis leak rate and re-operative rate in selected series

Author/year	Location	Sample size	Leak rate	Re-operative rate
Chude et al./2008 [29]	Greece	120 LAR	10%	2.5%
Rullier et al./2008 [11]	France	272 LAR	12%	4.8%
Karliczek et al./2009 [30]	Netherlands	191 Colorectal anastomosis	14%	NR
Ashraf et al./2013 [31]	UK	285 LAR	10%	5.6%
Caulfield et al./2013 [4]	USA	198 LAR	15%	NR
Senagore et al./2014 [32]	USA	258 Colorectal anastomosis	12%	7.4%
Mongin et al./2014 [33]	France	171 LAR	12%	7.6%
Leahy et al./2014 [34]	USA	245 Colorectal anastomosis	14%	NR
Shiomi et al./2015 [35]	Japan	936 LAR	13%	4.7%

LAR low anterior resection, *NR* not reported

less recognized consequence of AL is the effect on oncologic outcomes. Anastomotic leak has been shown in several studies and meta-analyses to significantly increase the risk for local recurrence, reduce disease-free survival rates, and increase long-term cancer-specific mortality rates [9, 10].

Despite research, technique modifications, and risk factor identification and optimization, the pathogenesis of AL has yet to be fully understood; similarly, rates of AL have been acceptably lowered. A multitude of risk factors have been identified for AL, not all of which are modifiable:

- *Distance from the anal verge*: It is a well-established fact that the AL rates after proctectomy is significantly higher compared to other types of bowel anastomosis. Furthermore, the closer the anastomosis is to the anal verge (AV), the higher the risk for AL. This fact has been demonstrated in a plethora of studies and reports [11–13]. In their study, Bertelsen et al. showed an odds ratio (OR) of 2 for AL when the anastomosis is at 10 cm from the AV [12]. This rises to OR of 3.6 at 7 cm from the AV, and OR of 5.4 for AL when the anastomosis is lower than 5 cm from the AV.
- *Neoadjuvant chemoradiation*: There have been conflicting data regarding the role of neoadjuvant chemoradiation as an independent risk factor for AL [14–17]. However, radiation is regarded by most surgeons as a risk factor for AL due to the established effects on tissue healing and vascular damage.

- *Presence of a diverting stoma*: A stoma may or may not reduce the AL rate; however, it definitely blunts the clinical significance and reduces the catastrophic sequelae of a devastating AL. Therefore, it is widely acceptable to divert high-risk pelvic anastomoses, especially those lower than 10 cm from the AV and in patients who had received neoadjuvant chemoradiation. A diverting stoma does, however, have implications on quality of life, and its reversal is not devoid of complications [18].
- *Tension on the anastomosis*: A tension-free anastomosis is regarded as a cornerstone of modern surgery. During restorative proctectomy, this goal may be achieved via splenic flexure mobilization and high ligation of the inferior mesenteric vein and artery.
- *Intraoperative leak testing*: It is common practice to intraoperatively test the anastomosis for leak. Testing can be performed in several manners, mostly via endoscopic evaluation of the anastomosis and examination for air leak. Ricciardi et al. evaluated 998 patients with left-sided colorectal anastomoses and without proximal diversion [19]. Of these, 825 were air leak tested, with positive intraoperative leak test found in 7.9% of cases. If the anastomosis was suture repaired alone, the rate of postoperative clinical leak was 12.2%, compared to 0% clinical leak rate if patients were diverted or the anastomosis was recreated following a positive intraoperative AL test.
- *Adequate anastomotic perfusion*: A major tenet of modern surgery is the creation of a

Table 19.2 Methods for evaluation of bowel perfusion

Technique	Laparoscopic surgery	Easy to use	Accurate	Objective	Reproducible	Cost effective
Color of the bowel	+	+	−	−	+/−	$
Marginal blood vessels	+	+	−	−	+/−	$
On table angiography [28]	+	−	+	+	+	$$$
Pulse oximetry [29]	−	+	−	+	+	$
Polarographic oxygen tension [11, 30]	−	−	+	−	+	$$
Doppler ultrasound [31]	−	+	+/−	+/−	+/−	$
Intravital microscopy	−	−	+/−	+/−	+/−	$$$ No human use
Spectrophotometry	−	−	+	+	+	$$
Bowel wall contractility	−	−	+/−	+	+/−	$$$
pH measurement	−	−	+/−	+	+	$$
Microdialysis	−	−	+/−	+/−	+/−	$$
Fluorescein fluorescence [4]	+/−	−	+/−	+	−	$$
Laser Doppler flowmetry [15]	+/−	−	+/−	+/−	+/−	$$
Near-infrared [24]	+	+	+	+	+	$

Used with permission from Ris et al. [20]. Copyright © Thieme Medical Publishers. $ = least cost effective; $$ = average cost effectiveness; $$$ = most cost effective

well-perfused anastomosis. Several measures have been routinely used to evaluate vasculature of the bowel prior to and after resection and also after anastomotic creation. These methods include evaluation of tissue color, palpation of mesenteric pulse, and the presence of bleeding edges of transected margins and other measures (Table 19.2) [20].

- A sufficiently well-perfused anastomosis still remains elusive to adequately evaluate AL. This problem has been reflected in several studies showing that the clinical judgment of the operating surgeon does underestimate the risk for AL when based on traditional assessments for tissue perfusion and anastomotic integrity [21, 22].
- Other risk factors include surgeon experience, male gender, tobacco smoking, obesity, steroid use, and malnutrition.

In recent years, the most promising new technology to try to achieve a significant reduction in AL is the use of indocyanine green (ICG)-based near-infrared fluorescence angiography (FA) to intraoperatively evaluate for adequate anastomotic perfusion. Other methods for tissue perfusion assessment have also been developed, including Doppler ultrasound, transabdominal laser Doppler flowmetry, and oxygen spectroscopy. However, such techniques have not been widely accepted due to complexity and problems with accuracy and reliability. ICG-based FA has been proven in several studies to allow intraoperative perfusion assessment in a simple, safe, precise, and reducible manner and with marginal effect on procedure length [23, 24].

Technical Aspects

Prior to surgery, patients are evaluated for allergy to shellfish or prior adverse reactions to ICG.

Just prior to colonic transection, and after the surgeon decides on the proximal site of division, an intravenous bolus of ICG (our routine is 3.5 mL) is administered followed immediately by 10 mL flush of water. Using a near-infrared (NIR) camera, the quality and distribution of florescence angiogram is evaluated to assess perfusion. When applicable, the resection point may be modified based on the FA findings (Video 19.1).

Following resection, the anastomosis is created in the usual fashion, following which another bolus of ICG is administered in order to evaluate the serosal surface of the anastomosis (Video 19.2) as well as the mucosal surface with a third administration of ICG, when possible (Video 19.3). The anastomosis is taken down and reperformed when signs of insufficient perfusion are evident. The dose of ICG in the application for bowel perfusion is in the range of 0.1–0.3 mg/kg [25].

Literature Review

There are an increasing number of publications showing AL risk reduction with the use of ICG-based IF. We will review the most significant and important publications.

The earliest and largest series regarding the use of ICG-based FA for AL risk reduction was by Kudszus et al. in 2010 [26]. The authors presented their early experience with FA to evaluate colorectal anastomoses. In their study, 332 patients underwent colorectal resections for cancer, and their anastomoses were evaluated using FA for perfusion, while 306 who did not undergo FA evaluation of their anastomosis served as the control group. After matching, the study and control groups each included 201 patients. Matching was performed for age, T-stage, type of resection, type of anastomosis, defunctioning stoma, need for blood intraoperatively, emergency surgery, and body mass index (BMI). Their findings included the following:

- The mean time required for intraoperative FA was 6.8 ± 2.6 min.
- 33/201 (16.4%) in the FA group had a change of planned resection site based on the results of the FA. In 28 patients, a clinically presumed well-vascularized colon was proven to be insufficiently perfused using FA, thus extending the resection margin. In another 5 patients, the clinical impression of malperfusion of the resection margins was not confirmed by FA; thus the resection margin was not extended. Importantly, no patients in this subgroup developed AL.

- The rate of surgical revision due to AL was lower in the FA group and was comparable to the rate noted in the control group: 3.5% vs. 7.5%, respectively. Although this difference did not reach statistical significance, there was significance in a subgroup of patients >70 years of age (4.3% vs. 11.9%, $p = 0.04$, risk reduction of 64%).
- In a subgroup analysis, the rate of revision during elective resections was 3.1% in the FA group compared to 7.7% in the control group ($p = 0.04$, risk reduction of 60%).
- After hand-sewn anastomosis, the rate of revision was 1.2% in the study group and 8.5% in the control group ($p = 0.03$, risk reduction of 84%).
- Hospital stay was significantly reduced in the study group (Wilcoxon test; $p = 0.01$).

The Pillar II study, by Jafari and colleagues [27], is another key study in the field of AL risk reduction using FA. This is a multicenter prospective case series of 139 patients who underwent laparoscopic left-sided colectomy or proctectomy. FA was successfully performed in 99% of patients. There was a change of surgical plan in 11 patients (7.9%), with the majority of changes occurring at the time of transection of the proximal margin (7%). The overall AL rate was very low at 1.4%, while none of the 11 who had a change in the surgical plan developed AL.

A subsequent publication by Ris et al. evaluated 504 patients who underwent a restorative elective colorectal operation in a prospective phase II trial [28]. Indications for surgery were neoplasia in 330 patients and benign disease in 174. The majority of patients (85.3%) underwent a laparoscopic procedure, with a conversion rate of 5.9%. ICG-based FA was successfully achieved in all patients. The median added operating time to each procedure was 4 min per ICG administration. FA resulted in a change in resection margin in 29 patients (5.8%), with no subsequent AL in these patients. The overall AL rate was low at 2.4%.

Conclusion

While the risk for AL is multifactorial and probably may not be totally eliminated, there has been much experience and evidence that ICG-based FA is very beneficial in the quest to lower the risk for AL. This method has been proven to be safe, easy to perform, readily reproducible, and effective in evaluation of bowel perfusion prior to and after creation of anastomosis. Thus, colorectal surgeons should be familiar with and encouraged to use this technique.

References

1. McDermott FD, Heeney A, Kelly ME, Steele RJ, Carlson GL, Winter DC. Systematic review of preoperative, intraoperative and postoperative risk factors for colorectal anastomotic leaks. Br J Surg. 2015. 2015;102(5):462–79.
2. Jafari MD, Wexner SD, Martz JE, McLemore EC, Margolin DA, Sherwinter DA, et al. Perfusion assessment in laparoscopic left-sided/anterior resection (PILLAR II): a multi-institutional study. J Am Coll Surg. 2015;220(1):82–92 e1.
3. Hammond J, Lim S, Wan Y, Gao X, Patkar A. The burden of gastrointestinal anastomotic leaks: an evaluation of clinical and economic outcomes. J Gastrointest Surg. 2014;18(6):1176–85.
4. Caulfield H, Hyman NH. Anastomotic leak after low anterior resection: a spectrum of clinical entities. JAMA Surg. 2013;148(2):177–82.
5. Ashburn JH, Stocchi L, Kiran RP, Dietz DW, Remzi FH. Consequences of anastomotic leak after restorative proctectomy for cancer: effect on long-term function and quality of life. Dis Colon Rectum. 2013;56(3):275–80.
6. Marinatou A, Theodoropoulos GE, Karanika S, Karantanos T, Siakavellas S, Spyropoulos BG, Toutouzas K, Zografos G. Do anastomotic leaks impair postoperative health-related quality of life after rectal cancer surgery? A case-matched study. Dis Colon Rectum. 2014;57(2):158–66.
7. Hallbook O, Sjodahl R. Anastomotic leakage and functional outcome after anterior resection of the rectum. Br J Surg. 1996;83(1):60–2.
8. Nesbakken A, Nygaard K, Lunde OC. Outcome and late functional results after anastomotic leakage following mesorectal excision for rectal cancer. Br J Surg. 2001;88(3):400–4.
9. Mirnezami A, Mirnezami R, Chandrakumaran K, Sasapu K, Sagar P, Finan P. Increased local recurrence and reduced survival from colorectal cancer following anastomotic leak: systematic review and meta-analysis. Ann Surg. 2011;253(5):890–9.
10. Lu ZR, Rajendran N, Lynch AC, Heriot AG, Warrier SK. Anastomotic leaks after restorative resections for rectal cancer compromise cancer outcomes and survival. Dis Colon Rectum. 2016;59(3):236–44.
11. Rullier E, Laurent C, Garrelon JL, Michel P, Saric J, Parneix M. Risk factors for anastomotic leakage after resection of rectal cancer. Br J Surg. 1998;85(3):355–8.
12. Bertelsen CA, Andreasen AH, Jorgensen T, Harling H. Anastomotic leakage after anterior resection for rectal cancer: risk factors. Color Dis. 2010;12(1):37–43.
13. Lipska MA, Bissett IP, Parry BR, Merrie AE. Anastomotic leakage after lower gastrointestinal anastomosis: men are at a higher risk. ANZ J Surg. 2006;76(7):579–85.
14. Stone HB, Coleman CN, Anscher MS, McBride WH. Effects of radiation on normal tissue: consequences and mechanisms. Lancet Oncol. 2003;4(9):529–36.
15. Tibbs MK. Wound healing following radiation therapy: a review. Radiother Oncol. 1997;42(2):99–106.
16. Enker WE, Merchant N, Cohen AM, et al. Safety and efficacy of low anterior resection for rectal cancer: 681 consecutive cases from a specialty service. Ann Surg. 1999;230(4):544–52.
17. Nisar PJ, Lavery IC, Kiran RP. Influence of neoadjuvant radiotherapy on anastomotic leak after restorative resection for rectal cancer. J Gastrointest Surg. 2012;16(9):1750–7.
18. Sharma A, Deeb AP, Rickles AS, Iannuzzi JC, Monson JR, Fleming FJ. Closure of defunctioning loop ileostomy is associated with considerable morbidity. Color Dis. 2013;15(4):458–62.
19. Ricciardi R, Roberts PL, Marcello PW, Hall JF, Read TE, Schoetz DJ. Anastomotic leak testing after colorectal resection: what are the data? Arch Surg. 2009;144(5):407–11; discussion 411–2
20. Ris F, Yeung T, Hompes R, Mortensen NJ. Enhanced reality and intraoperative imaging in colorectal surgery. Clin Colon Rectal Surg. 2015;28(3):158–64.
21. Karliczek A, Harlaar NJ, Zeebregts CJ, Wiggers T, Baas PC, Van Dam GM. Surgeons lack predictive accuracy for anastomotic leakage in gastrointestinal surgery. Int J Color Dis. 2009;24(5):569–76.
22. Markus PM, Martell J, Leister I, Horstmann O, Brinker J, Becker H. Predicting postoperative morbidity by clinical assessment. Br J Surg. 2005;92:101–6.
23. Boni L, David G, Mangano A, Dionigi G, Rausei S, Spampatti S, Cassinotti E, Fingerhut A. Clinical applications of indocyanine green (ICG) enhanced fluorescence in laparoscopic surgery. Surg Endosc. 2015;29(7):2046–55.
24. Boni L, Fingerhut A, Marzorati A, Rausei S, Dionigi G, Cassinotti E. Indocyanine green fluorescence angiography during laparoscopic low anterior resection: results of a case-matched study. Surg Endosc. 2017;31:1836–40. https://doi.org/10.1007/s00464–016–5181–6.
25. Foppa C, Denoya PI, Tarta C, Bergamaschi R. Indocyanine green fluorescent dye during bowel

surgery: are the blood supply "guessing days" over? Tech Coloproctol. 2014;18(8):753–8.

26. Kudszus S, Roesel C, Schachtrupp A, Höer JJ. Intraoperative laser fluorescence angiography in colorectal surgery: a noninvasive analysis to reduce the rate of anastomotic leakage. Langenbeck's Arch Surg. 2010;395(8):1025–30.

27. Jafari MD, Wexner SD, Martz JE, McLemore EC, Margolin DA, Sherwinter DA, Lee SW, Senagore AJ, Phelan MJ, Stamos MJ. Perfusion assessment in laparoscopic left-sided/anterior resection (PILLAR II): a multi-institutional study. J Am Coll Surg. 2015;220(1):82–92.

28. Ris F, Liot E, Buchs NC, Kraus R, et al. Multicentre phase II trial of near-infrared imaging in elective colorectal surgery. Br J Surg. 2018;105(10):1359–67.

29. Chude GG, Rayate NV, Patris V, Koshariya M, Jagad R, Kawamoto J, Lygidakis NJ. Defunctioning loop ileostomy with low anterior resection for distal rectal cancer: should we make an ileostomy as a routine procedure? A prospective randomized study. Hepatogastroenterology. 2008;55(86–87):1562–7.

30. Karliczek A, Benaron DA, Baas PC, Zeebregts CJ, Wiggers T, van Dam GM. Intraoperative assessment of microperfusion with visible light spectroscopy for prediction of anastomotic leakage in colorectal anastomoses. Color Dis. 2010;12(10):1018–25.

31. Ashraf SQ, Burns EM, Jani A, Altman S, Young JD, Cunningham C, Faiz O, Mortensen NJ. The economic impact of anastomotic leakage after anterior resections in English NHS hospitals: are we adequately remunerating them? Color Dis. 2013;15(4):e190–8.

32. Senagore A, Lane FR, Lee E, Wexner S, Dujovny N, Sklow B, Rider P, Bonello J. Bioabsorbable Staple Line Reinforcement Study Group. Bioabsorbable staple line reinforcement in restorative proctectomy and anterior resection: a randomized study. Dis Colon Rectum. 2014;57(3):324–30.

33. Mongin C, Maggiori L, Agostini J, Ferron M, Panis Y. Does anastomotic leakage impair functional results and quality of life after laparoscopic sphincter-saving total mesorectal excision for rectal cancer? A case-matched study. Int J Color Dis. 2014;29(4):459–67.

34. Leahy J, Schoetz D, Marcello P, Read T, Hall J, Roberts P, Ricciardi R. What is the risk of clinical anastomotic leak in the diverted colorectal anastomosis? J Gastrointest Surg. 2014;18(10):1812–6.

35. Shiomi A, Ito M, Maeda K, Kinugasa Y, Ota M, Yamaue H, Shiozawa M, Horie H, Kuriu Y, Saito N. Effects of a diverting stoma on symptomatic anastomotic leakage after low anterior resection for rectal cancer: a propensity score matching analysis of 1,014 consecutive patients. J Am Coll Surg. 2015;220(2):186–94.

Lymph Node Harvesting in Colorectal Cancer: The Role of Fluorescence Lymphangiography

Heidi Paine and Manish Chand

Lymph Node Harvest in Colorectal Cancer

Lymph node harvest in colon cancer is an independent prognostic factor for survival outcomes, with a correlation between number of regional lymph nodes harvested and prognosis irrespective of stage and tumor characteristics [1]. Indeed, lymph node yield acts as a surrogate marker for appropriate oncological surgery, and several international guidelines recommend procuring a minimum of 12 nodes in colectomy specimens for accurate staging [2, 3]. Despite this knowledge, there is presently no consensus on optimal technique or extent of mesenteric lymphadenectomy in colon cancer, and current strategies are largely guided by anatomical landmarks. Complete mesocolic excision (CME) has been

Electronic Supplementary Material The online version of this chapter (https://doi.org/10.1007/978-3-030-38092-2_20) contains supplementary material, which is available to authorized users.

H. Paine
Department of General Surgery, London Deanery, London, UK

M. Chand (✉)
Department of Surgery and Interventional Sciences, University College London Hospitals NHS Trust & GENIE Centre, University College London, London, UK
e-mail: m.chand@ucl.ac.uk

purported to achieve better oncological results and increase disease-free survival (DFS) when compared to "conventional" resection [4, 5]. CME involves dissection in the embryologically defined mesocolic planes to create an intact envelope of mesocolic fascia with central vessel ligation; all lymph nodes along the tumor-supplying vessels are contained within the specimen [5]. It aims to translate the "holy plane" principle of total mesorectal excision (TME) for rectal cancer onto the colon cancer stage. While the oncological rationale of taking an enclosed envelope of fascia with all its attendant lymph nodes in CME is sound, there is a lack of high-quality, large-scale evidence supporting its benefits in improved overall survival, and its use has not been widely recommended or adopted. Moreover, the extent of CME exposes retroperitoneal structures and major vessels not involved in conventional resections to potential damage. Despite previously demonstrating improved DFS for stage I-III adenocarcinoma with CME compared to conventional resection [4], Bertelsen and colleagues [6] reported higher incidences of intraoperative splenic and superior mesenteric vein injuries, as well as postoperative sepsis and respiratory failure in the CME group.

In contrast to colon cancer, rectal cancer surgery follows a standardized approach which was revolutionized by the universal adoption of the TME, first described in 1988 by Heald [7]. The principle of TME is based upon dissection in embryological anatomical planes with dissection of the mesorectum from the parietal plane, leading to a specimen with an intact coverage of both the rectal tumor and its main lymphatic drainage. This has seen survival from rectal cancer improve dramatically, largely due to reduction in local recurrence, to levels around 5%. Lymph node harvest *en bloc* with the specimen in rectal cancer is therefore less variable provided the TME plane is dissected, though the extent to which locoregional pelvic sidewall nodes are targeted and harvested differs between Eastern and Western practice, with Eastern practice favoring extended pelvic lymphadenectomy as standard. Reduced nodal counts within TME specimens, provided they are deemed to be complete according to Quirke grading [8], are often due to sampling error or distortion of architecture due to neoadjuvant chemoradiation.

Current Issues

The importance of lymph node harvest in reducing local recurrence in colorectal cancer is well established as previously mentioned. However, extensive D3 lymphadenectomy or CME in colon cancer and pelvic sidewall clearance in rectal cancer are technically demanding and physiologically insulting. To offer these universally would be to expose patients to great and often unnecessary morbidity; the prospect of being able to stratify patients into those requiring more extensive resection and lymph node harvest, as well as personalize lymphadenectomy to the tumor's specific lymphatic basin, is therefore an attractive one, and may be achievable with the advent of fluorescence lymphangiography.

Current Status of ICG Fluorescence Lymphangiography in Colorectal Surgery

Fluorophores and Their Use in Colorectal Cancer

Fluorescence-guided surgery (FGS) is an increasingly studied area with applications identified to aid intraoperative decision making across surgical specialties. Fluorescence imaging involves illumination of the tissue of interest, which emits light at longer wavelengths. When this is carried out within the near-infrared spectrum (NIR), interference from background fluorescence from compounds present in the human body such as water and hemoglobin is minimized, allowing focused visualization of the tissue of interest. Within the NIR spectrum (700–900 nm), tissue is illuminated with an excitation wavelength of 750–800 nm, and fluorescence emitted at wavelengths >800 nm. Several camera models for multiple surgical modalities (open, laparoscopic, robotic) are available with filters at the specific wavelength required for NIR FGS.

Indocyanine Green Fluorescence

Indocyanine green (ICG) is a fluorophore approved for clinical use and is the most commonly used agent displaying NIR fluorescence in FGS. ICG is a heptamethine cyanine fluorophore with peak excitation and emission wavelengths of 807 nm and 822 nm, respectively. It is 98% plasma protein-bound and remains within the lymphatic and circulatory vasculature once taken up into the microcirculation [9], rendering it highly suited for use in NIR fluorescence angiography and lymphangiography. It has a favorable safety profile, though should be avoided in patients with iodine sensitivity. Tissue penetration of ICG is around 15 mm [10] and is favorable for tissue visualization when compared to visible light and blue dye. When injected intravenously it undergoes hepatic excretion with a serum half-life of 3–5 minutes; interstitial intestinal injection is associated with much longer periods of visualization of ICG.

The application of ICG FGS in colorectal surgery has to date focused on fluorescence angiography, with implications on tissue transection margins, formation of healthy anastomoses, and the need for diverting stomas. This chapter covers a newer area of ICG FGS research, fluorescence lymphangiography, considering its applications in lymph node harvest.

Fluorescence Lymphangiography

Due to its low molecular size and weight (775 Da), ICG is rapidly taken up by the lymphatic spaces and efferent channels when injected submucosally or subserosally in the intestine, before traveling to, and depositing in, lymph nodes [9]. Injection of ICG at the peri-tumoral site reveals the lymphatic basin of the tumor when viewed in NIR mode, and may also identify both the sentinel node as well as any aberrant nodes outside the typical or planned limits of resection. The implications of this lymph node mapping are multiple; visualization of the lymphatic basin could help to guide mesocolic resection margins to include the entire lymphatics of the tumor and maximize the yield of locoregional lymph nodes likely to harbor macro- or micro-metastases. This is especially novel in patients in whom aberrant lymph nodes are identified outside the planned field of resection, allowing real-time decisions to be made to either include these in the specimen or berry-pick these nodes for analysis. In addition, fluorescence lymphangiography has the potential to guide surgeons on which patients require more extensive lymphadenectomy and pelvic sidewall clearance in rectal cancer; this personalized approach may reduce unnecessary morbidity associated with these procedures and support decisions for extensive surgery in appropriate patients. Finally, lymph node histology is an important component of cancer staging which impacts both prognosis and further therapy. Detection of sentinel nodes for detailed immunohistochemical analysis could have implications for upstaging and subsequent adjuvant therapy for patients in whom this would not previously have been offered.

Lymphatic Basin Mapping and Guiding Resection Margins

Lymph node basin mapping intraoperatively can help guide resection margins by ensuring the lymphatics of a tumor are included in the specimen, and multiple studies have demonstrated the feasibility of ICG fluorescence lymphangiography (ICG FL) in successfully identifying the lymphatic basin of tumors. Nishigori and colleagues [11] reported lymph flow visualization intraoperatively in 18 out of 21 patients (85.7%) undergoing laparoscopic colorectal resections, identifying inadequate injection into the submucosa as the cause of failure in the remaining 3 patients. In four patients (23.5%), identification of lymph flow and main node basins changed the surgical plan with respect to the ligature of the root of the central blood vessel and the mesocolic division line. More recent studies have reported similar findings with respect to lymphatic mapping, and the positive histology of aberrant nodes identified by ICG FL may have clinical implications on staging and prognosis. Chand [12] and Noguera et al. [13] demonstrated lymphatic basin visualization in 100% patients in both studies, and nodes outside the planned resection field were seen in 20% and 30% of patients, respectively, leading to extension of lymphadenectomy. Two of two [12] and one of three [13] of these aberrant nodes were found to be positive on histopathology. Importantly, multiple studies of lymphatic mapping using ICG fluorescence have successfully demonstrated delineation of the lymphatic basin with TIII/IV tumors alongside those with early stage disease [11–13].

In addition to ensuring that the lymphatic basin is incorporated into the resection specimen, ICG FL could have an application in personalizing surgery for patients with tumors in anatomical locations known to have variable lymphatic drainage, such as flexural or transverse colon cancers. Carcinoma around the splenic flexure for example has several lymphatic drainage roots, with drainage to the left branch of the middle colic artery (lt-MCA), left colic artery (LCA), and left accessory aberrant colic artery area (LAACA) when present. CME for splenic flexural colon cancer may therefore involve ligation of both the MCA at its origin as well as the ascending branch of the LCA (and LAACA if it exists) to ensure removal of potentially involved nodes. Watanabe and colleagues [14] used ICG FL to map the lymphatic drainage of splenic flexure tumors in 31 patients. The prevalent direction of lymph flow was LCA in 25.8% cases, lt-MCA

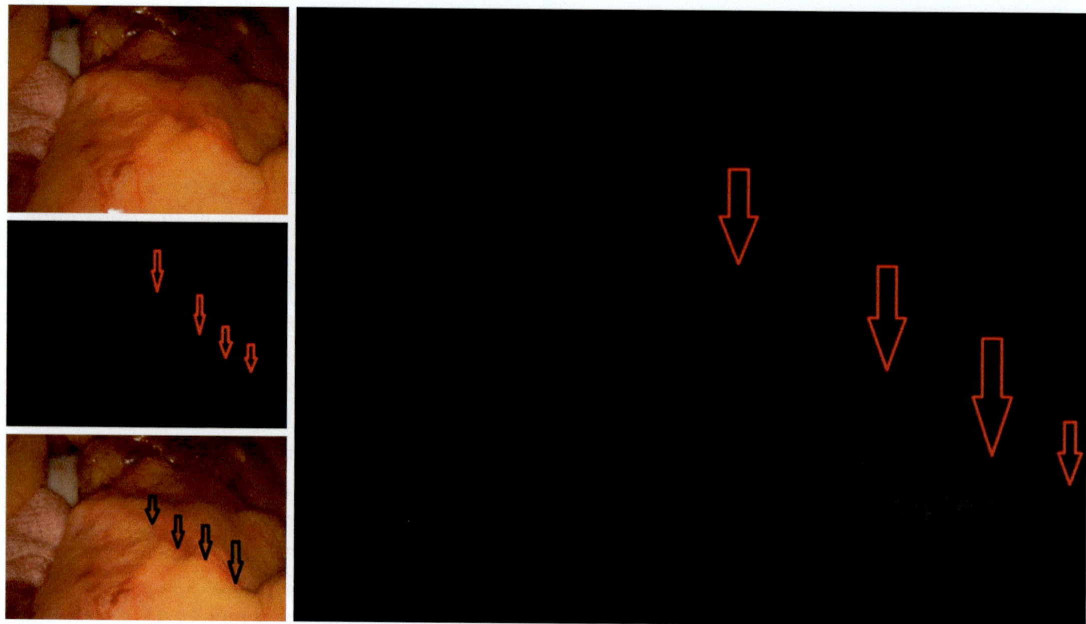

Fig. 20.1 Delineation with ICG fluorescence lymphangiography of the ileocolic watershed area between the colonic mesentery of the right colon and the small bowel mesentery of the terminal ileum. Shown under white light *(black arrows)* and near-infrared light *(red arrows)*

in 19.4% cases, LAACA in 12.9% cases, root of the IMV which did not accompany the artery in 16.1% cases, and the LAACA plus LCA (16.1%) or lt-MCA (9.7%). No case exhibited lymph flow to both the LCA and lt-MCA. In six cases lymph node metastases were observed; all the positive nodes existed in the lymph flow areas outlined with ICG FL. This technique helps to clarify appropriate central vessels to be ligated and guide mesocolic division. The authors propose that in splenic flexure tumors without widespread lymph node involvement, it may not be necessary to ligate both the LCA and lt-MCA if ICG FL is employed to delineate the lymphatic basin on an individualized basis. A similar study has shown feasibility of ICG FL in delineating lymphatic drainage in right-sided colonic tumors, where a watershed area exists in the ileocecal region at the confluence between the terminal ileum and its small bowel mesentery and the right mesocolic mesentery. Peri-tumoral injection of ICG following mobilization and ileocolic artery ligation delineated precisely the lymphatic drainage of the tumor within the ileocolic mesenteric watershed area, identifying the appropriate line of

mesenteric division [15] (Fig. 20.1). This technique allows personalization of surgery in areas with variable lymphatic drainage, and may be of similar benefit in patients undergoing re-operative surgery for malignancy in whom lymphatic channels have been interrupted.

Sentinel Nodes: Detection and Analysis

Sentinel lymph node (SLN) mapping has become well established in cancers such as breast and melanoma, but its role in colorectal cancer has not been fully elucidated. The sentinel node is the first lymph node in the orderly progression of drainage from the primary tumor. Given that the sentinel node is the most likely to harbor metastases, its positivity indicates the likely lymph node involvement and has implications on need for extensive lymphadenectomy as well as staging, prognosis, and adjuvant therapy. Furthermore, identification of sentinel nodes may facilitate targeted, detailed immunohistochemical analysis. While hematoxylin and eosin (H&E) staining is widely employed for lymph node analysis in resection specimens, more detailed immunohistochemistry such as reverse transcription polymerase chain reaction (RT-PCR) exists with a greater sensitivity for demonstrating micrometastases [16]. This is not routinely applied to all nodes due to time and expense but may be considered practical in evaluation of a small number of sentinel nodes. Historically, sentinel node identification has been conducted with dyes such as methylene blue, radioisotope tracers, or a combination of both. These have limitations; dyes have been associated with high false-negative rates and reduced tissue contrast and carry a small but significant risk of anaphylaxis. Radioisotope use can increase detection rates, but high radioactivity at injection sites may interfere with gamma probe detection of nodes in close tumor proximity. In addition, their use requires expensive equipment and radiation protection measures which are not readily available at all institutions [17]. Identification of sentinel nodes using ICG FL is an exciting application which overcomes some of the issues of traditional methods and may be of value in colorectal cancer, albeit in a staging capacity.

Kusano and colleagues [18] described one of the first series of ICG FL sentinel node detection in colorectal cancer. In all 26 patients undergoing open resection, one or more sentinel nodes and the lymphatic basin were clearly visualized. Accuracy, positive, and negative predictive values of sentinel lymph node biopsy (SLNB) were 82.6%, 100%, and 81%, respectively. Similarly, in a series of 18 patients with colorectal cancer or high-grade dysplastic lesions not amenable to endoscopic resection, Cahill et al. [9] demonstrated detection of sentinel node and lymphatic drainage basins in every case. In four cases, aberrant fluorescing nodes were seen outside the conventional resection field (all negative on histology). Sentinel node status was found to accurately predict the oncological status of the mesocolon in every case, identifying three patients with mesocolic nodal metastases, and correctly excluding mesocolic basin node involvement in the remaining 15. Similar work by Hirche and colleagues [17] in 26 patients with colon cancer reported a 96% detection rate of

sentinel nodes, with clear demonstration of lymphatic basin in each case. ICG FL identified metastatic SLN involvement in 9 out of 11 patients (sensitivity 82%). Two cases had a negative SLN but positive non-SLN, corresponding to an 18% false-negative rate.

A recent meta-analysis of ICG FL in detection and analysis of sentinel nodes in colorectal cancer, encompassing 248 patients from 12 studies, reported a pooled SLNB sensitivity of 71% and specificity of 84.6% [19]. A high degree of heterogeneity was present with respect to administration dose and protocol as well as stage of cancer, prompting subgroup analysis. This demonstrated an association between stage of cancer and performance of ICG FL. In studies with a high percentage (>50%) of early stage cancers (I/II), median sensitivity, specificity, and accuracy were all 100%. Where early stage tumors did not comprise the majority, median sensitivity, specificity, and accuracy rates were 76%, 87.2%, and 68.8%, respectively. This finding of improved sensitivity in early stage tumors mirrors that seen in studies involving conventional methods of SLNB such as blue dye and radiolabeled tracers; [20, 21] it is thought that in larger tumors, transmural extension can destroy efferent lymphatic channels, while longitudinal advancement can involve additional lymphatic deltas, resulting in increased false-negative rates. It may also be the case that in large tumors, circumferential injection renders the central area unmapped. Though this finding questions the role for sentinel node biopsy in TIII/IV disease, it is encouraging that it should perform most accurately in patients most likely to be suitable for localized resection, and in whom the decision to offer adjuvant therapy is greatly influenced by nodal status.

Certain factors have been identified that influence detection of SLN using conventional blue dye or radioisotope methods, including body mass index (BMI), mesocolic adiposity, and lymphovascular invasion. [9, 10] ICG FL has been shown in early studies to at least match detection and accuracy parameters of conventional techniques while improving upon some of these limitations. A prospective study of 20 colon cancer patients undergoing colectomy compared ICG FL with blue dye (BD) [22]. Similar detection rates were noted for both groups (95%), and overall correlation between the two techniques was 80%. Overall sensitivity was higher for ICG than BD (57% vs. 43%), and in particular ICG showed higher sensitivity in patients with BMI >25 than BD. This is perhaps due to superior tissue contrast of ICG over BD enabling detection through increased mesocolic adiposity, and multiple ICG FL studies have demonstrated clear sentinel node and lymphatic basin mapping in patients with high BMI (>25) [9, 14]. Lymphovascular invasion has also been reported to interfere with conventional methods of SLN identification; promising results from ICG FL work have shown detection of SLN even in advanced tumors [9, 12].

Sentinel Nodes: Upstaging

Despite the recommendation for a minimum of 12 nodes collected for accurate staging, in daily clinical practice the nodal yield varies, with more than 50% of resection specimens containing fewer than 12 nodes [23]. This relates to clinically significant understaging in colorectal cancer. Identification of sentinel nodes could allow targeted, detailed analysis with techniques offering greater sensitivity than conventional methods, such as serial sectioning and additional immunohistochemistry or RT-PCR, which has been shown to lead to upstaging in colorectal cancer. A prospective study of 268 colorectal cancer patients using BD for SLN identification reported that of 141 patients classified as N0 by routine H&E staining who underwent step sections and immunohistochemistry of the SLN, 7 revealed micrometastases (with a further 23 revealing isolated tumor cells, which are of undetermined prognostic significance in colorectal cancer) [24]. A subsequent systematic review of sentinel lymph node mapping in colorectal cancer by van der Zaag et al. [21] found a 7.7% upstaging from stage I/II to III in a combined 928 patients from 10 studies based on a finding of micrometastases on RT-PCR or serial sectioning and staining of nodes histologically classified as N0. This is a clinically sig-

nificant group given that upstaging from stage I/II to III alters the decision to offer adjuvant therapy.

Overall, the utility of sentinel node biopsy in colorectal cancer remains unclear. While the ability to identify and analyze sentinel nodes in real time may guide lymphadenectomy extent, ongoing issues exist with high false-negative rates. However, the high sensitivity of ICG FL in sentinel node biopsy in early stage tumors is encouraging; with screening programs and advanced diagnostics, colorectal cancer is being diagnosed at an earlier stage, and moreover, these are the patients in whom accurate staging is crucial for decisions regarding adjuvant therapy. Importantly, ICG FL improves upon conventional SLN mapping techniques in patients with high BMI, which is increasingly becoming the predominant demographic in the West. Despite the uncertainty surrounding biopsy of sentinel nodes, there may be an emerging role for their detection to guide targeted, detailed immunohistochemistry of a defined group of nodes, potentially leading to upstaging with clinically significant implications on adjuvant therapy. Use of ICG FL for this purpose, with its improved performance over conventional techniques especially in the prevailing demographic of patient, is an exciting prospect.

Identifying Pelvic Sidewall Nodes in Rectal Cancer

ICG fluorescence lymphangiography has a potential application in mapping of pelvic sidewall (PSW) nodes in rectal cancer. It has been shown that up to 7% of patients undergoing TME will have involved pelvic sidewall nodes, and lateral lymph node metastasis is thought to be a major cause of locoregional recurrence in rectal cancer treated with preoperative chemoradiotherapy and curative resection [25]. Despite this, pelvic sidewall clearance involves high morbidity including sexual and urinary dysfunction, with the clinical benefits of offering this as standard unquantified. Should ongoing randomized trials prove distinct benefit of pelvic sidewall basin clearance on survival, lymphatic mapping may guide precise nodal clearance, reducing morbidity. Kazanowski and colleagues [26] demonstrated feasibility of pelvic sidewall node mapping. They injected five patients with low rectal tumors with submucosal ICG at the tumor site via proctoscopy at commencement of resection. In all five cases, pathology confirmed the presence of lymph node tissue; none had cancer cells evident on pathological processing.

There is also potential for sentinel node identification and analysis in pelvic side wall clearance, though as in colon cancer, the role of the sentinel node here remains unclear. The recent FILM study [27] demonstrated the superiority of ICG over BD injected at the tumor site in identifying pelvic sidewall nodes in cervical and uterine cancer; moreover, all metastatic sentinel nodes were detected by ICG FL. Though conducted in non-GI cancer, this high-quality evidence may have implications on accurate sentinel node identification in a range of oncological surgery. Noura and colleagues [28] injected ICG submucosally at the tumor site in 25 patients with low rectal cancer. Lateral sentinel nodes were detected in 23 patients (92%), and upon pelvic sidewall nodal resection and analysis, negative predictive value of the sentinel nodes identified by ICG was 100%. Sentinel lymph node identification and analysis could therefore have a potential application in stratifying patients into those requiring or not requiring pelvic sidewall clearance, minimizing morbidity in cases unlikely to show survival benefit. Of note, a report that 15% of patients with negative pelvic sidewall nodes on standard H&E staining have micrometastases in these nodes on RT-PCR [26] highlights the need to consider use of RT-PCR in further work on ICG in pelvic sidewall mapping.

One interesting proposal to localize PSW nodes with greater accuracy and minimize morbidity of resection, particularly in patients with increased BMI, is to conjugate fluorophores with a radioisotope such as Tc-99. Dual targeting of the nodes using a combination of methods can help mitigate the limitations of fluorescence alone—chiefly, lack of depth penetration, which is important in the fatty sidewall. The authors are currently setting up a feasibility study to investigate this practice.

Variations in Technique

Wide variation in the technique of ICG FL is evident between studies. Methods of injection, timing of ICG administration, and doses and concentrations of ICG are not standardized. Within the literature, ICG concentration ranges from 0.5 to 5 mg/mL and doses from 0.2 to 5 mL, administered in up to four injections at the peri-tumoral site. Method and anatomical layer of injection varies, from subserosally at laparoscopy via either rigid or flexible needle, to submucosally via proctoscope or colonoscopy, or both. Timing of injection ranges from 7 days prior to surgery to intraoperatively; where ICG is injected intraoperatively, optimal lymphatic basin visualization is reported from 5 to 40 minutes. A recent meta-analysis by Emile and colleagues [19] encompassing 248 patients found preoperative administration had the highest sensitivity while intraoperative injection had the highest specificity. With respect to injection site, they noted the highest sensitivity, specificity, and accuracy to be achieved following combined submucosal and subserosal ICG injection. The low sensitivity of subserosal injection alone was proposed to be largely due to lack of tactile feedback in the setting of injecting during laparoscopic surgery, preventing the tip of the needle reaching the submucosal plane where the lymphatic network is located. While the heterogenous nature of the literature renders drawing clear conclusions about the ideal protocol difficult, encouraging results from recent studies identifying and confirming feasible protocols are emerging. Chand and colleagues [12] recently conducted a feasibility study of ICG FL in colorectal cancer and compared doses and concentrations commonly used in the literature to date. They identified the optimal to be a 1 mL dose of 5 mg/10 mL concentration, which was injected submucosally at four peri-tumoral sites (Fig. 20.2). NIR mode was employed between 30 and 40 minutes following injection and demonstrated localization of the primary tumor alongside mapping of its lymphatic basin (Fig. 20.3). Further similar work comparing other variables including timing and site of injection will pave the way for much needed standardized protocols for ICG fluorescence lymphangiography, which is crucial in elucidating its applications in colorectal cancer (Video 20.1).

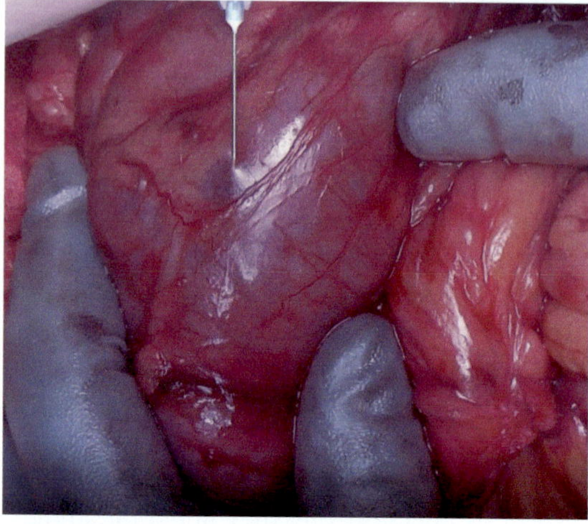

Fig. 20.2 Intraoperative submucosal injection of indocyanine green

Safety Profile

ICG has been used and studied for many years in other disciplines of medicine with applications such as determining cardiac output, hepatic function, and ophthalmic angiography. Its use in colorectal surgery is relatively new and has largely focused on fluorescence angiography to assess anastomotic perfusion. Its established safety profile from multiple studies in these areas has been mirrored in the newer field of fluorescence lymphangiography, and no studies to date have reported any adverse outcomes from ICG administration for this purpose.

Limitations

The current body of literature demonstrates technical feasibility of ICG in lymphatic mapping in colorectal cancer, and the potential implications of this in guiding resection, personalizing surgery, and improving staging are far reaching. However, limitations of the technique have been identified in early work, and further optimization

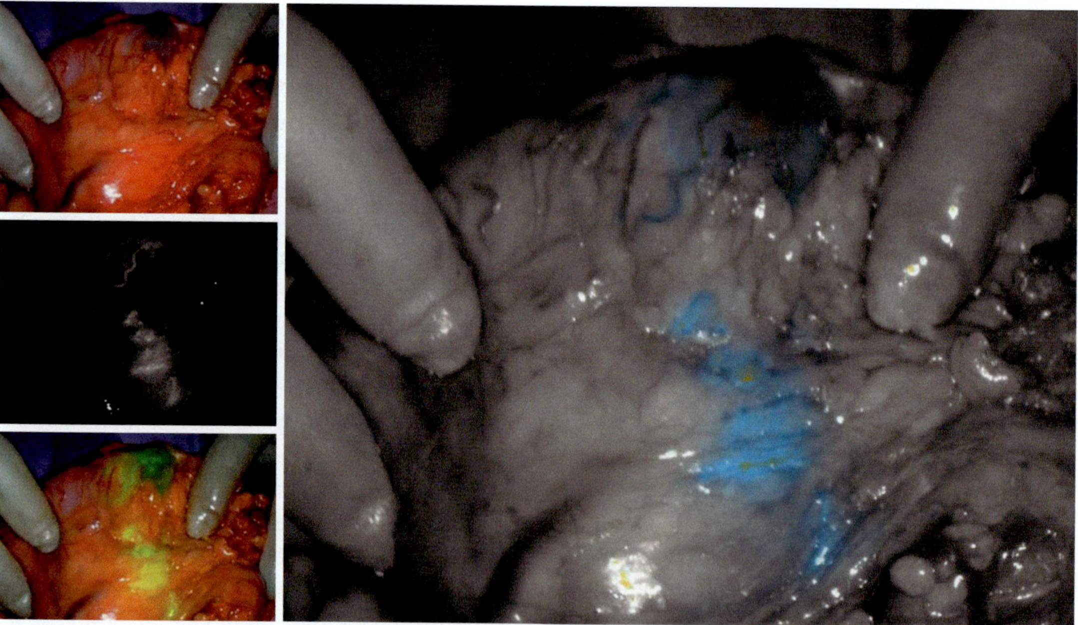

Fig. 20.3 Demonstration of the primary colonic tumor and its associated lymphatic channels using ICG fluorescence imaging under white light and near-infrared light

of ICG FL techniques are required. Furthermore, larger, less heterogenous studies will enable the true impact of this adjunctive procedure to be elucidated.

Technical Factors

Several technical factors have been identified which impact performance of ICG in lymphatic mapping. Chand et al. [12] proposed an effect from excess India ink (from endoscopic tattooing) and peri-tumoral inflammation from tattooing which limited complete visualization of the lymphatic basin in some patients. Given that ICG persists in tissue for at least 8 days following interstitial injection [29], some have proposed an additional role for ICG in endoscopic tumor tattooing instead of India ink. This may overcome the issues identified with India ink interference, while also allowing both tumor tattooing and fluorescence lymphangiography to take place in one rather than two sittings.

While tissue penetration of ICG is superior to blue dyes, it is limited to a few millimeters (approximately 15 mm), and this may limit its visualization in patients with very high BMI, as is becoming increasingly prevalent in the West, or in areas difficult to access such as deep in the pelvis. Some groups have proposed investigation of new, more fluorescent dyes, though ICG is one of very few fluorophores approved for use in clinical practice. An option to overcome this is dual modality lymphatic mapping with ICG and radioisotopes. This would integrate the advantages of both modalities, with quantitative detection and unlimited depth of detection of radioisotope tracers combined with the high spatial resolution and functional molecular imaging potential of targeted fluorophores [30]. Dual modality agents are currently being evaluated in other solid tumors such as renal cell carcinomas.

A further limitation is the tendency of ICG to "wash out" the circulation or not remain in lymph nodes long enough to be detected. The addition of colloid leads to preferential binding to intracellular components of the nodes, allowing for a longer time period for detection. Conjugated agents such as Nanocol have been described in various cancers in the body [31]. Making more stable and longer-lasting compounds will no doubt help improve accuracy in identifying lymphatics and nodes.

Cancer-Specific Factors

Cancer-specific factors have also been found to impact the performance of ICG FL and may limit its applicability to colorectal cancer as a whole, highlighting the need for further work to identify those patients in whom ICG FL carries most benefit. One such factor is the stage of tumor, which influences the performance of sentinel node biopsy. Irrespective of conventional technique or ICG, a high false-negative rate has been reported in SLNB in colorectal cancer, precluding its standardized use to guide the extent of resection and lymphadenectomy akin to that employed in breast cancer and melanoma. However, subgroup analysis in studies using ICG FL has demonstrated high sensitivity in early stage cancers, and therefore this may represent a limitation of the technique only in patients with stage III/IV disease. Importantly, high tumor stage and associated lymphovascular invasion has been found not to affect SLN detection rates with ICG, and thus the role of ICG FL in identification of SLN for detailed immunohistochemical testing and accurate staging may be more universally applicable.

A second consideration is the impact of neoadjuvant treatment in ICG FL. This is yet to be fully explored, and the majority of patients in studies to date have not received neoadjuvant therapy. Discrepancies in performance of ICG FL in rectal cancer have been postulated to be a result of a pathological response in the tumor and metastatic lymph nodes elicited by neoadjuvant therapy. Two trials have investigated the role of ICG fluorescence for lymph node mapping in rectal cancer with discordant results. Handgraaf and colleagues [32] studied five patients with low rectal cancer, 90% of whom received neoadjuvant chemo- or radiotherapy. Of 83 nodes resected (21 fluorescent), 1 contained a micrometastasis; this was not fluorescent with ICG, yielding a sensitivity of 0%.

In contrast, Noura et al. [28] included 25 patients with low rectal cancer, none of whom underwent neoadjuvant therapy. They reported no false-negatives, yielding a sensitivity of 100%. Neoadjuvant therapy may therefore limit the use of ICG FL in colorectal cancer, and future work should include subgroup analysis of patients with and without neoadjuvant therapy to quantify any effect of this.

Heterogeneity of Current Literature

The current body of work displays high levels of heterogeneity with respect to technique and patient demographics, and the corresponding heterogeneity in sensitivity, specificity, and accuracy render generalization of results and clinical recommendation difficult. Future work will need to address this heterogeneity, and several areas are clear targets. Firstly, identification of a standardized protocol for ICG injection in terms of dose, concentration, timing, and mode of injection is crucial and will enable direct comparison of performance of ICG FL. Secondly, it is becoming clear that ICG FL may have different roles in early versus late stage colorectal cancer, as well as in colon versus rectal cancer, and in patients with or without neoadjuvant therapy. Recognition of this and inclusion of relevant patients in studies to reflect the diverse demographic and pathology of colorectal cancer patients, and subsequent subgroup analysis, is key in delineating and personalizing the role of ICG FL and maximizing its clinical application.

Future Research

Identifying Pathological Nodes

Though fluorescence lymphangiography in colorectal cancer is in its infancy and clearly larger trials are required, the favorable safety profile of ICG and early promising results herald exciting prospects for future applications of the technique. Fluorescence lymphangiography has predominantly been used to identify lymphatic drainage of a tumor, allowing targeted analysis of

sentinel nodes and inclusion of entire lymphatic basins in resections. An exciting prospect is the ability to not only delineate lymphatics but to discriminate normal nodes from those harboring micrometastases, allowing surgeons to tailor resections to each patient's specific lymphatic involvement pattern and minimize morbidity associated with extensive lymphadenectomy in those without nodal involvement. Liberale and colleagues [33] have reported the ability to identify pathological nodes from colorectal cancer based on the degree of fluorescence following ICG injection in two patients. Following injection of intravenous ICG, four fluorescing lymph nodes were identified whose signal-to-background ratio (SBR) was around two. No other areas of fluorescence were seen, and macroscopically normal lymph nodes within the specimen demonstrated the same fluorescence as surrounding fatty tissue (SBR = 1). Of the total nodes harvested (n = 27), histopathological examination revealed the four fluorescent nodes to be malignant; all non-fluorescent lymph nodes (n = 23) were tumor-free. In one patient the pathologic nodes correlated to preoperative imaging; the second patient had no nodes detected preoperatively, with the metastatic node being detected as the only area of fluorescence on systematic exploration of the abdominal cavity. The increased fluorescence of involved nodes has been proposed to be due to the "enhanced permeability and retention (EPR) effect," describing the tendency of abnormal tumor vasculature to be permeable to macromolecules [34].

Cancer-Specific Fluorophores

Another possible future application of ICG FL is the development of cancer-specific fluorophores. Fluorophores such as ICG can be conjugated to ligands to target specific cell types expressing receptors for these; when viewed with NIR equipment, these conjugates enable identification of the primary tumor alongside metastases. In colorectal cancer, anti-carcinoembryonic antigen (CEA) antibody conjugated to a fluorophore (DyLight 650 nm; a cynanine fluorophore similar to ICG) has been shown in a mouse model to accurately detect and delineate colorectal cancer liver metastases, and subsequent resection of these under NIR navigation resulted in smaller residual tumor area and longer overall and disease-free survival compared to those mice operated on under bright light [35]. Boogerd and colleagues recently conducted a pilot study using a fluorescent anti-CEA monoclonal antibody (SGM-101) and demonstrated safety and feasibility in detecting both primary and recurrent colorectal cancer lesions [36]. Other similar monoclonal antibodies are also being investigated for this purpose, such as Bevacizumab-800CW which is a monoclonal antibody to VEGF (VEGF-A has been shown to be expressed in 79–96% colorectal cancer lesions) [29]. This work is still in the preclinical phase, and with respect to fluorescence lymphangiography would rely on proof of concordant expression of a receptor between the primary colorectal tumor and its lymph node metastases. The development of cancer-specific fluorophores is an exciting prospect for intraoperative real-time identification of lymph node metastases in colorectal cancer.

Conclusion

Lymph node status is intimately related to staging and prognosis of colorectal cancer, and lymph node harvest plays a crucial role in preventing locoregional recurrence and prolonging disease-free survival. The advent of fluorescence-guided surgery and development of NIR viewing technologies has already shown great promise in fluorescence angiography with potential to reduce anastomotic leak and stoma formation rates. A new application of fluorescence-guided surgery is lymphangiography; to date its safety and feasibility in identifying tumor lymphatic basins and sentinel nodes have identified benefits such as guiding resection margins, detection of positive aberrant lymph nodes, and upstaging of patients. Future work, which should include standardized protocols for ICG injection, will aim to further validate this technique in subgroups of patients

and design targeted cancer-specific fluorophores. ICG fluorescence lymphangiography is an exciting addition to the fluorescence surgery toolkit, with the potential to minimize morbidity and optimize survival with personalized colorectal resection surgery for every patient.

References

1. Chen SL, Bilchik AJ. More extensive nodal dissection improves survival for stages I to III of colon cancer: a population-based study. Ann Surg. 2006;244:602–210.
2. NCNN Clinical Practice Guidelines in Oncology (NCNN Guidelines). Colon Cancer, version 1.2019. https://www.nccn.org/professionals/physician_gls/pdf/colon.pdf. Accessed Mar 2019.
3. NQF #0225: At least 12 regional lymph nodes are removed and pathologically examined for resected colon cancer. Commission on Cancer, American College of Surgeons. https://www.facs.org/~/media/files/quality%20programs/cancer/ncdb/measure%20specs%20colon.ashx. Accessed Mar 2019.
4. Bertelsen CA, et al. Disease-free survival after complete mesocolic excision compared with conventional colon cancer surgery: a retrospective, population-based study. Lancet Oncol. 2015;16:161–8.
5. Hohenberger W, Weber K, Matzel K, Papadopoulos T, Merkel S. Standardized surgery for colonic cancer: complete mesocolic excision and central ligation – technical notes and outcome. Color Dis. 2009; 11:354–64.
6. Bertelsen CA, et al. Short-term outcomes after complete mesocolic excision compared with 'conventional' colonic cancer surgery. Br J Surg. 2016;103:581–9.
7. Heald RJ. The 'Holy Plane' of rectal surgery. J R Soc Med. 1988;81:503–8.
8. Quirke P, et al. Effect of the plane of surgery achieved on local recurrence in patients with operable rectal cancer: a prospective study using data from the MRC CR07 and NCIC-CTG CO16 randomised clinical trial. Lancet Oncol. 2009;373:821–8.
9. Cahill RA, et al. Near-infrared (NIR) laparoscopy for intraoperative lymphatic road-mapping and sentinel node identification during definitive surgical resection of early-stage colorectal neoplasia. Surg Endosc. 2012;26:197–204.
10. Ankersmit M, van der Pas MHGM, van Dam DA, Meijerink WJHJ. Near infrared fluorescence lymphatic laparoscopy of the colon and mesocolon. Color Dis. 2011;13(Suppl 7):70–3.
11. Nishigori N, et al. Visualization of lymph/blood flow in laparoscopic colorectal cancer surgery by ICG fluorescence imaging (Lap-IGFI). Ann Surg Oncol. 2016;23(Suppl 2):266–74.

12. Chand M, et al. Feasibility of fluorescence lymph node imaging in colon cancer: FLICC. Tech Coloproctol. 2018;22:271–7.

13. Noguera J, Castro L, Garcia L, Mosquera C, Gomez A. Lymphadenectomy guided by indocyanine-green (ICG) in colorectal cancer: a pilot study. J Surg Tech Proc. 2019;3:1023.

14. Watanabe J, et al. Evaluation of lymph flow patterns in splenic flexural colon cancers using laparoscopic real-time indocyanine green fluorescence imaging. Int J Color Dis. 2017;32:201–7.

15. Keller DS, et al. Using fluorescence lymphangiography to define the ileocolic mesentery: proof of concept for the watershed area using real-time imaging. Tech Coloproctol. 2017;21:757–60.

16. Koyanagi K, et al. Prognostic relevance of occult nodal micrometastases and circulating tumour cells in colorectal cancer in a prospective multicenter trial. Clin Cancer Res. 2008;14:7391–6.

17. Hirche C, et al. Ultrastaging of colon cancer by sentinel node biopsy using fluorescence navigation with indocyanine green. Int J Color Dis. 2012;27:319–24.

18. Kusano M, et al. Sentinel node mapping guided by indocyanine green fluorescence imaging: a new method for sentinel node navigation surgery in gastrointestinal cancer. Dig Surg. 2008;25:103–8.

19. Emile SH, et al. Sensitivity and specificity of indocyanine green near-infrared fluorescence imaging in detection of metastatic lymph nodes in colorectal cancer: systematic review and meta-analysis. J Surg Oncol. 2017;116:730–40.

20. Cahill RA, et al. Sentinel node biopsy for the individualization of surgical strategy for cure of early-stage colon cancer. Ann Surg Oncol. 2009;16:2170–80.

21. Van der Zaag ES, et al. Systemiatic review of sentinel lymph node mapping procedure in colorectal cancer. Ann Surg Oncol. 2012;19:3449–59.

22. Liberale G, et al. Ex vivo detection of tumoral lymph nodes of colorectal origin with fluorescence imaging after intraoperative intravenous injection of indocyanine green. J Surg Oncol. 2016;114:348–53.

23. Mitchell PJ, et al. Multicentre review of lymph node harvest in colorectal cancer: are we understanging colorectal cancer patients? Int J Color Dis. 2009;24:915–21.

24. Bembenek AE, et al. Sentinel lymph node biopsy in colon cancer: a prospective multicenter trial. Ann Surg. 2007;245:858–63.

25. Kim TH, et al. Lateral lymph node metastasis is a major cause of locoregional recurrence in rectal cancer treated with preoperative chemoradiotherapy and curative resection. Ann Surg Oncol. 2008;15:729–37.

26. Kazanowski M, Al Furajii H, Cahill RA. Near-infrared laparoscopic fluorescence for pelvic side wall delta mapping in patients with rectal cancer- 'PINPOINT' nodal assessment. Color Dis. 2015;17:32–5.

27. Frumovitz M, et al. Near-infrared fluorescence for detection of sentinel lymph nodes in women with cervical and uterine cancers (FILM): a randomised, phase 3, multicentre, non-inferiority trial. Lancet Oncol. 2018;19:1394–403.

28. Noura S, et al. Feasibility of a lateral region sentinel node biopsy of lower rectal cancer guided by indocyanine green using a near-infrared camera system. Ann Surg Oncol. 2010;17:144–51.

29. Cahill RA, Ris F, Mortensen NJ. Near-infrared laparoscopy for real-time intra-operative arterial and lymphatic perfusion imagin. Color Dis. 2011;13:12–7.

30. Zhang RR, et al. Beyond the margins: real-time detection of cancer using targeted fluorophores. Nat Rev Clin Oncol. 2017;14:347–64.

31. Chand M, Keller DS, Devoto L, McGurk M. Furthering precision in sentinel node navigational surgery for oral cancer: a novel triple targeting system. J Fluoresc. 2018;28:483–6.

32. Handgraaf HJ, et al. Intraoperative fluorescence imaging to localize tumors and sentinel lymph nodes in rectal cancer. Minim Invasive Ther Allied Technol. 2016;25:48–53.

33. Liberale G, et al. Fluorescence imaging after intraoperative intravenous injection of indocyanine green for detection of lymph node metastases in colorectal cancer. Eur J Surg Oncol. 2015;41:1256–60.

34. Maeda H, et al. Tumour vascular permeability and the EPR effect in macromolecular therapeutics. J Control Release. 2000;65:271–84.

35. Hiroshima Y, et al. Effective luorescence-guided surgery of liver metastasis using a fluorescent anti-CEA antibody. J Surg Oncol. 2016;114:951–8.

36. Boogerd LSF, et al. Safety and effectiveness of SGM-101, a fluorescent antibody targeting carcinoembryonic antigen, for intraoperative detection of colorectal cancer: a dose-escalation pilot study. Lancet Gastroenterol Hepatol. 2018;3:181–91.

The Role of Near-Infrared Fluorescence Imaging in the Assessment of Peritoneal Carcinomatosis from Colorectal Cancer

Gennaro Galizia, Andrea Mabilia,
Francesca Cardella, Annamaria Auricchio,
Nicoletta Basile, Silvia Erario, Giovanni Del Sorbo,
Paolo Castellano, and Eva Lieto

Introduction

Peritoneal carcinomatosis (PC) is a severe onco-logical condition originating from the mesothe-lium (primary PC) or, more frequently, from gastrointestinal or gynecological tumors (secondary PC). Every year, peritoneal carcinomatosis affects about 25,000 people in Italy [1].

This condition is interpreted as a terminal stage of disease and, if not treated, allows a median survival of ≤ 6 months after diagnosis [2, 3]. Indeed, peritoneal involvement is considered

Electronic Supplementary Material The online version of this chapter (https://doi.org/10.1007/978-3-030-38092-2_21) contains supplementary material, which is available to authorized users.

G. Galizia (✉)
Department of Translational Medical Sciences,
Division of Surgical Oncology of the Gastrointestinal Tract, University of Campania 'Luigi Vanvitelli' –
School of Medicine, Naples, Italy
e-mail: gennaro.galizia@unicampania.it

A. Mabilia · F. Cardella · A. Auricchio · N. Basile
S. Erario · G. Del Sorbo · P. Castellano · E. Lieto
Division of Surgical Oncology of the Gastrointestinal Tract, University of Campania "Luigi Vanvitelli",
Naples, Italy

the most serious event in tumor progression [4]. Since it is difficult to treat it, peritoneal diffusion is often the main cause of morbidity and mortality due to tumors affecting the peritoneal serosa. Even in patients resected for intra-abdominal carcinoma, PC is the most frequent cause of death [5–7]. Interestingly, PC often develops as a "local" disease in the absence of hematogenous or distant metastases [8]. Particularly, peritoneal metastases occur in 30–40% of patients with colorectal carcinoma (CRC), and they are the only metastases in 25% of patients [9, 10].

In abdominal neoplasms, peritoneal dissemination may be present at the time of diagnosis, but, more often, it occurs as a life-threatening condition after surgical treatment of the primary tumor [5].

In gastric cancer, 10–20% of patients who are candidates for potentially curative resection and 40% of those in advanced stages have peritoneal involvement at the time of abdominal exploration [11]. Furthermore, 20–50% of patients undergoing potentially curative surgery will show a peritoneal recurrence in the future [12]. In the case of advanced gastric cancer, the intracavitary spread of neoplastic cells is responsible up to 54% of deaths due to recurrence after surgery [13]. The greatest risks of peritoneal recurrence have been

E. M. Aleassa, K. M. El-Hayek (eds.), *Video Atlas of Intraoperative Applications of Near Infrared
Fluorescence Imaging*, https://doi.org/10.1007/978-3-030-38092-2_21

demonstrated in patients with diffuse or mixed histologic carcinoma (69% at 5 years) and, even more so, those with positive peritoneal cytology at the time of the resective intervention (80% at 5 years) [14, 15]. In addition, the peritoneal cavity is the only place of diffusion in the 40–60% of the recurrences of gastric cancer [16].

The PC originating from colorectal cancer is frequently a metachronous disease, and only 10–15% of colorectal cancer patients show PC at the time of primary diagnosis; however, as observed in gastric cancer, peritoneum is involved up to 50% of cases in colorectal cancer patients who develop tumor recurrence after potentially curative surgery of the primary tumor [17], and, in 10–35% of the cases is the only site of tumor relapse [18]. The mucinous carcinomas of the colon and the carcinoma of the appendix, especially if there is a positive peritoneal cytology, show the highest rates of peritoneal dissemination [12].

Pathogenic Mechanisms

The pathogenic mechanisms that regulate carcinomatosis are multifactorial, but essentially consist of:

1. Peritoneal dissemination of free tumor cells, which exfoliate as a result of the direct invasion of the serosa of the organ involved by primary neoplasm [19] and subsequent implantation on the peritoneal surface through molecules of cell adhesion [5, 8]
2. Passage of malignant cells through the lymphatic lacunae and venous vessels of the peritoneum [19]
3. Insemination after trauma and surgical manipulation [19]

In particular, in low-grade malignant tumors it is assumed that the PC originates from a transparietal spread, and that the dissemination follows a migration path called "neoplastic redistribution." This migration is governed by a "non-random" redistribution process that is not dependent from the intrinsic biological aggressiveness of the tumor but primarily is related to physical mechanisms, such as the effect of gravity in relation to the site of the primary tumor, and the presence or less of intra-abdominal fluid (ascites, mucus, etc.) [5, 8, 20], as well as the characteristic viscosity of the same. Tumor cells, which move freely within the peritoneal cavity, generally aggregate into well-defined areas due to gravity concentrating in the normal reabsorption sites of the peritoneal fluids, such as the lymphatic lacunae of the small and large omentum and the diaphragm, in particular of the right hemidiaphragm. This generally involves the development of disease, especially in the pelvis, in the subphrenic space, in the parietocolic groove and in Morrison's pouch [5, 8], or in anfractuous regions where the peritoneal fluid circulates at low flow. When the tumor does not produce fluids, the malignant cells have more limited motility and implant more frequently near the site of the primary tumor. While a liquid vehicle is present within the abdominal cavity, sites more distant than the primary tumor may also be affected, such as the Treitz ligament and the small omentum in the case of ovarian carcinoma. Likewise, as a result of physical mechanisms, the PC does not occur, at least in the initial stages, on the mesenteric surface and on the serosa of the small intestine due to the active peristaltic movements. In contrast, relatively fixed intestinal areas, such as the duodenum and the ileocecal and rectum-sigmoid conjunctions, are often infiltrated by carcinomatosis.

Treatment

Just as the metastatic involvement of the liver by CRC is currently considered susceptible of hepatic resection for curative purposes, the treatment of PC could be considered as potentially curative considering that, in selected cases and within certain limits, the involvement of the peritoneal serosa may represent the extreme margin of diffusion of the neoplasm.

In the last 20 years, the growing and renewed interest in the malignant tumors of the peritoneum, and the increase of the knowledge on the biology of these neoplasms, has led to the search for new and increasingly aggressive therapeutic techniques. There is sufficient consent that the only potentially curative treatment in primary and metastatic peritoneal carcinomatosis is cytoreductive surgery (CS) associated with hyperthermic intraperitoneal chemotherapy (HIPEC) with a 5-year survival rate ranging from 30% to 48% in selected cases [21, 22].

The HIPEC was introduced in 1980 for the treatment of the PC and was initially used alone [23]. Since 1995 some procedures of peritonectomy were associated [24] in several world centers which have reported their experiences using different HIPEC protocols showing encouraging results [2]. This innovative and aggressive treatment modality, directed to the entire abdominal-pelvic area, is able, despite the high rate of morbidity, to significantly reduce and sometimes completely eliminate carcinomatosis, improving long-term survival [24, 25]. The logic that underlies the HIPEC is essentially based on both the direct cytotoxicity of hyperthermia on neoplastic cells, increased rate of the cytotoxicity of some chemotherapeutic agents determined by hyperthermia itself, and, finally, pharmacokinetic advantage obtained by the administration of intraperitoneal chemotherapy [5, 6].

The plasma-peritoneum-barrier (i.e., a physiologic barrier that limits the resorption of drugs from the peritoneal cavity into the blood) guarantees, at the regional site, high concentrations of some cytostatic drugs (including cisplatin, mitomycin c, oxaliplatin, adriblastine) limiting systemic toxicity. Multimodal treatment combining HIPEC and cytoreductive surgery (CRS) with peritonectomy [24] finds space in the treatment of primary peritoneal malignant tumors (abdominal sarcomatosis, peritoneal mesothelioma) [26], pseudomyxoma peritonei, and CR peritoneal carcinomatosis from colorectal [27, 28], ovarian [29], and gastric carcinoma [13]. On the contrary, HIPEC is contraindicated in the case of peritoneal carcinomatosis from neoplasia showing high biological aggressiveness (pancreatic adenocarcinoma and neoplasia of the esophagus), extra-abdominal metastasis, extensive retroperitoneal or lymph node disease, coexistence of important pathologies (cardiorespiratory, neurological, and renal), multiple and diffuse or otherwise unresectable hepatic metastases, previous side effects, and poor response after systemic chemotherapy.

Prognostic Factors

To define the extent of cytoreduction, Jaquet and Sugarbaker [30] introduced the so-called completeness of cytoreduction (CCR) score which provides an assessment of the amount of residual disease after cytoreductive surgery. CCR-0 indicates that no macroscopic disease remains after cytoreduction. CCR-1 indicates that tumor nodules with a diameter of less than 2.5 mm remain after surgery. Finally, CCR-2 and CCR-3 indicate that tumor nodules between 2.5 mm and 2.5 cm, and tumor nodules with a diameter greater than 2.5 cm remain after surgical treatment, respectively.

Since PC should be considered as a regional metastasis and being impossible to remove all microscopic residues, the concept of radicality is relative, so that not only the complete cytoreduction, CCR-0, but also CCR-1 (residual tumor ≤2.5 mm) is deemed acceptable [31]. To assess the extension of the resection in the PC treatment, the CCR score appears to be the most reliable system compared to the R (resection) stage that is traditionally used for primary neoplasms in the tumor node metastasis staging system [4]. In PC, it is generally believed that it is not possible to obtain an R0 state, and therefore CCR-0 is equivalent to R1 (no gross residual disease). R2a indicates that minimal tumor nodules of less than 5 mm remain. R2b indicates that coarse tumor nodules exceeding 5 mm and up to 2 cm remain. R2c indicates that it remains an extended disease of over 2 cm [28].

The diagnosis of peritoneal carcinomatosis is challenging, both pre- and intraoperatively. The gold standard for PC staging is still the direct laparotomic or laparoscopic visualization. Computed tomography (CT) and positron emission tomography (PET) provide the best results before surgery, but underestimation of the disease phase is frequently reported [32]. During laparotomy, surgeons depend on visual inspection and palpation to determine PC extension and extent of resection. However, some subclinical peritoneal lesions may escape intraoperative detection. The peritoneal cancer index (PCI) is of fundamental importance in treatment planning and is closely correlated with the prognosis after CS + HIPEC [5]. The Peritoneal Cancer Index (PCI) is the most accepted metric to quantify the extent of peritoneal disease and is evaluated with the utmost accuracy at the time of surgery, as it has been shown that sensitivity in the detection of peritoneal disease by computerized tomographic scan (CT) turns out to be 41.1% and the specificity 89%. PCI is calculated by evaluating the size of peritoneal lesions in each of the 13 abdomino-pelvic regions. The lesion size (LS) is evaluated with a score of 0–3 for each of the 13 regions and summed to obtain a score from 0 to 39. In patients with PC from CRC, a PCI of 10–20 means extensive carcinomatosis and therefore a worse prognosis. It is believed that only palliative cure should be offered to such patients [17, 33–35].

Intraoperative Fluoroscopy and Indocyanine Green

As outlined above, one of the most critical trouble in PC treatment is represented by both correct diagnosis of peritoneal nodules and identification of smaller lesions. In recent years, new technologies have allowed surgeons to better address such limitations [36, 37]. Intraoperative fluoroscopy (FI) is a recently introduced imaging modality that can improve PC detection [38]. Indocyanine green (ICG), a near-infrared (NIR) contrast agent becoming fluorescent if excited by light with a wavelength of 800–900 nm, has been recently proposed for FI due to its special affinity for the cancerous tissue [39, 40]. Approximately 95% of the ICG molecules bind rapidly to intravascular macromolecules, such as albumin and lipoproteins, after intravenous injection. Since in tumor tissue neoangiogenesis is responsible for the presence of immature and permeable vessels, the ICG, like these macromolecules, permeates the endothelial lesions and is retained in the cancerous tissue due to the altered lymphatic drainage

(permeability and advanced retention [EPR]) of the lesion [41, 42]. The extravascular ICG accumulation is responsible for the hyperfluorescence observed in the tumor tissue in contrast to the surrounding normal tissue [41, 42].

The detection of tumor tissue depends on the tumor-background relationship (TBR), which is the ratio between the intensity of the fluorescence, expressed in arbitrary units, of the tumor tissue and of the surrounding normal tissue [43]. The ICG has a half-life of 150–180 s, is metabolized by the liver microsomes, and excreted through the bile. Overall, its toxicity can be classified as low. Occasionally, in 1 out of 42,000 cases, mild side effects have been reported in humans such as sore throats and hot flashes. Effects such as anaphylactic shock, hypotension, tachycardia, dyspnea, and urticaria have occurred only in individual cases [44]. The mortality rate is 1:300,000.

Currently ICG is a non-specific fluorescent probe registered and approved by the FDA for optical imaging in clinical settings [45]. ICG is recognized as a safe and economical NIR fluorescent probe. The properties of the ICG, which is a water-soluble amphiphilic molecule with a molecular weight of 775 Dalton and a hydrodynamic diameter of 1.2 nm, make it an excellent vascular and lymphatic contrast agent when injected intravenously (IV) and in the system lymphatic (e.g., by subcutaneous injection), respectively. The intravascular compartmentalization of the ICG before its rapid clearance explains its angiographic properties. Therefore, ICG is used in ophthalmology for retinoscopy and in plastic surgery to evaluate the vascularization of the reconstruction flap [46–48]. Furthermore, as it is excreted exclusively from the liver into the bile, it can also be used to evaluate liver function in cirrhotic patients before undergoing liver surgery [49, 50], or during cholecystectomy as a cholangiographic agent [51–53]. Moreover, in colorectal surgery for oncological and non-oncological indications, ICG-FI is expected to become a useful application for the evaluation of the vascularization of colorectal anastomoses [54–57]. After subcutaneous injection, free ICG is a small molecule that can rapidly enter the small lymphatic vessels and serves as a good marker of the lymphatic system. Recently, ICG-FI has emerged as a potential tool in surgical oncology for detection of sentinel lymph nodes (SLN) in various cancers such as breast [58], skin [59], gastric [60], and colorectal cancers [61–67]. Furthermore, FI after IV injection of ICG has been described as a novel imaging technique to assist surgeons in the intraoperative detection of hepatocellular carcinoma (HCC) [68, 69], cholangiocarcinoma [70], hepatoblastoma [71], and hepatic metastases [72]. Several reviews have reported the role of optical imaging using ICG [38, 73–78], but none of these has specifically focused on the role of ICG-FI for the detection of carcinomatosis in colorectal cancer. ICG-FI represents a wide potential field for the clinical application of this emerging imaging technique.

FI-guided surgery with ICG (ICG-FI), both in vivo (ICG-IF intraoperative) and ex vivo (on the ICG-FI table), seems to be particularly suitable for detecting PC in which superficial lesions are present. However, data on ICG-guided surgery in PC CRC treatment are still poor and the technique has not yet been standardized for this use.

Our Experience

At the Division of Surgical Oncology of the University of Naples "Luigi Vanvitelli," a prospective study was conducted to evaluate the role of ICG-FI in the improvement of outcome in patients affected by peritoneal carcinomatosis from CRC and undergoing CS + HIPEC (Video 21.1). Inclusion criteria for CS + HIPEC were age of 18–70 years, PCI $\leq$20 at preoperative diagnosis, tumor limited to the peritoneal cavity without other distant metastases, and absence of serious comorbidity with the performance status $\leq$1. Overall, seven patients with PC from CRC were admitted. Three patients were excluded from surgical treatment due to high PCI (29 and 31, respectively), or poor general conditions (one patient). Ultimately, four patients underwent surgical exploration. All patients had previously been successfully submitted to a potentially curative resection for stage III colorectal adenocarcinoma. All patients underwent adjuvant chemotherapy with 5-fluorouracil plus oxaliplatin, and they were followed at 3-month intervals until tumor recurrence [79].

All operations were performed through open median relaparotomy. After clinical exploration of the entire peritoneal cavity and evaluation of the feasibility of CC-0 or CC-1 cytoreduction and localization of metastatic nodules, a dose of 0.25 mg/kg ICG (PULSION Medical Systems SE, FeldKirchen, Germany) was injected intravenously. FI-guided imaging was performed in vivo on the entire peritoneal cavity using Fluobeam® (Fluoptics Imaging Inc., Cambridge, MA, USA), an open system for in vivo infrared fluorescence imaging. At Fluobeam® examination, the peritoneum appears as a large gray area striped with very thin bright lines corresponding to vascular structures. With black and white vision, a hyperfluorescent peritoneal nodule appeared as a well-defined area of intense bright light with clear margins (Fig. 21.1a). This area, with the color vision allowed by Fluobeam®, appeared as a red area with ultraviolet margins (Fig. 21.1b). Visible and/or palpable nodules showing no clear dissimilarity from the gray peritoneal serosa (with black and white vision) or colors ranging from green to ultraviolet were defined as hypofluorescent nodules. All peritoneal sites were checked again at the end of surgical resection to evaluate residual fluorescence. Finally, all specimens were observed ex vivo with Fluobeam® to confirm their previous appearance and investigate the margins of resected tissue.

HIPEC was performed through a closed technique by using oxaliplatin (400 mg/m^2) in 5 L of 5% glucose solution for 30 min at 42 °C.

Patient characteristics are reported in Table 21.1. A cytoreductive surgery classified as CCR-0 followed by HIPEC was performed in all patients. No patient had serious postoperative complications and all were discharged on postoperative days 9–11. Peritoneal exploration was performed at a median time of 50 min after ICG injection (range 30–60; IQR 35–60 min). The ICG-FI required on average 20 min (range 10–30, IQR 15–25 min), and all images collected by

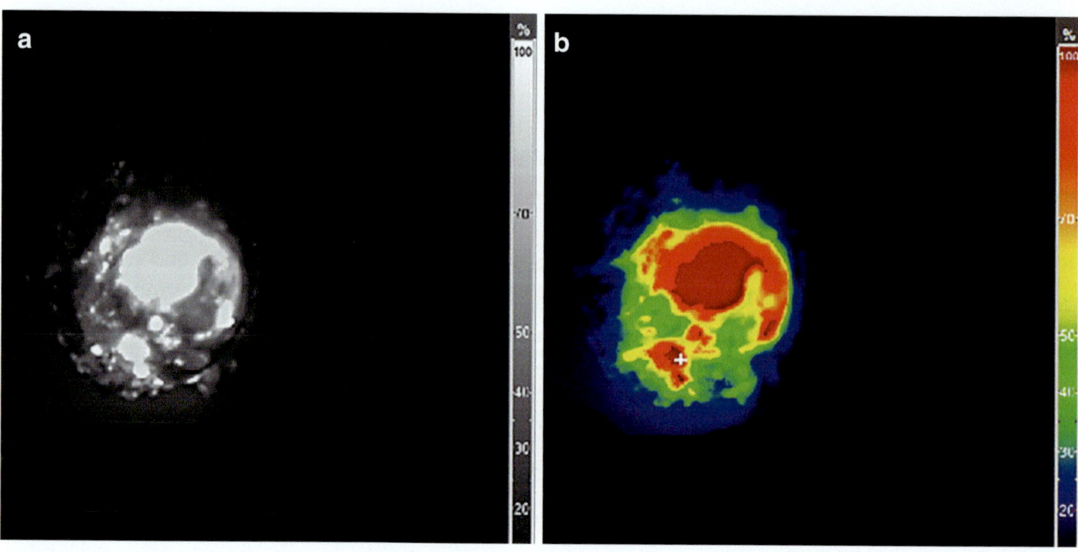

Fig. 21.1 (**a**) Patient #3. ICG-FI guided surgery (black and white vision). Hyperfluorescent nodule visible as an intense bright light surrounded by a gray area. (**b**) Same case (color vision). The nodule appeared as a red area with ultraviolet margins. (From Lieto et al. [79]; used with permission)

Table 21.1 Clinicopathological characteristics

	Patient #1	Patient #2	Patient #3	Patient #4
Age (years)	62	67	64	59
Gender	Female	Male	Male	Female
Primary tumor				
Site	Right colon	Rectum	Left colon	Right colon
TNM stage	pT3N2aM0	pT4aN0M0	pT4aN1bM0	pT4aN1bM0
Grade	well differentiated/G1	undifferentiated/G3	moderately differentiated/G2	moderately differentiated/G2
Time to relapse (months)	13	26[a]	15	15
Number of nodules	25	2	24	18
Preoperative diagnosis	12 (48%)	1 (50%)	10 (42%)	7 (39%)
Intraoperative diagnosis[b] – ICG-FI	6 (24%) 7 (28%)	// 1 (50%)	8 (33%) 6 (25%)	8 (44%) 3 (17%)
Peritoneal Cancer Index				
Before ICG-FI	12	2	9	6
After ICG-FI	15	3	12	8

ICG-FI indocyanine green fluorescence imaging
From Lieto et al. [79]; used with permission
[a]13 months after CS + HIPEC for previous peritoneal carcinomatosis
[b]Visual and palpatory diagnosis

Fluobeam® were converted into pictures and videos. The operation time ranged from 240 to 360 min (median 280 min, IQR 250–330 min).

A total of 69 nodules were collected (median diameter 2.7 cm, range 0.2–5.0 cm, IQR 1.2–3.8 cm). With conventional techniques, such as CT and PET scans, 30 nodules had been preoperatively discovered (median diameter 3.8 cm, range 1.5–5.0 cm, IQR 3.5–4.4 cm). At intraoperative exploration further 22 peritoneal nodules (median diameter 2.3 cm, interval 1.3–3.1 cm, IQR 1.8–2.8 cm) were identified by the surgical team. Out of these 52 nodules, 47 (90%) were hyperfluorescent on examination with Fluobeam®. Finally, ICG-FI identified 17 additional hyperfluorescent nodules with a median diameter of 0.5 mm (range 0.2–0.7 cm, IQR 0.3–0.6 cm) (Fig. 21.2). All samples were also examined with Fluobeam® ex vivo, namely on the table in the operating room. There was a complete correspondence between in vivo and

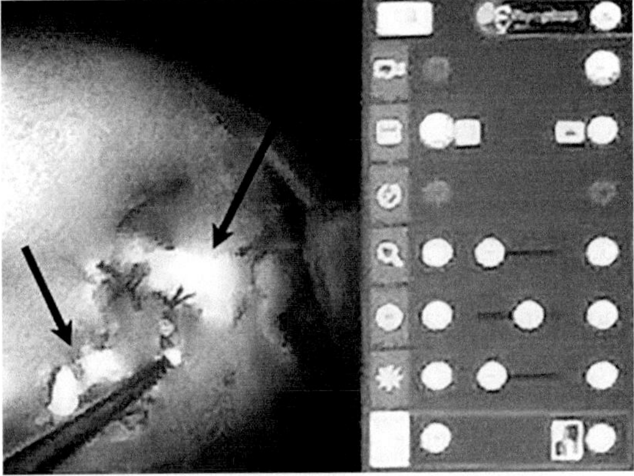

Fig. 21.2 Patient #1. Diffuse pelvic peritoneal carcinomatosis (hyperfluorescent areas–black arrows) clearly visible. In addition, ICG-FI revealed a hyperfluorescent peritoneal nodule (visible between the two branches of the surgical clamp). (From Lieto et al. [79]; used with permission)

ex vivo observations (Fig. 21.3a, b). In addition, a hypofluorescent tissue boundary was identified around each lesion. Postoperative histopathology showed that two nodules detected in the intraoperative phase and two nodules detected intraoperatively were not metastatic. Of the 64 hyperfluorescent nodules, 1 (false-positive) was non-cancerous; of the remaining 5 hypofluorescent nodules, 2 (false-negatives) turned out to be metastatic tissues. In all cases, the hypofluorescent tissue around each lesion was negative for metastatic tissue. Of the 65 metastatic peritoneal nodules, the ICG-FI allowed to identify 16 nodules not diagnosed with conventional procedures, adding a 25% diagnostic improvement. Overall, the sensitivity of current diagnostic procedures (CT and PET) was 43.1% preoperatively and 76.9% intraoperatively (visual examination and palpation). With the ICG-FI sensitivity increased to 96.9%, ICG-FI showed the highest specificity and positive and negative predictive values. The accuracy of the test, that is, the global prognostic performance of the procedure, was 43.4%, 75.3%, and 95.6%

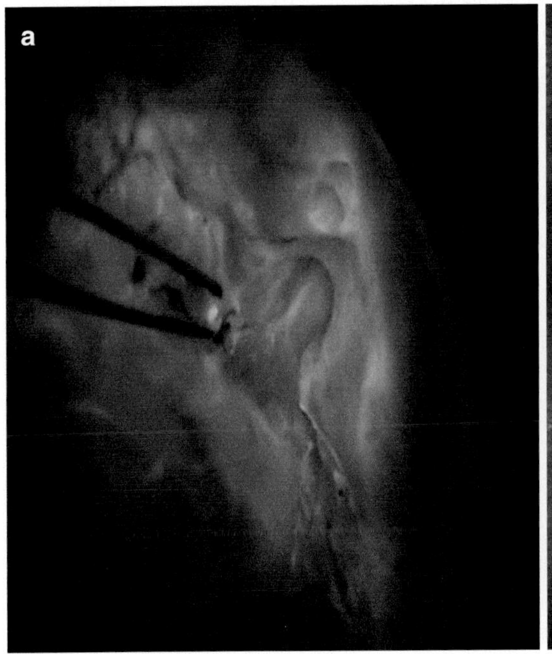
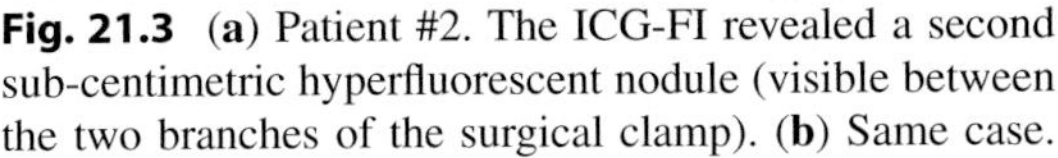
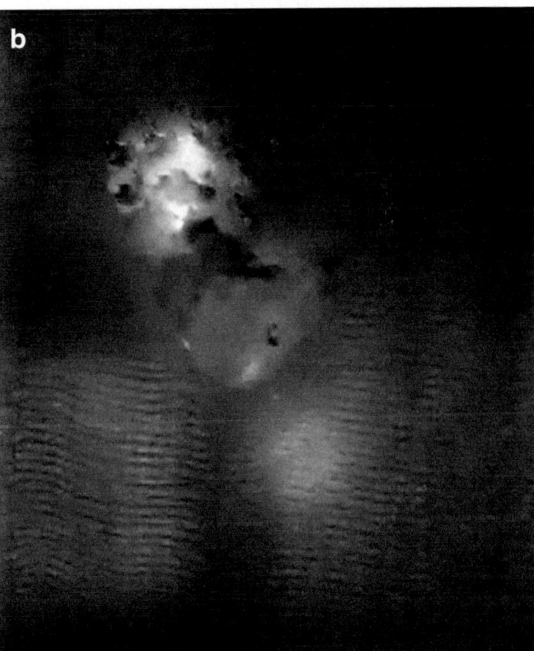

Fig. 21.3 (a) Patient #2. The ICG-FI revealed a second sub-centimetric hyperfluorescent nodule (visible between the two branches of the surgical clamp). (b) Same case. ICG-FI guided surgery ex vivo, on the table, to confirm the radicality of the surgical resection. (From Lieto et al. [79]; used with permission)

for preoperative, intraoperative, and ICG-FI, respectively (Table 21.2).

Prior to ICG-FI, median PCI was 7 (range 2–12, IQR 4–10), but after ICG-FI, PCI increased significantly to a median of 10 (range 3–15, IQR 5–13; $p < 0.001$). However, the worsening of PCI did not prevent a complete cytoreduction in all patients.

Cytological examination of the peritoneal liquid was positive for malignant cells in three out four cases before HIPEC and negative in all cases after HIPEC.

Considerations

Cytoreductive surgery achieving CCR-0 or at least CC-1 cytoreduction should be the *gold standard* in the treatment of primary and metastatic peritoneal carcinomatosis, including PC from colorectal cancer. A technique that improves intraoperative detection of PC nodules would help to achieve complete cytoreduction and avoid resection of non-cancerous lesions. Despite the limited number of patients and PC nodules that are limitations of the present study, our results with intraoperative ICG-FI appear promising. Using this imaging technique, it was possible to correctly map the metastatic areas with a sensitivity of 97%, a test accuracy of 95.6%, and an improvement of almost 25% in the identification of the disease. Particularly, the 16 malignant lesions identified intraoperatively with Fluobeam® had not been detected during conventional abdominal exploration.

In 2016, Liberale et al. and Barabino et al., both from Europe, have reported their results in 17 and 10 patients, respectively, showing PC from colorectal cancer [33, 40]. Our results differ from those reported by Barabino [40]. In contrast to our results showing that the PCI score has improved significantly from 7 (with conventional methods) to 10 (with PCI-FI), Barabino et al. reported a non-significant difference between conventional and ICG-FI-guided surgery [40]. They also reported false-positive and false-negative rates of 40% and 27%, respectively, while our rates were 25% and 3%, respectively. The explanation of the authors of these high per-

centages includes preoperative chemotherapy and the limitations of the EPR effect of ICG. However, Barabino and colleagues administered ICG 24 h before surgery and it could have impaired their results. In our experience, 50 min after ICG intravenous injection, the intraoperative view with Fluobeam® of the fluorescent areas in the abdomen was optimal. Our decision to perform the intraoperative injection of the fluorescent probe was influenced by our previous experience with ICG-FI guided surgery for liver cancers [80]. In order to consistently reduce physiological hepatic uptake and allow the drug to concentrate in the tumor, the injection of ICG had been performed 24 h before surgery [81, 82]. In these cases, no peritoneal fluorescence occurred at the time of the operation. Interestingly, as in our observations, Liberale et al. did not detect fluorescence in peritoneal metastatic nodules in the first two patients who received ICG 24 h before surgery. In contrast, in the remaining patients who received ICG intraoperative injection, all peritoneal nodules were hyperfluorescent [33]. Establishing the optimal ICG dosage and injection times are important for the standardization of the technique. Some authors [42] propose a dose of 0.5 mg/kg 12–24 h before surgery, others [33] a total dose of 5 mg administered intraoperatively. In the case of the PC, in which numerous, small, hypervascularized nodules are to be detected, an intraoperative ICG injection is suitable since the ICG disappears from the plasma at a rate of 18–25% per minute [83].

A new interesting tool is represented by prophylactic HIPEC in CRCs at high risk of developing peritoneal metachronous carcinomatosis, such as tumors invading serosa (pT4a) or with positive peritoneal lavage [84]. In these patients, current clinical and imaging techniques do not have sufficient diagnostic sensitivity [85], and ICG-FI-guided surgery could identify small undiagnosed peritoneal metastatic nodules. Furthermore, this technique would be an excellent tool to improve sensitivity for second-level laparoscopy in high-risk patients and could be practice-changing.

Although all the available studies show some limitations particularly related to the small number

Table 21.2 Diagnostic performance of pre- and intraoperative conventional technology and ICG-FI pathological examination

		Positive	Negative	Total	Sensitivity % (95% CI)	Specificity % (95% CI)	PPV % (95% CI)	NPV % (95% CI)	Diagnostic accuracy % (95% CI)
Pre-operative	Positive	28	2	30	43.1	50.0	93.3	5.1	43.4
	Negative	37	2	39	(31.1–55.1)	(34.5–65.5)	(84.3–100)	(2.9–7.2)	(31.7–55.1)
	Total	65	4	69					
Intra-operative	Positive	50	2	52	76.9	50.0	96.1	11.7	75.3
	Negative	15	2	17	(64.8–86.5)	(34.5–65.5)	(90.8–100)	(6.8–16.5)	(65.1–85.4)
	Total	65	4	69					
ICG-FI	Positive	63	1	64	96.9	75.0	98.4	60.0	95.6
	Negative	2	3	5	(89.3–99.5)	(61.5–88.4)	(95.3–100)	(46.4–73.5)	(90.7–100)
	Total	65	4	69					

From Lieto et al. [79]; used with permission

True positive (TP): positive both at pathological examination and diagnostic tools

True negative (TN): negative both at pathological examination and diagnostic tools

False positive (FP): positive at diagnostic tools and negative at pathological examination

False negative (FN): negative at diagnostic tools and positive at pathological examination

Sensitivity: TP/TP + FN; Specificity: TN/TN + FP; PPV (positive predictive value): TP/TP + FP;

NPV (negative predictive value): TN/TN + FN; Diagnostic accuracy: TP + TN/all cases of investigated patients, ICG-FI-guided surgery appears to be a promising tool to improve the radicality of CS in PC originating from CRC. Further studies are needed to standardize the technique and determine its role in this patient population.

References

1. Pontiggia P, Pontiggia E. Immunità e ipertermia nella cura dei tumori. ETS edizioni 8; 2016.
2. Glehen O, Mohamed F, Gilly FN. Peritoneal carcinomatosis from digestive tract cancer: new management by cytoreductive surgery and intraperitoneal chemohyperthermia. Lancet Oncol. 2004;5:219–28.
3. Chua TC, Yan TD, Saxena A, et al. Should the treatment of peritoneal carcinomatosis by cytoreductive surgery and hyperthermic intraperitoneal chemotherapy still be regarded as a highly morbid procedure: a systematic review of morbidity and mortality. Ann Surg. 2009;249:900–7.
4. Jessup MJ, Goldberg RM, Asara EA, et al. Colon and rectum. In: American Joint Committee on Cancer, editor. AJCC cancer staging manual. 8th ed. Berlin: Springer; 2017. p. 251–74.
5. Sugarbaker PH. Intraperitoneal chemotherapy and cytoreductive surgery for the prevention and treatment of peritoneal carcinomatosis and sarcomatosis. Semin Surg Oncol. 1998;14:254–61.
6. Van der Speeten K, Stuart OA, Sugarbaker PH. Pharmacokinetics and pharmacodynamics of perioperative cancer chemotherapy in peritoneal surface malignancy. Cancer J. 2009;15(3):216–24.
7. Ferlay J, Soerjomataram I, Dikshit R, et al. Cancer incidence and mortality worldwide: sources, methods and major patterns in GLOBOCAN 2012. Int J Cancer. 2015;136:359–86.
8. Sugarbaker PH. Observations concerning cancer spread within the peritoneal cavity and concepts supporting an ordered pathophysiology. Cancer Treat Res. 1996;82:79–100.
9. Chu DZ, Lung NP, Thompson C, et al. Peritoneal carcinomatosis in non-gynecologic malignancies: a prospective study of prognostic factors. Cancer. 1989;63:364–7.
10. Sadeghi B, Arvieux C, Glehen O, et al. Peritoneal carcinomatosis in non-gynecologic malignancies: results of EVOCAPE 1 multicentric prospective study. Cancer. 2000;88:358–63.
11. Kodera Y, Yamamura Y, Shimizu Y, et al. Peritoneal washing cytology: prognostic value of positive findings in patients with gastric carcinoma undergoing a potentially curative resection. J Surg Oncol. 1999;72:60–4.
12. Roviello F, Marrelli D, Neri A, et al. Treatment of peritoneal carcinomatosis by cytoreductive surgery and intraperitoneal hyperthermic chemoperfusion (IHCP): postoperative outcome and risk factors for morbidity. World J Surg. 2006;30:2033–40.
13. Fujimoto S, Takahashi M, Mutou T, et al. Successful intraperitoneal hyperthermic chemoperfusion for the prevention of postoperative peritoneal recurrence in patients with advanced gastric carcinoma. Cancer. 1999;85:529–34.
14. Marrelli D, Roviello F, De Manzoni G, Italian Research Group for Gastric Cancer, et al. Different patterns of recurrence in gastric cancer depending on Lauren's histological type: longitudinal study. World J Surg. 2002;26:1160–5.
15. Roviello F, Marrelli D, de Manzoni G, Italian Research Group for Gastric Cancer, et al. Prospective study of peritoneal recurrence after curative surgery for gastric cancer. Br J Surg. 2003;90:1113–9.
16. Al-Shammaa HA, Li Y, Yonemura Y. Current status and future strategies of cytoreductive surgery plus intraperitoneal hyperthermic chemotherapy for peritoneal carcinomatosis. World J Gastroenterol. 2008;14:1159–66.
17. Portilla AG, Sugarbaker PH, Chang D. Second look surgery after cytoreductive and intraperitoneal chemotherapy for peritoneal–29 carcinomatosis from colorectal cancer: analysis of prognostic features. World J Surg. 1999;23:23–9.
18. Sadeghi B, Arvieux C, Glehen O, et al. Peritoneal carcinomatosis from non-gynecologic malignancies: results of the EVOCAPE 1 multicentric prospective study. Cancer. 2000;88:358–63.
19. Stewart JH 4th, Shen P, Levine EA. Intraperitoneal hyperthermic chemotherapy for peritoneal surface malignancy: current status and future directions. Ann Surg Oncol. 2005;12(10):765–77.
20. Yonemura Y, Endo Y, Yamaguchi T, et al. Mechanisms of the formation of the peritoneal dissemination in gastric cancer. Int J Oncol. 1996;8(4):795–802.
21. Glehen O, Kwiatkowski F, Sugarbaker PH, et al. Cytoreductive surgery combined with preoperative intraperitoneal chemotherapy for the management of peritoneal carcinomatosis from colorectal cancer: a multi-institutional study. J Clin Oncol. 2004;22:3284–92.
22. Blackham AU, Russell GB, Stewert JH 4th, et al. Metastatic colorectal cancer: survival comparison of hepatic resection versus cytoreductive surgery and hyperthermic intraperitoneal chemotherapy. Ann Surg Oncol. 2014;21:2667–74.
23. Spratt JS, Adcock RA, Muskovin M, et al. Sistema di somministrazione clinica per la chemioterapia ipertermica intraperitoneale. Cancer Res. 1980;40:256–60.
24. Sugarbaker PH. Peritonectomy procedures. Ann Surg. 1995;221:29–42.
25. Esquivel J, Sugarbaker PH. Second aspect surgery in patients with peritoneal dissemination from appendicular neoplasia: analysis of prognostic factors in 98 patients. Ann Surg. 2001;234:198–205.
26. Deraco M, Nonaka D, Baratti D, et al. Prognostic analysis of clinicopathologic factors in 49 patients with diffuse malignant peritoneal mesothelioma treated with cytoreductive surgery and intraperitoneal hyperthermic perfusion. Ann Surg Oncol. 2006;13:229–37.

27. Moran B, Baratti D, Yan TD, et al. Consensus statement on the loco-regional treatment of appendiceal mucinous neoplasms with peritoneal dissemination (pseudomyxoma peritonei). J Surg Oncol. 2008;98:277–82.

28. Esquivel J, Sticca R, Sugarbaker P, Society of Surgical Oncology Annual Meeting, et al. Cytoreductive surgery and hyperthermic intraperitoneal chemotherapy in the management of peritoneal surface malignancies of colonic origin: a consensus statement. Society of Surgical Oncology. Ann Surg Oncol. 2007;14:128–33.

29. Raspagliesi F, Kusamura S, Campos Torres JC, et al. Cytoreduction combined with intraperitoneal hyperthermic perfusion chemotherapy in advanced/recurrent ovarian cancer patients: the experience of National Cancer Institute of Milan. Eur J Surg Oncol. 2006;32:671–5.

30. Jaquet P, Sugarbaker PH. Clinical research methodologies in diagnosis and staging of patients with peritoneal carcinomatosis. Cancer Treat Res. 1996;82:359–74.

31. Begossi G, Gonzales-Moreno S, Ortega Perez G, et al. Cytoreduction and intraperitoneal chemotherapy for the management of peritoneal carcinomatosis, sarcomatosis and mesothelioma. Eur J Surg Oncol. 2002;28:80–7.

32. Dromain C, Leboulleux S, Auperin A, et al. Staging of peritoneal carcinomatosis: enhanced CT vs. PET/CT. Abdom Imaging. 2008;33:87–9.

33. Liberale G, Vankerckhove S, Caldon MG, et al. Fluorescence imaging after indocyanine green injection for detection of peritoneal metastases in patients undergoing cytoreductive surgery for peritoneal carcinomatosis from colorectal cancer: a pilot study. Ann Surg. 2016;264:1110–5.

34. Sugarbaker PH. Successful management of microscopic residual disease in large bowel cancer. Cancer Chemother Pharmacol. 1999;43:15–25.

35. Berthet B, Sugarbaker TA, Chang D, et al. Quantitative methodologies for selection of patients with recurrent abdominopelvic sarcoma for treatment. Eur J Cancer. 1999;3:413–9.

36. Kim S, Lim YT, Soltesz EG, et al. Near-infrared fluorescent type II quantum dots for sentinel lymph node mapping. Nat Biotechnol. 2004;22:93–7.

37. Schaafsma BE, Mieog JSD, Hutteman M, et al. The clinical use of indocyanine green as a near-infrared fluorescent contrast agent for image-guided oncologic surgery. J Surg Oncol. 2011;104:323–32.

38. Polom K, Murawa D, Rho Y, et al. Current trends and emerging future of indocyanine green usage in surgery and oncology: a literature review. Cancer. 2011;117:4817–22.

39. Fox IJ, Wood EH. Indocyanine green: physical and physiologic properties. Proc Staff Meet Mayo Clin. 1960;35:732–44.

40. Barabino G, Klein JP, Porcheron J, et al. Intraoperative near-infrared fluorescence imaging using indocyanine green in colorectal carcinomatosis surgery: proof of concept. Eur J Surg Oncol. 2016;42:1931–7.

41. Maeda H, Wu J, Sawa T, et al. Tumor vascular permeability and the EPR effect in macromolecular therapeutics: a review. J Control Release. 2000;65:271–84.

42. Bekheit M, Vibert E. Fluorescent-guided liver surgery: Paul Brousse experience and perspectives. In: Dip FD, editor. Fluorescence imaging for surgeons: concepts and applications, vol. 11. Cham: Springer; 2015. p. 117–26.

43. Frangioni J. In vivo near-infrared fluorescence imaging. Curr Opin Chem Biol. 2003;7:626–34.

44. Sabapathy MV, Mentam J, Jacob PM, et al. Non invasive optical imaging and in vivo cell tracking of indocyanine green labeled human stem cells transplanted at superficial or in-depth tissue of SCID. Stem Cells Int. 2015;2015:606415. https://doi.org/10.1155/2015/606415.

45. FDA. Product Insert: Indocyanine Green (IC-GreenTM); 2016. http://www.accessdata.fda.gov/drugsatfda_docs/label/2006/011525s017bpdf.

46. Stanga PE, Lim JI, Hamilton P. Indocyanine green angiography in chorioretinal diseases: indications and interpretation: an evidence-based update. Ophthalmology. 2003;110:15–23.

47. Holm C, Tegeler J, Mayr M, et al. Monitoring free flaps using laser-induced fluorescence of indocyanine green: a preliminary experience. Microsurgery. 2002;22:278–87.

48. Munabi NC, Olorunnipa OB, Goltsman D, et al. The ability of intra-operative perfusion mapping with laser-assisted indocyanine green angiography to predict mastectomy flap necrosis in breast reconstruction: a prospective trial. J Plast Reconstr Aesthet Surg. 2014;67:449–55.

49. Makuuchi M, Kosuge T, Takayama T, et al. Surgery for small liver cancers. Semin Surg Oncol. 1993;9:298–304.

50. Nanashima A, Abo T, Tobinaga S, et al. Indocyanine green retention rate at 15 minutes by correlated liver function parameters before hepatectomy. J Surg Res. 2011;169:119–25.

51. Ishizawa T, Bandai Y, Kokudo N. Fluorescent cholangiography using indocyanine green for laparoscopic cholecystectomy: an initial experience. Arch Surg. 2009;144:381–2.

52. Ishizawa T, Bandai Y, Ijichiet M, et al. Fluorescent cholangiography illuminating the biliary tree during laparoscopic cholecystectomy. Br J Surg. 2010;97:1369–77.

53. Ishizawa T, Tamura S, Masuda K, et al. Intraoperative fluorescent cholangiography using indocyanine green: a biliary road map for safe surgery. J Am Coll Surg. 2009;208:1–4.

54. Hellan M, Spinoglio G, Pigazzi A, et al. The influence of fluorescence imaging on the location of bowel transection during robotic left-sided colorectal surgery. Surg Endosc. 2014;28:1695–702.

55. Boni L, Fingerhut A, Marzorati A, et al. Indocyanine green fluorescence angiography during laparoscopic low anterior resection: results of a case-matched study. Surg Endosc. 2017;31:1836–40.

56. Boni L, David G, Dionigi G, et al. Indocyanine green-enhanced fluorescence to assess bowel perfusion during laparoscopic colorectal resection. Surg Endosc. 2016;30:2736–42.

57. Jafari MD, Wexner SD, Martz JE, et al. Perfusion assessment in laparoscopic left-sided/anterior resection (PILLAR II): a multi-institutional study. J Am Coll Surg. 2015;220:82–92.

58. Kitai T, Inomoto T, Miwa M, et al. Fluorescence navigation with indocyanine green for detecting sentinel lymph nodes in breast cancer. Breast Cancer. 2005;12:211–5.

59. Tanaka R, Nakashima K, Fujimoto W, et al. Sentinel lymph node detection in skin cancer using fluorescence navigation with indocyanine green. J Dermatol. 2009;36:468–70.

60. Nimura H, Narimiya N, Mitsumori N, et al. Infrared ray electronic endoscopy combined with indocyanine green injection for detection of sentinel nodes of patients with gastric cancer. Br J Surg. 2004;91:575–9.

61. Nagata K, Endo S, Hidaka E, et al. Laparoscopic sentinel node mapping for colorectal cancer using infrared ray laparoscopy. Anticancer Res. 2006;26:2307–12.

62. Kusano M, Tajima Y, Yamazaki K, et al. Sentinel lymph node mapping guided by indocyanine green fluorescence imaging: a new method for sentinel lymph node navigation surgery in gastrointestinal cancer. Dig Surg. 2008;25:103–8.

63. Noura S, Ohue M, Seki Y, et al. Feasibility of a lateral region sentinel lymph node biopsy of lower rectal cancer guided by indocyanine green using a near-infrared camera system. Ann Surg Oncol. 2010;17:144–51.

64. Hirche C, Mohr Z, Kneif S, et al. Ultrastaging of colon cancer by sentinel node biopsy using fluorescence navigation with indocyanine green. Int J Colorectal Dis. 2012;27:319–24.

65. Cahill RA, Anderson M, Wang LM, et al. Near-infrared (NIR) laparoscopy for intraoperative lymphatic road-mapping and sentinel node identification during definitive surgical resection of early-stage colorectal neoplasia. Surg Endosc. 2012;26:197–204.

66. Van der Pas MH, Ankersmit M, Stockmann HB, et al. Laparoscopic sentinel lymph node identification in patients with colon carcinoma using a near-infrared dye: description of a new technique and feasibility study. J Laparoendosc Adv Surg Tech A. 2013;23:367–71.

67. Liberale G, Vankerckhove S, Galdon MG, et al. Sentinel lymph node detection by blue dye versus indocyanine green fluorescence imaging in colon cancer. Anticancer Res. 2016;36:4853–8.

68. Ishizawa T, Fukushima N, Shibahara J, et al. Real-time identification of liver cancers by using indocyanine green fluorescent imaging. Cancer. 2009;115:2491–504.

69. Gotoh K, Yamada T, Ishikawa O, et al. A novel image-guided surgery of hepatocellular carcinoma by indocyanine green fluorescence imaging navigation. J Surg Oncol. 2009;100:75–9.

70. Harada N, Ishizawa T, Muraoka A, et al. Fluorescence navigation hepatectomy by vizualization of localized cholestasis from bile tumor infiltration. J Am Coll Surg. 2010;210:2–6.

71. Yamamichi T, Oue T, Yonekura T, et al. Clinical application of indocyanine green (ICG) fluorescent imaging of hepatoblastoma. J Pediatr Surg. 2015;50:833–6.

72. Yokoyama N, Otani T, Hashidate H, et al. Real-time detection of hepatic micrometastases from pancreatic cancer by intraoperative fluorescence imaging: preliminary results of a prospective study. Cancer. 2012;118:2813–9.

73. Frangioni JV. New technologies for human cancer imaging. J Clin Oncol. 2008;26:4012–21.

74. Velde EA, Veerman T, Subramaniam V, et al. The use of fluorescent dyes and probes in surgical oncology. Eur J Surg Oncol. 2009;36:6–15.

75. Rao J, Dragulescu-Andrasi A, Yao H. Fluorescence imaging in vivo: recent advances. Curr Opin Biotechnol. 2007;18:17–25.

76. Gioux S, Choi HS, Frangioni JV. Image-guided surgery using invisible near-infrared light: fundamentals of clinical translation. Mol Imaging. 2010;9:237–55.

77. Xiong L, Gazyakan E, Yang W, et al. Indocyanine green fluorescence-guided sentinel node biopsy: a meta-analysis on detection rate and diagnostic performance. Eur J Surg Oncol. 2014;40:843–9.

78. Lim C, Vibert E, Azoulay D, et al. Indocyanine green fluorescence imaging in the surgical management of liver cancers: current facts and future implications. J Visc Surg. 2014;151:117–24.

79. Lieto E, Auricchio A, Cardella F, et al. Fluorescence-guided surgery in the combined treatment of peritoneal carcinomatosis from colorectal cancer: preliminary results and considerations. World J Surg. 2018;42:1154–60.

80. Lieto E, Galizia G, Cardella F, et al. Indocyanine green fluorescence imaging-guided surgery in primary and metastatic liver tumors. Surg Innov. 2018;25:62–8.

81. Miyashiro I, Miyoshi N, Hiratsuka M, et al. Detection of sentinel node in gastric cancer surgery by indocyanine green fluorescence imaging: comparison with infrared imaging. Ann Surg Oncol. 2008;15:1640–3.

82. Takahashi H, Zaidi N, Berber E. An initial report on the intraoperative use of indocyanine green fluorescence imaging in the surgical management of liver tumors. J Surg Oncol. 2016;114:625–9.

83. Faybik P, Hetz H. Plasma disappearance rate of indocyanine green in liver dysfunction. Transplant Proc. 2006;38:801–2.

84. Honoré C, Goéré D, Souadka A, et al. Definition of patients presenting a high risk of developing peritoneal carcinomatosis after curative surgery for colorectal cancer: a systematic review. Ann Surg Oncol. 2013;20:183–92.

85. Cortes-Guiral D, Elias D, Cascales-Campos PA, et al. Second-look surgery plus hyperthermic intraperitoneal chemotherapy for patients with colorectal cancer at high risk of peritoneal carcinomatosis: does it really save lives. World J Gastroenterol. 2017;23:377–81.

M. Al-Taher, J. van den Bos, B. Knapen,
N. D. Bouvy, and L. P. S. Stassen

Indications

Although surgical procedures are performed to improve a medical condition, the risk for iatrogenic injury is always part of the operation. During colorectal, urologic, and gynecologic surgery, ureteric injury is a feared complication. In order to prevent such iatrogenic damage, the surgeon must be aware of the exact location of the ureter.

Ureteric injury can result in pain, intra-abdominal sepsis, systemic infection, abscesses, urinoma, ureteral stricture, ureteric fistula, renal failure, and even loss of the ipsilateral renal unit [1–3]. The majority of ureteral injuries are often found only after other, more profound injuries are addressed, which may lead to worse outcomes.

Previous pelvic operations, infection, and inflammatory bowel disease are among the known risk factors for iatrogenic ureteral injury during laparoscopy, but most ureteral injuries occur in patients lacking these risk factors [4]. In earlier studies, an incidence of 0.1–7.6% of iatrogenic ureteral injury has been reported during colorectal and gynecologic surgery in which more than 80% of cases were unrecognized intraoperatively [5–7]. Failure to identify the relevant anatomy is the main factor leading to ureteral damage [8]. In an earlier study, Assimos et al. [7] compared the incidence of iatrogenic ureteral injuries between the pre-laparoscopic and laparoscopic era and found that the incidence of iatrogenic ureteral injuries was significantly greater in the latter. Thus, the early detection and prevention of ureteral injury have become even more important. Now laparoscopic surgery is the standard of care in the majority of pelvic surgical procedures. Therefore, a technique or method that improves visualization of the ureter by the surgeon would be beneficial in preventing ureteral damage.

A method to detect the ureters pre-operatively is by the use of retrograde pyelography or urologic computed tomography [9]. However, intraoperative visualization would be more desirable since the anatomy changes during surgery. A method used in open surgery to assist in manually identifying the ureters is by placement of ureteral stents. However, laparoscopic pelvic surgery is increasingly performed and tactile

Electronic Supplementary Material The online version of this chapter (https://doi.org/10.1007/978-3-030-38092-2_22) contains supplementary material, which is available to authorized users.

M. Al-Taher and J. van den Bos contributed equally with all other contributors.

M. Al-Taher (✉) · J. van den Bos · B. Knapen
N. D. Bouvy · L. P. S. Stassen
Department of Surgery, Maastricht University
Medical Center, Maastricht, The Netherlands
e-mail: m.taher@zuyderland.nl

feedback is strongly reduced when using laparoscopic instruments as compared to open surgery. In laparoscopic surgery ureteral stent placement is therefore less helpful. Moreover, stent placement as a procedure itself can cause complications to the ureter [10–12].

Intraoperative fluorescence ureteral identification with preoperative optical dye administration is a new technique for easier and earlier intraoperative visualization of the ureter and could therefore improve the safety and efficiency of laparoscopic colorectal surgery [13, 14]. In fluorescence imaging, a near infrared (NIR) fluorescent dye is administered intravenously and is excited by a specific light source and detected by the use of a laparoscope with near-infrared (NIR) imaging properties.

However, at present no dye for ureteral identification is commercially available for use in the human setting. Methylene blue (MB) is a registered dye with fluorescent characteristics that is excreted by the kidneys and would therefore be applicable for ureter imaging. Unfortunately, the results of clinical experiments so far give conflicting results. These may be due to the characteristics of the dye itself with only a weak fluorescent signal or the currently available laparoscopic equipment. The latter refers to a disadvantage of MB: this dye is excited at 600 nm, which is a different wavelength than most other dyes like indocyanine green in other indications which is excited at around 800 nm. The use of MB therefore demands specifically developed equipment. The equipment used in the experiments with MB was experimental and is not available commercially for laparoscopic use so far.

Three experimental dyes are now available which are cleared by the kidneys and therefore excreted through urine with excitation around 800 nm and therefore applicable with the usual equipment. The first of these dyes was IRDye® 800CW (LI-COR Biotechnology, Lincoln, United States). Because of its high cost, two other dyes have been developed: IRDye® 800NOS and IRDye® 800BK. Their price is in the range of that of ICG which can be considered affordable for daily practice.

The present chapter describes and illustrates the use of these dyes in an experimental setting in pigs.

Surgeries particularly at risk are obviously surgeries concerning the area near the ureters: pelvic surgery including rectal cancer surgery, low anterior resection, but possibly also gynecological surgery.

Therefore, in these surgeries NIR ureter imaging is most required.

Technical Description of the Procedure(s)

In the experiments described in this chapter, the dye to illuminate the ureter is administered intravenously. Another application is the use through ureteral stents that are introduced with cystoscopy. In the following, only applications using intravenously (IV) administered dyes are described and the more invasive ureteral stenting technique is not described further. In current literature, several IV administered dyes have been tested for ureter visualization.

In 2007, the first use of NIR imaging for ureter visualization was described by Tanaka et al. in 2007. In pigs, IRDye® 800CW (earlier referred to as CW-800-CA) was injected in several concentrations. An NIR imaging system prototype was used to detect the fluorescent signal. Illumination of the ureters in both rats and pigs was obtained at 10 minutes post injection until 60 minutes post injection [14].

In 2013, Schols et al. published a second article on the use of this dye for ureter visualization in pigs. A low dose of 0.25 mg IRDye® 800CW was injected in the first pig and 3 mg in the second. In the first pig, no ureter fluorescence was observed, but in the second pig both ureters could be clearly visualized from 10 minutes onward after IV administration of the dye [15].

Korb et al. showed comparable results after systemic administration of 30, 60, or 120 µg/kg injection of IRDye® 800CW in pigs. An optimal signal was reached by 30 minutes and with a dose of 60 µg/kg [16].

MB as a dye for ureteral imaging was described in several studies. In 2010, Matsui et al. published a study on female Yorkshire pigs that were included for open surgery and laparoscopic surgery. The FLARE™ image guided surgery system was used for the open surgery setting, and for the laparoscopic setting a prototype was used. Animals were divided into three subgroups: slow infusion over 5 minutes with 0.01 mg/kg MB diluted in 30 mL saline, pretreatment with 10 mg intravenous furosemide 1 hour prior to MB injection, and injection with a higher dose of 0.5 mg/kg MB. In all included animals the ureter could be identified from 10 up to 75 minutes after MB administration, with a higher fluorescence to background ratio in the third group. No added value of the use of furosemide was found. In the laparoscopic setting, a dose of 0.1 mg/kg did not provide sufficient fluorescence intensity, but after intravenous injection of 1 mg/kg MB the ureters could be readily identified from 10 to 30 minutes post injection [13].

The first described in-human use of MB for ureter visualization was in 2013 by Verbeek et al. In their article, the intravenous administration of several concentrations of MB followed by NIR imaging using the mini-FLARE™ system was assessed. In all included 12 patients, the ureter could be visualized 10 minutes after infusion with MB, with a higher fluorescence intensity achieved when administering a higher dose of MB [17].

A second article on the in-human use of MB showed less favorable results. The injected dose of MB in this study ranged between 0.125 and 1 mg/kg. The ureter was successfully detected in 5 out of the 10 patients, in whom the highest doses were administered (0.75–1 mg/kg), but the fluorescent signal was only picked up after the ureter was already visible in the conventional white light mode. Therefore, the technique was considered to be of no added value in these patients [18].

Most recently, Barnes et al. used MB for ureter visualization in 40 patients in a dose ranging from 0.25 to 1 mg/kg. Of the 69 ureters analyzed, 64 were seen under fluorescence of which 14 were seen earlier with fluorescence than white light. Fluorescence was deemed useful in 13 cases, whereas in 10 cases, the fluorescence revealed the ureter to be in a different location than expected. The highest signal to background ratio was found when using 0.75 mg/kg [19].

Friedman-Levi and colleagues used ICG loaded into liposomes, enabling IV administration and renal excretion. In the liposomal-ICG treated animals, the ureters could be visualized, up to 90 minutes after administration. However, background fluorescence was quite bright using this technique diminishing the discrimination of the ureter [20].

Verbeek et al. assessed the use of ZW800–1 conjugated to the cyclic RDG-peptide to both visualize the ureter and colorectal cancer in mice. ZW800 has an absorption peak at 772 nm and emission peak at 788 nm. The Flare system was used to detect the fluorescent signal. With these dyes both the experimentally induced tumors and the ureters could be visualized using cRDG-ZW800–1 [21].

De Valk et al. recently published an article describing the first in-human use of ZW800–1. After a low dose injection of this dye, the ureters were clearly visible up to 3 hours after injection, without observable toxicity [22].

Dip et al. described the use of IV sodium fluorescein in rats for ureteral imaging after laparotomy. A 530 nm excitation light was used to visualize the fluorescent signal. Using this light, the peristaltic movement of the ureters was seen in all rats [23].

A new dye, UreterGlow, with emission at 800 nm and excitation at 830 nm was tested by Mahalingam et al. in mice using a commercially available NIR system. Ureter identification with white light was achieved in none of the pigs, but within 15 minutes after injection of the fluorescent dye, both ureters could be clearly visualized for up to 2 hours without background fluorescence [24].

Regarding the Presented Video

Video 22.1 is derived from a study that has been reported before in a peer-reviewed journal [25]. This study was approved by the local animal ethics committee, and the experiments were conducted at the central animal facilities of Maastricht University (Maastricht, the Netherlands). Animals were used in compliance with the regulations of the Dutch legislation concerning animal research. A pig model was chosen because of the similarities between pig anatomy and human anatomy and because of earlier successful application of NIR imaging in pigs [15]. The experiments were done in three female Dutch landrace pigs (each weighing 40 kg). After surgery, the pigs were sacrificed by the veterinarian-anesthesiologist.

Laparoscopic Fluorescence Imaging System

A commercially available laparoscopic fluorescence imaging system (Karl Storz SE & Co. KG, Tuttlingen, Germany) was used. This system with a xenon based light source enables both excitation and detection of all three dyes used in this experiment: IRDye® 800CW (λEX/EM = 775/796 nm), IRDye® 800BK (λEX/EM = 774/790 nm), and IRDye® 800NOS (λEX/EM = 767/786 nm). A food pedal allows the surgeon to switch easily between the white and NIR light imaging modalities. The same NIR imaging settings were used for all three dyes tested. All procedures were digitally recorded with the built-in recording equipment.

Characteristics of the Dyes

The characteristics of the dyes used (IRDye® 800CW, IRDye® 800BK, IRDye® 800NOS) have been previously described [26].

Preparation of the Dyes

The dyes were prepared and used following instructions of the manufacturer. They were diluted in sterile phosphate buffered saline (PBS) solution to a concentration of 1 mg/mL. In this dilution, 6 mg of each dye was prepared for intravenous injection in one pig.

Surgical Technique and Assessment

The surgical procedures were performed under general anesthesia. Premedication consisted of intramuscular injection of azaperone 3 mg/kg, ketamine 10 mg/kg, and atropine 0.05 mg/kg. Anesthesia was induced with intravenous thiopental 10–15 mg/kg. After intubation, the pigs were maintained under anesthesia with isoflurane and oxygen.

Surgical residents performed a laparoscopic partial excision of the bicornuate uterus, mimicking a laparoscopic appendectomy. These procedures were strictly supervised by two expert endoscopic gastrointestinal surgeons. One dye was tested per animal, using a 6 mg dose (1 mg/mL) which was intravenously administered.

Fluorescence imaging was initiated immediately after the intravenous administration of the dye. Further imaging was performed intermittently in fluorescence mode and white light mode. Intraoperatively, it was systematically documented whether the ureters could be identified in fluorescence mode by filling in a registration form. The attending surgeon was consulted to reach agreement on the identification of the ureters. A structure was defined as "identified" if its localization was confirmed with absolute certainty by the experienced surgeon.

Interpretation

All three dyes enabled clear and satisfactory visualization of the anatomical course of both ureters, in which the highest fluorescence intensity compared to the background was found in the pigs in which IRDye® 800BK and IRDye® 800CW were used.

The first identification of the ureters occurred within minutes after dye administration in all three pigs because of vascular imaging of the wall of the organ. At this time, also other structures are illuminated such as the uterus, bowel wall, and lymph nodes. No peristaltic movement of fluorescent dye through the ureter is yet visualized. This occurs in IRDye® 800BK, IRDye® 800CW, and IRDye® 800NOS 35, 10, and

45 minutes after dye administration, respectively, when the ureters become visible through excretion of the dyes in the urine. The ureters remained fluorescent during pulsatile movement of the ureter for 3.5 hours after administration.

Pitfalls

Despite the promising results, the findings of this study have to be interpreted with caution. Since each dye was only tested in vivo at one specific dosage and each dye was only tested in one pig, further experiments are needed to determine optimal dosing and timing of the dyes which are dependent on the pharmacokinetic properties of the dyes. The ureter wall thickness of pigs is slightly less than the thickness of the ureter wall in humans; therefore, the use of NIR in humans might give different results [27].

Before visible pulsatile flow occurs, NIR highlights the ureter and other well vascularized structures because of intravascular presence of the dye. In this phase, the ureter might be confused with other structures. When the dye appears in the urine, the ureter is easy to distinguish from the surrounding vascularized structures. These structures have lost most fluorescence at that time because of washout, while the remaining pulsatile movement of urine through the ureter is quite characteristic. The relationship with peristalsis has one slight drawback, as the signal is not present permanently and the surgeon must wait for the ureter to make these peristaltic movements. In addition, adequate renal function is required for sufficient excretion of the fluorescent dye into the urine.

No adverse reactions as a result of the administration of the dyes were observed.

A transient decrease in measured SpO_2 oxygen saturation is displayed. This is due to the measurement method, in which the color of the blood is used, which changes after administration of the dyes.

Of course, one should be aware that the present results were obtained in an experimental setting, studying pigs. Two clinical studies are being performed evaluating the use in the human setting. One of these studies focuses on the safety and efficacy of IRDye® 800BK in laparoscopic bowel resection and laparoscopic donor nephrectomy (NCT03387410). The second clinical trial currently performed is a dose-escalation study in gynecological surgery (NCT03106038). The information and video presented in this chapter should be regarded as indicative of what the use in the clinical setting could be like, but the results of these trials will determine whether these expectations were justified.

References

1. da Silva G, Boutros M, Wexner SD. Role of prophylactic ureteric stents in colorectal surgery. Asian J Endosc Surg. 2012;5(3):105–10.
2. Abboudi H, Ahmed K, Royle J, Khan MS, Dasgupta P, N'Dow J. Ureteric injury: a challenging condition to diagnose and manage. Nat Rev Urol. 2013;10(2):108–15.
3. Esparaz AM, Pearl JA, Herts BR, LeBlanc J, Kapoor B. Iatrogenic urinary tract injuries: etiology, diagnosis, and management. Semin Intervent Radiol. 2015;32(2):195–208.
4. Delacroix SE Jr, Winters JC. Urinary tract injuries: recognition and management. Clin Colon Rectal Surg. 2010;23(3):221.
5. Park JH, Park JW, Song K, Jo MK. Ureteral injury in gynecologic surgery: a 5-year review in a community hospital. Korean J Urol. 2012;53(2):120–5.
6. Palaniappa NC, Telem DA, Ranasinghe NE, Divino CM. Incidence of iatrogenic ureteral injury after laparoscopic colectomy. Arch Surg. 2012;147(3):267–71.
7. Assimos DG, Patterson LC, Taylor CL. Changing incidence and etiology of iatrogenic ureteral injuries. J Urol. 1994;152(6 Pt 2):2240–6.
8. Zhang X, Wang Z, Zhou H, Liang J, Zhou Z. Analysis of ureteral injuries for laparoscopic rectal cancer surgery. J Laparoendosc Adv Surg Tech A. 2014;24(10):698–701.
9. Brandes S, Coburn M, Armenakas N, McAninch J. Diagnosis and management of ureteric injury: an evidence-based analysis. BJU Int. 2004;94(3):277–89.
10. Delacroix SE Jr, Winters JC. Urinary tract injures: recognition and management. Clin Colon Rectal Surg. 2010;23(2):104–12.
11. Speicher PJ, Goldsmith ZG, Nussbaum DP, Turley RS, Peterson AC, Mantyh CR. Ureteral stenting in laparoscopic colorectal surgery. J Surg Res. 2014;190(1):98–103.
12. Beraldo S, Neubeck K, Von Friderici E, Steinmuller L. The prophylactic use of a ureteral stent in laparoscopic colorectal surgery. Scand J Surg. 2013;102(2):87–9.

13. Matsui A, Tanaka E, Choi HS, Kianzad V, Gioux S, Lomnes SJ, et al. Real-time, near-infrared, fluorescence-guided identification of the ureters using methylene blue. Surgery. 2010;148(1):78–86.
14. Tanaka E, Ohnishi S, Laurence RG, Choi HS, Humblet V, Frangioni JV. Real-time intraoperative ureteral guidance using invisible near-infrared fluorescence. J Urol. 2007;178(5):2197–202.
15. Schols RM, Lodewick TM, Bouvy ND, van Dam GM, Dejong CH, Stassen LP. Application of a new dye for near-infrared fluorescence laparoscopy of the ureters: demonstration in a pig model. Dis Colon Rectum. 2014;57(3):407–11.
16. Korb ML, Huh WK, Boone JD, Warram JM, Chung TK, de Boer E, et al. Laparoscopic fluorescent visualization of the ureter with intravenous IRDye800CW. J Minim Invasive Gynecol. 2015;22(5):799–806.
17. Verbeek FP, van der Vorst JR, Schaafsma BE, Swijnenburg RJ, Gaarenstroom KN, Elzevier HW, et al. Intraoperative near infrared fluorescence guided identification of the ureters using low dose methylene blue: a first in human experience. J Urol. 2013;190(2):574–9.
18. Al-Taher M, van den Bos J, Schols RM, Bouvy ND, Stassen LP. Fluorescence ureteral visualization in human laparoscopic colorectal surgery using methylene blue. J Laparoendosc Adv Surg Tech A. 2016;26(11):870–5.
19. Barnes TG, Hompes R, Birks J, Mortensen NJ, Jones O, Lindsey I, et al. Methylene blue fluorescence of the ureter during colorectal surgery. Surg Endosc. 2018;32(9):4036–43.
20. Friedman-Levi Y, Larush L, Diana M, Marchegiani F, Marescaux J, Goder N, et al. Optimization of liposomal indocyanine green for imaging of the urinary pathways and a proof of concept in a pig model. Surg Endosc. 2018;32(2):963–70.
21. Verbeek FP, van der Vorst JR, Tummers QR, Boonstra MC, de Rooij KE, Lowik CW, et al. Near-infrared fluorescence imaging of both colorectal cancer and ureters using a low-dose integrin targeted probe. Ann Surg Oncol. 2014;21(Suppl 4):S528–37.
22. de Valk KS, Handgraaf HJ, Deken MM, Sibinga Mulder BG, Valentijn AR, Terwisscha van Scheltinga AG, et al. A zwitterionic near-infrared fluorophore for real-time ureter identification during laparoscopic abdominopelvic surgery. Nat Commun. 2019;10(1):3118.
23. Dip FD, Nahmod M, Anzorena FS, Moreira A, Sarotto L, Ampudia C, et al. Novel technique for identification of ureters using sodium fluorescein. Surg Endosc. 2014;28(9):2730–3.
24. Mahalingam SM, Dip F, Castillo M, Roy M, Wexner SD, Rosenthal RJ, et al. Intraoperative ureter visualization using a novel near-infrared fluorescent dye. Mol Pharm. 2018;15(8):3442–7.
25. van den Bos J, Al-Taher M, Bouvy ND, Stassen LPS. Near-infrared fluorescence laparoscopy of the ureter with three preclinical dyes in a pig model. Surg Endosc. 2019;33(3):986–91.
26. van den Bos J, Al-Taher M, Hsien SG, Bouvy ND, Stassen LPS. Near-infrared fluorescence laparoscopy of the cystic duct and cystic artery: first experience with two new preclinical dyes in a pig model. Surg Endosc. 2017;31(10):4309–14.
27. Al-Taher M, van den Bos J, Schols RM, Kubat B, Bouvy ND, Stassen LPS. Evaluation of a novel dye for near-infrared fluorescence delineation of the ureters during laparoscopy. BJS Open. 2018;2(4):254–61.

Wojciech Polom, Karol Polom, and Marcin Matuszewski

Indications

Radical cystectomy with pelvic lymphadenectomy and urinary diversion is a method of choice for the treatment of muscle invasive bladder cancer (MIBC) [1]. Bladder cancer is the ninth most common malignancy worldwide with 430,000 new cases and more than 165,100 deaths annually [2]. In the case of MIBC, radical cystectomy (RC) is a treatment method of choice. This method increases life expectancy by approximately 50% [3, 4]. Moreover, data suggest that cisplatin-based combination neoadjuvant chemotherapy (NAC) improves the 5-year survival rate [5, 6]. The extent of lymphadenectomy and the number of lymph nodes removed during the operation are a subject of debate. Standard lymphadenectomy involves the removal of nodal tissue cranially up to the common iliac bifurca-

tion, with the ureter as the medial border, including the internal iliac, presacral, obturator fossa, and external iliac nodes [7]. Extended lymphadenectomy adds all lymph nodes in the region of the aortic bifurcation, and presacral and common iliac vessels medial to the crossing ureters [8, 9]. A superextended lymphadenectomy extends cranially to the level of the inferior mesenteric artery [10, 11]. No doubt this issue requires further studies. Cancer recurrence and spread of the tumor cells to the lymph nodes have a significant independent prognostic value for patients' survival [12, 13] and it has been widely explored in other malignancies. In many studies, sentinel lymph node biopsy has been proved to be encouraging; moreover, fluorescence methods of sentinel lymph nodes detection in different cancers has been described [14–16]. It has been shown that in patients with bladder cancer after NAC, the SLNB procedure can be performed regardless of the pT stage, but sentinel node detection played no role in nodal staging [17]. In the meta-analysis of Tee et al., based on 13 studies of sentinel lymph node biopsy after neoadjuvant chemotherapy in initially biopsy-proven node-positive breast cancer patients, the authors proved that the identification rate was 19%, the false negative rate was 14%, and, importantly, the false negative rate was higher when it was based on single mapping [18]. Among well-defined methods of identifying the sentinel lymph nodes, fluorescence seems to be especially interesting; it

Electronic Supplementary Material The online version of this chapter (https://doi.org/10.1007/978-3-030-38092-2_23) contains supplementary material, which is available to authorized users.

W. Polom (✉) · M. Matuszewski
Department of Urology, Medical University of Gdansk, Gdansk, Pomorskie, Poland
e-mail: wojciech.polom@gumed.edu.pl

K. Polom
Department of Oncological Surgery, Medical University of Gdansk, Gdansk, Pomorskie, Poland

does not use radioactivity, it is cheap, easy to use, and harmless both for the patient and for the medical staff.

The number of studies into applications of real-time near infrared fluorescence image-guided surgery is growing [19, 20]. This technique requires the use of fluorophore and special equipment for its detection. Fluorophore is used as an indicator substance that can be detected with the use of special equipment. From among the fluorescent dyes approved by the Food and Drug Administration, Indocyanine green (ICG) is the most widely used and is suitable for use with near infrared (NIR) camera systems. What should be noted is that ICG does not bind specifically to any target after injection. ICG injected into the bladder wall flows through lymphatic vessels to lymphatic nodes. Near infrared light source (laser) is needed for the excitation of the fluorescent dye. The laser is combined with a camera—a detector of fluorescence that records its absorption. Thus, the visualized tissue can be more easily detected and removed—the aim for the use of this system is to improve surgical precision and patient's safety. This is especially useful in the case of laparoscopic and robotic procedures where the near infrared system is integrated with standard robotic or laparoscopic optics providing the surgeon with enhanced vision of different structures. Another advantage may be that better visualization of the tissue that has to be removed can reduce the extent of the resection, which is important in the minimally invasive approach. Finally, it is also possible to visualize important structures that are not to be resected.

The fluorescence-guided surgical technique in bladder cancer is still under development and requires further investigation [21, 22]. Some of the solutions investigated in studies conducted into other malignancies can also be tested for bladder cancer [4, 23]. This chapter offers a few indications for the use of near infrared fluorescence imaging performed during cystectomy. The first one is detection of a possible lymphatic tumor spread during the extirpative part of the procedure, which is possible after cystoscopic injection of the fluorescent dye around the tumor into the bladder wall (Fig. 23.1).

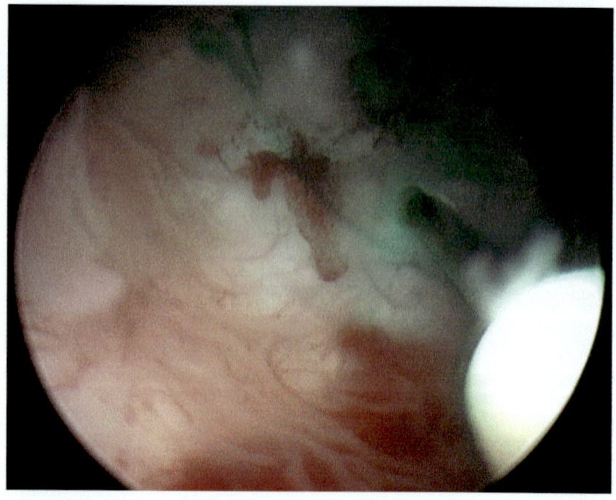

Fig. 23.1 Injection of fluorescent dye indocyanine green (ICG) during cystoscopy into the healthy bladder wall around the tumor site with the use of Williams needle

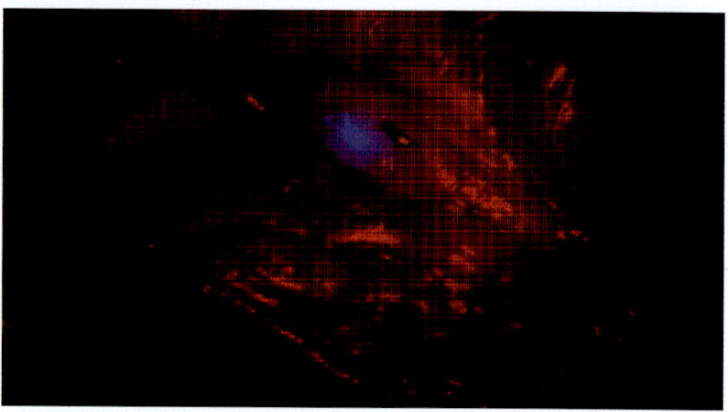

Fig. 23.2 Fluorescent lymph node stained by indocyanine green (ICG) in the common iliac region. Position of the sentinel lymph node is marked with the clip during surgery

The fluorescent dye is taken up from the injection site by the lymphatic tissue and through the lymphatic vessels, and thus may potentially identify bladder lymphatic drainage and mark first lymph nodes draining the lymph from the tumor, that is, sentinel lymph nodes (Fig. 23.2).

This technique can help the surgeon improve lymph node dissection, dissect lymph nodes outside standard template otherwise missed, and potentially improve the oncological outcome. Another interesting application utilizes the fact that after the intravenous injection of ICG during the surgery it is easier to identify mesenteric vasculature, which helps avoid ischemia during urinary diversion preparation with the use of the ileum.

Technical Description of the Procedure(s)

The fluorescent-based technique of sentinel lymph nodes biopsy in muscle invasive bladder cancer is still under development and should be performed in parallel with the standard radioactive technique. To improve cancer staging and decrease morbidity associated with lymph node dissection, the sentinel lymph node biopsy has been introduced in different malignancies [4, 23]. Recently it was adopted in the case of bladder cancer [24]. Significantly, a technique employing hybrid radioactive-fluorescent tracer has been recently proposed in different cancers with promising results [25]. The procedure involves injecting a radiotracer and a fluorescent agent (in the case of hybrid tracer injection, their mixture) into the bladder wall around the tumor site. Intraoperative localization of the first nodes that drain the lymph from the tumor is performed with the use of hand-held gamma probe. The estimation of the lymphatic outflow and of the position of the first lymph nodes with the use of fluorescent agent, indocyanine green (ICG), and near infrared camera has to be deemed an additional method employed to improve intraoperative visualization of lymph vessels and lymph nodes [25] (Fig. 23.3).

The exclusion criteria for this procedure include: allergy to the ICG or iodine or shellfish, pregnancy and lactation period, metastatic cancer, former surgery in the pelvic region, any previous radiotherapy in the pelvic region, and lymph node metastases found on ultrasound or CT (cN+) [24]. Indications for this procedure after neoadjuvant chemotherapy are currently under debate [17].

Sentinel Node Biopsy and Visualization of Lymphatic Structures

First, induction of anesthesia is performed, and the patient is placed in low-lithotomy position. The procedure consists of preoperative rigid or flexible cystoscopy with tracer injection into the bladder wall. An 18-gauge cystoscopic needle is used for tracer injection. For tumors localized in the bladder's triangle, dome, left, right, and back wall, rigid cystoscope should be used. In the case of tumors placed on the front wall of the bladder and its bladder neck, flexible cystoscope should be preferred for better visualization of the tumor. This allows injection of the tracer around the inconveniently located tumors. Please see Video 23.1 Indocyanine green (ICG) injection in cystoscopy.

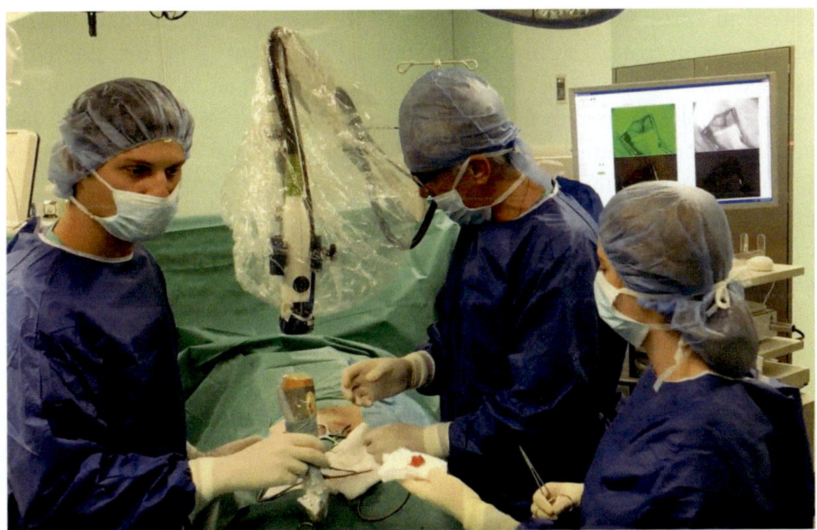

Fig. 23.3 Application of both systems—a radio-guided, hand-held gamma probe and a fluorescent—NIR camera for the detection of tracer-marked lymph nodes

Technique of Parallel Injection of Radiotracer—99m-Technetium and Fluorescent Agent—Indocyanine Green (ICG)

Four doses of the radioactive tracer—99m-Technetium with radioactivity of 5 mCi/ 1 mL—are injected during cystoscopy aimed at the submucosa and superficial detrusor muscle to avoid its perforation circumferentially around the tumor into the healthy tissue and to avoid injection into the scar tissue after transurethral bladder tumor resection (TURBT). See Video 23.2 Injection site bladder. This may affect the outflow of the tracer. The injections are preferred to be performed at 3, 6, 9, and 12 o'clock positions around the tumor at least 12 hours before the surgery. Then, optionally, a single-photon emission computed tomography (SPECT/CT) lymphoscintigraphy can be done to document the visualization of the radioactive lymph nodes before the surgery. This allows for a better preparation of the surgeon for the lymphadenectomy procedure and visualize potentially nonstandard lymphatic outflow and localization of the radioactive lymph nodes outside the standard lymphadenectomy regions, which is observed in some patients [24]. The ICG injection is performed just before the surgery in the same manner, using cystoscopy before the operation. In this case, 10 mg (5 mg/ mL) per dose is injected in the same manner as the radiocolloid the previous day. The ICG is dissolved in water for the injection. In a different method, both tracers are mixed together in one syringe just before injection into the bladder wall. This allows to skip the second cystoscopy and the second injection of the fluorescent agent. It is recommended that the bladder should not be empty after administering the tracer. The outflow of urine from the Foley catheter before the cystectomy should be blocked for some time to allow the bladder to expand naturally with urine. It is important not to leave the bladder empty and not to overflow it either. In this condition, lymphatic vessels are open and this allows the tracer to flow from the injection sites to the first lymph nodes. During the surgery, initial assessment under NIR and white light is performed to assess the ability of fluorescent agent—ICG—to mark the area of the tumor. The surgeon performing the cystectomy can localize this site with high accuracy guided by the infrared image provided by the NIR camera to dissect tissues in this region more carefully and to possibly widen the resection in the tumor site so as not to leave any potentially remaining tumor behind. Please see Video 23.3 Sentinel lymph nodes identification. The dissection of the bladder starting on both lateral sites is conducted from the anterior abdominal wall inferior-superior to expose the surface of the iliac vessels to the level of the aortic bifurcation. During the whole procedure, continuous systematic examination of the operative field conducted by a NIR camera is performed to visualize the flow of the ICG in lymphatic vessels to lymph nodes. Fluorescent lymph nodes are marked. Mobilization of the ureters, transposition of the left ureter behind sigmoid mesentery, and bowel preparation with vascular pedicle preparation are performed next. Localization of the radioactive lymph nodes is assessed with the precise use of a hand-held gamma probe. After removing both the tracer-marked fluorescent and radioactive lymph nodes, lymphadenectomy is performed from the aortic bifurcation distally to the endopelvic fascia. If tracer-marked lymph nodes are found outside the standard lymphadenectomy templates, extended lymph node dissection is possible, but should be performed with caution. Nodal packets are sent separately for standard permanent pathologic examination. The nodes marked by tracers are sent for pathologic examination and are examined according to the sentinel lymph node protocol for metastases and micrometastases (Fig. 23.4). Please see Video 23.4 Sentinel lymph node after excision.

This technique allows performance of sentinel lymph node biopsy with the use of hybrid tracer. This compound is a conjunction of radioactive 99 m-technetium and indocyanine green. The connection between both compounds is highly durable by covalent binding and its creation requires special preparation. This compound is characterized by the simultaneous presence of both properties: radioactivity and fluorescence. With the use of this hybrid tracer, only one injection

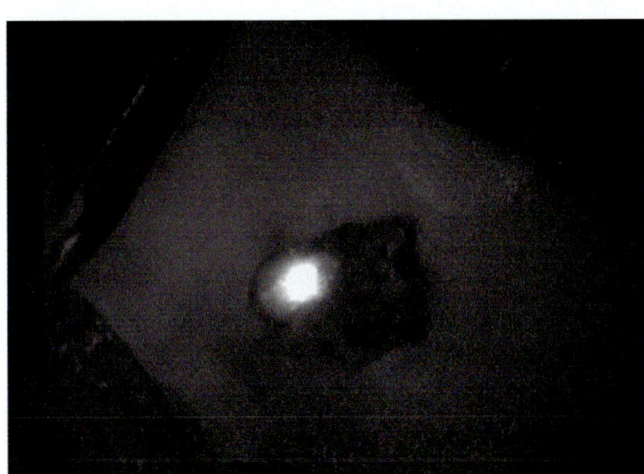

Fig. 23.4 Sentinel lymph node after excision seen in gray scale with the use of a NIR camera. Technique with the use of hybrid radioactive—fluorescent tracer (99m-technetium-indocyanine green)

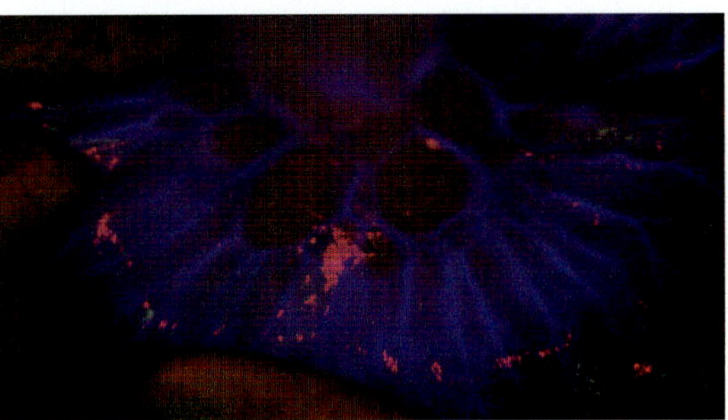

Fig. 23.5 Mesenteric live angiography for identification of mesenteric arcades after intravenous ICG injection

procedure is performed in the same manner as described in the case of single tracer. Both detection systems—gamma camera and near infrared camera are used for lymph nodes identification. Cystectomy procedure remains the same as described above.

Angiography of Mesenteric Vessels

Ileal conduit is performed with the use of distal ileum at least 15 cm proximal to the ileocecal valve. During bowel preparation, 2 mL (2.5 mg/mL) of ICG is additionally administered intravenously to perform life mesenteric angiography for identification of mesenteric arcades. This technique allows to maximally preserve the blood supply to the ileal conduit with additional benefit of safe preparation of the mesentery. If a NIR camera for open surgery is used, it can be held by the surgeon or it can be attached to a special arm connected to the camera set allowing it to be placed near the operating field covered in sterile covers. In the case of laparoscopic or robotic NIR camera use, the view can be switched from normal endoscopic to fluorescent-guided image or overlay of the fluorescent filter on the real image can be used with the special filter installed in the camera set. Those images can be switched with the use of the button on the camera head or a foot switch depending on the used camera set (Fig. 23.5).

Interpretation

Customization of the diagnosis and treatment of different cancers has been recently gaining approval. In the case of bladder cancer, due to numerous variables such as tumor position in the bladder, the number of tumors, as well as complicated lymphatic drainage of the tumor, it is of great importance to treat every patient individually. While performing the SLNB procedure with ICG, one has to be aware of the downsides of both the substance and the technique [12, 26]. On the one hand, ICG is valuable in visualization of the lymphatic drainage and in visualization of SLNs. On the other, the depth of fluorescence penetration through the tissue, especially in obese patients, is relatively small; currently it is about 1–3 cm, which makes it difficult to detect SLNs that are located deeper in the adipose tissue. It is likely that thanks to using hybrid ICG-99m-technetium dyes, it will be possible to improve this parameter and eliminate the drawbacks of this substance in the future [27].

New diagnostic and visualization methods applied during diagnosis as well as intraoperatively create better, more effective treatment options. This allows identifying patients with a nonstandard course of the disease, in whom additional information prior to surgery can affect the extent of the applied procedure.

The treatment of MIBC patients is still evolving, especially in the case of minimally invasive approaches such as laparoscopic and robotic techniques of cystectomy and extensive pelvic lymph node dissection. Interpretation of new findings and results of new imaging techniques during operation are of great importance, but it must be noted that they have to be interpreted with caution and should not affect standard treatment protocol for the patient.

Interpretation of Injection of ICG into the Bladder Wall and Interpretation of Visualization of Injection Site During Surgery

Injection of ICG is performed with the use of cystoscope before the surgical procedure. It is important to assess injection sites very carefully. We recommend injecting the tracer around the tumor into the healthy tissue, avoiding injection into the tumor and avoiding injection into scar tissue after the TURBT procedure. Injections should be performed superficially under the mucosa to avoid bladder puncture. During the surgery after exposure of the bladder, the surgeon, guided by the image with the use of an NIR camera, can clearly identify the place where the injections were performed and where the tumor is located. This allows them to prepare tissues with more caution to avoid unintentional bladder rupture in the place where the tumor is located. What is more, visualization of the place where the tumor is located allows for wider preparation of tissues near the bladder wall, especially in the case of invading the muscle bladder wall and serosa of the bladder. This technique provides a good chance to achieve clear surgical margins.

Interpretation of Sentinel Lymph Node Biopsy Procedure with the Use of ICG and NIR Camera

After cystoscopic ICG injection into the bladder wall, the fluorescent tracer spreads through the lymphatic vessels to the lymph nodes. The flow of the tracer is fast, so the surgeon does not have to wait for its spread during the surgery, and so the injection can be performed just before or even during the surgery.

A NIR camera detects fluorescent lymphatic vessels as well as lymphatic nodes. In the case of bladder cancer, lymphatic outflow is complex, so the number of the first nodes that drain the lymph from the tumor site can vary. ICG is a small particle, so it flows rapidly through the lymphatic system and its spread from the first to the second and next lymphatic nodal stations can be observed. Because of ICG's small particle size, the number of sentinel lymph nodes can vary when compared to the radiotracer technique with the use of bigger compound 99m-technetium nanocolloid [21].

Interpretation of Mesenteric Fluorescence Angiography After Intravenous ICG Injection for Identification of Mesenteric Arcades in Preparation of ILEAL Conduit

The creation of urinary ileostomy is one of the elements of the cystectomy procedure in a selected group of patients that allows the urine outflow outside the abdominal cavity after bladder excision. The Ileal conduit uses a segment of the distal ileum for the diversion of urinary flow from ureters. The mesentery of this segment is incised and prepared in a careful manner. During bowel preparation, the segment is resected from the intestine with the blood supply intact. Large vessels of the mesentery must be spared during this process to prevent damage of the ileal conduit and digestive anastomosis. This can be achieved with the use of the transluminatory technique in which a satellite lamp is used at right angles to the bowel, allowing the identification of large vessels. This technique is impossible to perform in the case of laparoscopy and robotic procedures. The fluorescent technique for identification of mesenteric vessels consists of an intravenous ICG injection, the use of a NIR camera during bowel preparation, and assessment of the vascularization of ileal segment. After the intravenous injection of ICG, the surgeon can perform live fluorescent angiography. In this case, a clear picture of mesenteric vessels is revealed. First, arteries are identified, then veins. This technique allows for the selection of the right vessels for closure during ileal segment preparation. Please see Video 23.5 Ileal conduit angiography.

Pitfalls

Near infrared fluorescence applications in the case of bladder cancer are still under development. New techniques are being described and the use of fluorescent agents and near infrared camera systems are being standardized. As in every new procedure, a learning curve needs to be performed in the best way to avoid pitfalls and adverse events. We describe our problems and doubts while using fluorescent agent ICG in the case of bladder cancer.

First of all, the procedures with the use of a fluorescent agent for bladder tumor visualization, the SLNB procedure, and live angiography are additional procedures for standard cystectomy and lymphadenectomy. They require additional time to perform before, during, and after the surgery. They cause extra costs because of the use of additional equipment and extended pathological examination.

Considering the use of the near infrared camera systems, it must be noted that some of them require turning off the operating light during their use, and some of them also require turning off the light in the operating room. This was a disadvantage of the early systems because it was almost impossible to continue the surgical procedure. However, most of the newly developed systems do not require such conditions and they can be used with the lights on. As for the laparoscopic and robotic systems, the intensity of the light can be controlled according to the surgeon's needs. Some systems are designed for open surgeries, others for open and laparoscopic ones. It is good to choose the system adequately for the needs of the operating team and the performed procedures. In open procedures, especially in pelvic lymphadenectomy, the position of the camera has to be adjusted because of its suggested position—15 cm in front of the target site. This minimizes the operating field and clear view of the

operating field, especially for the assisting surgeon. In the case of new robotic systems, NIR cameras are added as standard equipment, which eliminates the problem with camera positioning. Please see Video 23.6 Camera position during open procedure.

Another problem that may arise during the procedure is the injection of ICG outside the bladder wall and spilling of the fluorescent agent in the case of unintentional puncture of the bladder and injecting the marker out of its wall into the peritoneal cavity. This should be particularly noted in the case of female patients, the elderly, or men who have been diagnosed with bladder trabeculation in which the bladder wall is much thinner than normal. If the marker is spilled, the operating field is contaminated with ICG, which does not interfere with the cystectomy and standard lymphadenectomy itself, but makes it difficult or impossible to identify the appropriate sentinel lymph nodes. Please see Video 23.7 Indocyanine green (ICG) spillage and field contamination. Moreover, during the SLNB procedure, when an exact lymph node is dissected, contamination of the surrounding tissues with ICG can appear. It is useful to close the lymph vessels on both sides of the lymph node with clips before its removal to avoid this problem (Fig. 23.6).

In some cases, there is no outflow of the fluorescent agent to the lymph nodes. This occurs mainly in the case of locally advanced disease, after wide and deep TURBT procedure or in the case of lymph nodes metastases blocking the

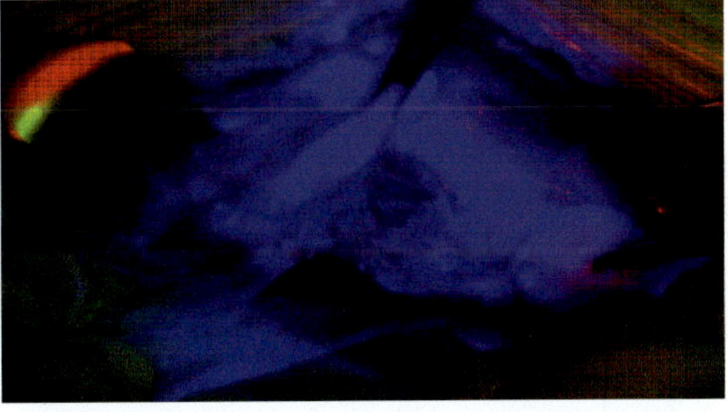

Fig. 23.6 Spillage of a fluorescent agent and operating field contamination after unintentional puncture of the bladder and injecting indocyanine green (ICG) out of its wall into the peritoneal cavity

flow of lymph with ICG. In those cases, the SLNB procedure is impossible to perform.

In the case of patients with obesity, there are some limitations to this technique. Penetration of the laser light, fluorescent dye excitation, and infrared visualization might be difficult because of excessive fat tissue. It is proven that the NIR camera system can detect fluorescence at a shallow depth [28]. In those cases, fat tissue preparation is recommended to allow the exposure of the lymphatic tissue and the bladder wall.

The surgeon using additional substance injected to the patient's body must be aware of anaphylactic reaction. ICG is a safe drug with no deaths reported after its use; however, in some cases anaphylactic reaction was reported. Some adverse events were associated with comorbidities including preexisting drug allergy, severe asthma, and shellfish allergy [29]. It is advised to be prepared for such possibilities during and after the surgery.

There are some limitations to injecting the tracer into the bladder wall in the case of bladder cancer. Some patients are diagnosed with multifocal tumors. Some tumors are very big, often involving the greater part of the bladder, making it impossible to find healthy tissue for injecting the tracer. Some tumors also bleed heavily, making the injection of the tracer hard to perform.

In the case of patients with MIBC after neoadjuvant chemotherapy, SLNB is under investigation and the results of such studies should be viewed with caution [17]. There are still no data of SLNB with the use of fluorescent agent in this group of patients. Future studies are required to prove its efficacy.

Fluorescence techniques in the case of bladder cancer are recently added to the patient's management. They are very promising and their additional value to image-guided surgery requires further research in order to test and prove their usefulness.

References

1. Stenzl A, Cowan NC, De Santis M, Kuczyk MA, Merseburger AS, Ribal MJ, et al. Treatment of muscle-invasive and metastatic bladder cancer: update of the EAU guidelines. Eur Urol. 2011;59(6):1009–18.
2. Torre LA, Bray F, Siegel RL, Ferlay J. Interpretation of model in modelling ecological niche.pdf. 2015;65(2):87–108.
3. Witjes JA, Compérat E, Cowan NC, De Santis M, Gakis G, Lebret T, et al. EAU guidelines on muscle-invasive and metastatic bladder cancer: summary of the 2013 guidelines. Eur Urol. 2013;65(4):778–92.
4. Van der Pas MHGM, Meijer S, Hoekstra OS, Riphagen II, De Vet HCW, Knol DL, et al. Sentinel-lymph-node procedure in colon and rectal cancer: a systematic review and meta-analysis. Lancet Oncol. 2011;12(6):540–50.
5. Vale CL. Neoadjuvant chemotherapy in invasive bladder cancer: update of a systematic review and meta-analysis of individual patient data. Eur Urol. 2005;48(2):202–5.
6. Yin M, Joshi M, Meijer RP, Glantz M, Holder S, Harvey HA, et al. Neoadjuvant chemotherapy for muscle-invasive bladder cancer: a systematic review and two-step meta-analysis. Oncologist [Internet]. 2016;21(6):708–15. Available from: http://theoncologist.alphamedpress.org/lookup/doi/10.1634/theoncologist.2015-0440.
7. Simone G, Papalia R, Ferriero M, Guaglianone S, Castelli E, Collura D, et al. Stage-specific impact of extended versus standard pelvic lymph node dissection in radical cystectomy. Int J Urol. 2013;20(4):390–7.
8. Holmer M, Bendahl P-O, Davidsson T, Gudjonsson S, Mansson W, Liedberg F. Extended lymph node dissection in patients with urothelial cell carcinoma of the bladder: can it make a difference? World J Urol. 2009;27(4):521–6.
9. Poulsen AL, Horn T, Steven K. Radical cystectomy: extending the limits of pelvic lymph node dissection improves survival for patients with bladder cancer confined to the bladder wall. J Urol. 1998;160(6 Pt 1):2015–9; discussion 2020.
10. Zlotta AR. Limited, extended, superextended, mega-extended pelvic lymph node dissection at the time of radical cystectomy: what should we perform? Eur Urol. Switzerland. 2012;61:243–4.
11. Zehnder P, Studer UE, Skinner EC, Dorin RP, Cai J, Roth B, et al. Super extended versus extended pelvic lymph node dissection in patients undergoing radical cystectomy for bladder cancer: a comparative study. J Urol. 2011;186(4):1261–8.
12. Billy GG. NIH Public Access. 2015;6(9):790–5.
13. Davison KK, Birch LL. NIH Public Access. 2008;64(12):2391–404.
14. Polom K, Murawa D, Rho Y-S, Nowaczyk P, Hunerbein M, Murawa P. Current trends and emerging future of indocyanine green usage in surgery and oncology: a literature review. Cancer. 2011;117(21):4812–22.
15. Polom K, Murawa D, Rho YS, Spychala A, Murawa P. Skin melanoma sentinel lymph node biopsy using real-time fluorescence navigation with indocyanine green and indocyanine green with human serum albumin. Br J Dermatol. England. 2012;166:682–3.

16. Polom K, Murawa D, Nowaczyk P, Rho YS, Murawa P. Breast cancer sentinel lymph node mapping using near infrared guided indocyanine green and indocyanine green—human serum albumin in comparison with gamma emitting radioactive colloid tracer. Eur J Surg Oncol. 2012;38(2):137–42.

17. Rosenblatt R, Johansson M, Alamdari F, Sidiki A, Holmström B, Hansson J, et al. Sentinel node detection in muscle-invasive urothelial bladder cancer is feasible after neoadjuvant chemotherapy in all pT stages, a prospective multicenter report. World J Urol. 2017;35(6):921–7.

18. Tee SR, Devane LA, Evoy D, Rothwell J, Geraghty J, Prichard RS, et al. Meta-analysis of sentinel lymph node biopsy after neoadjuvant chemotherapy in patients with initial biopsy-proven node-positive breast cancer. Br J Surg [Internet]. 2018;105(12):1541–52. Available from: http://doi.wiley.com/10.1002/bjs.10986.

19. Menon M, Hemal AK, Tewari A, Shrivastava A, Shoma AM, El-Tabey NA, et al. Nerve-sparing robot-assisted radical cystoprostatectomy and urinary diversion. BJU Int. 2003;92(3):232–6.

20. Parekh DJ, Messer J, Fitzgerald J, Ercole B, Svatek R. Perioperative outcomes and oncologic efficacy from a pilot prospective randomized clinical trial of open versus robotic assisted radical cystectomy. J Urol [Internet]. 2013;189(2):474–9. Available from: https://doi.org/10.1016/j.jur0.2012.09.077.

21. Polom W, Markuszewski M, Cytawa W, Czapiewski P, Lass P, Matuszewski M. Fluorescent versus radioguided lymph node mapping in bladder cancer. Clin Genitourin Cancer [Internet]. 2017;15(3):e405–9. Available from: https://doi.org/10.1016/j.clgc.2016.11.007.

22. Manny TB, Hemal AK. Fluorescence-enhanced robotic radical cystectomy using unconjugated indocyanine green for pelvic lymphangiography, tumor marking, and mesenteric angiography: the initial clinical experience. Urology [Internet]. 2014;83(4):824–9. Available from: https://doi.org/10.1016/j.urology.2013.11.042.

23. Markuszewski M, Polom W, Cytawa W, Czapiewski P, Lass P, Matuszewski M. Comparison of real-time fluorescent indocyanine green and99mTc-nanocolloid radiotracer navigation in sentinel lymph node biopsy of penile cancer. Clin Genitourin Cancer [Internet]. 2015;13(6):574–80. Available from: https://doi.org/10.1016/j.clgc.2015.06.005.

24. Polom W, Markuszewski M, Cytawa W, Lass P, Matuszewski M. Radio-guided lymph node mapping in bladder cancer using SPECT/CT and intraoperative γ-probe methods. Clin Nucl Med. 2016;41(8):e362–7.

25. van den Berg NS, Buckle T, KleinJan GH, van der Poel HG, van Leeuwen FWB. Multispectral fluorescence imaging during robot-assisted laparoscopic sentinel node biopsy: a first step towards a fluorescence-based anatomic roadmap. Eur Urol [Internet]. 2017;72(1):110–7. Available from: https://doi.org/10.1016/j.eurur0.2016.06.012.

26. Zelken JA, Tufaro AP. Current trends and emerging future of indocyanine green usage in surgery and oncology: an update. Ann Surg Oncol. 2015;22:1271–83.

27. Van Der Poel HG, Buckle T, Brouwer OR, Valdés Olmos RA, Van Leeuwen FWB. Intraoperative laparoscopic fluorescence guidance to the sentinel lymph node in prostate cancer patients: clinical proof of concept of an integrated functional imaging approach using a multimodal tracer. Eur Urol. 2011;60(4):826–33.

28. Hawrysz DJ, Sevick-Muraca EM. Developments toward diagnostic breast cancer imaging using near-infrared optical measurements and fluorescent contrast agents. Neoplasia [Internet]. 2000;2(5):388–417. Available from: http://linkinghub.elsevier.com/retrieve/pii/S147655860080010X.

29. Chu W, Chennamsetty A, Toroussian R, Lau C. Anaphylactic shock after intravenous administration of indocyanine green during robotic partial nephrectomy. Urol Case Rep [Internet]. 2017;12:37–8. Available from: https://doi.org/10.1016/j.eucr.2017.02.006.

Wojciech Polom, Karol Polom, and Marcin Matuszewski

Indications

There is no radiological imaging technique that can detect micro-metastases in lymph nodes in the case of penile cancer. For intermediate and high-risk pT1 tumors as well as T2-T4 tumors invasive nodal staging is recommended [1, 2]. There are two standard methods of invasive nodal staging—a dynamic sentinel lymph node biopsy (DSNB) and a modified inguinal lymphadenectomy (mILND) [3]. In the case of DSNB, 99m-technetium (99mTc) nanocolloid is injected around the tumor site into the healthy tissue one day before the surgery. The intraoperative assessment is performed with the use of a hand-held gamma probe. In some cases, methylene blue (MB) is injected in the same manner as an additional dye in order to better visualize sentinel lymph nodes (SLNs) during their excision. The

identification of the lymph nodes stained by MB is performed by the surgeon with the naked eye, without any additional tools for visualization. This method is standardized and is routinely used [4]. Sensitivity of DSLNB is reported to be as high as 88% and increases to 90% when MB is added as a second dye for better lymph nodes visualization [5]. mILND is an alternative option where the medial superficial inguinal lymph nodes and the lymph nodes from the central zone are removed from both groins [5]. Neither method of invasive staging provides absolute certainty that metastatic lymph nodes have been excised and may overlook micro-metastatic disease that can lead to regional recurrence. Identification of the right lymph node during its biopsy can cause some problems for the surgeon. Better visualization of the sentinel lymph node (SLN) can help to locate it during the operation, especially in difficult cases or in patients with obesity, in whom they are placed deeper and may be hard to distinguish from the fat tissue. Lately, the near-infrared fluorescence image-guided surgery has been getting much interest as it may help in the diagnosis, staging, and treatment of different malignancies including penile cancer. The potential benefit of the use of this new method in the case of DSLNB in penile cancer is still under investigation. Recent research has shown that this method can be used safely and efficiently in this indication when compared to standard techniques with the routinely used radiotracers [6].

Electronic Supplementary Material The online version of this chapter (https://doi.org/10.1007/978-3-030-38092-2_24) contains supplementary material, which is available to authorized users.

W. Polom (✉) · M. Matuszewski
Department of Urology, Medical University of Gdansk, Gdansk, Pomorskie, Poland
e-mail: wojciech.polom@gumed.edu.pl

K. Polom
Department of Oncological Surgery, Medical University of Gdansk, Gdansk, Pomorskie, Poland

© Springer Nature Switzerland AG 2020
E. M. Aleassa, K. M. El-Hayek (eds.), *Video Atlas of Intraoperative Applications of Near Infrared Fluorescence Imaging*, https://doi.org/10.1007/978-3-030-38092-2_24

Technical Description of the Procedure(s)

The technique with the use of indocyanine green (ICG) and near-infrared fluorescence (NIRF) camera in the case of DSLNB in penile cancer patients is not a standard method and must be approached with caution. This technique is still under development and because of the low incidence of penile cancer, there are only a few publications describing its use as a single agent [6, 7] or as a hybrid tracer [8]. As for now it should be used as an addition to the radio-guided technique, which is recommended by the European Urological Association. During the procedure, the patient is placed on the operating table in supine position with both legs rotated outside to allow access to the penis and both groin regions. The open technique is used for DSLNB as the standard in which skin incision is performed above the region identified preoperatively by gamma probe detection of the radioactivity of the radiotracers. In this area sentinel lymph node containing radioactive agent is detected. Laparoscopic and robotic approaches are not used during DSLNB but are used in the case of groin lymphadenectomy when metastatic lymph nodes are found. In this case, three ports and one assist port are placed in a V configuration below the tip of femoral triangle.

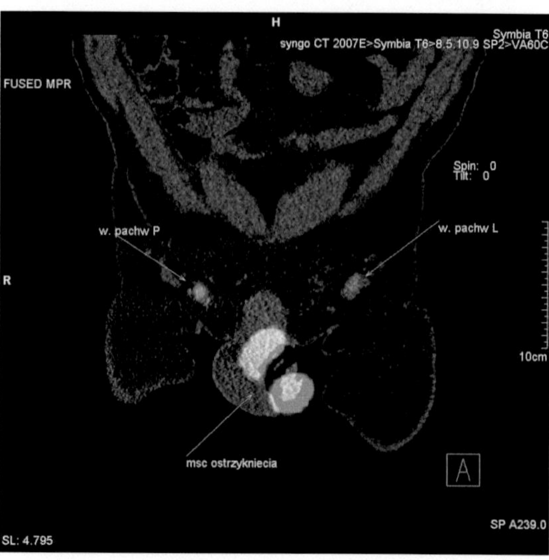

Fig. 24.1 SPECT/CT lymphoscintigraphy after the radioactive tracer 99m-technetium injection. Injection sites of the tracer and radioactive lymph nodes are clearly visible

The results are transferred to the surgeon in the operating theater and an intraoperative localization of radioactive lymphatic nodes is performed with the use of a hand-held gamma probe. After their identification, the skin is incised above the region of radioactivity, tissues are dissected, and SLNS are identified. Then their excision is performed, lymphatic vessels located and identified with the naked eye, and finally the site is closed and ligated.

Radio-Guided Technique

Before the planned operation 99mTc-nanocolloid is given in four intradermal injections into the healthy tissue at the lesion site. The activity of 1 mCi in 1 mL is recommended for injection. Approximately 1 hour after its injection, a single-photon emission computerized tomography—computed tomography (SPECT-CT) lymphoscintigraphy—is planned and performed, followed by the reconstruction and fusion of images. Any activity of the radiotracer detected in the groin region, a part of the site where tracer was administered, is considered for SLNS (Fig. 24.1).

Fluorescent Technique

In the case of the fluorescent technique, it is of great importance to inject the fluorescent dye at a different time scheme than the radiotracer. The ICG particle is small and can flow easily through the lymphatic system. An injection performed during the procedure allows for live lymphatic outflow visualization and identification of first lymph nodes. When injected in the same scheme as the radiotracer the day before surgery, more fluorescent lymph nodes are expected to be found. Preoperatively, ICG is injected intradermally into the healthy penile tissue proximally to the tumor mass (0.5 mL of 2 mg/kg concentration). Video 24.1 presents the injection technique and lymphatic route identification (Fig. 24.2).

Lymphatic vessels and first lymph nodes draining the lymph from the tumor are visualized with the use of a near-infrared (NIRF) camera. Lymphatic outflow of ICG is seen immediately after its injection. Lymph nodes can be visualized approximately 15 minutes after administrating the tracer [7]. This technique is presented in Video 24.2. In the open technique, skin incision is performed above the fluorescent region where SLN is detected (Fig. 24.3).

In patients with obesity, identification of fluorescent lymph nodes before skin incision and tissue preparation is in many cases uncertain. In those cases, we recommend to turn off the surgical light or even the lights in the operating room and perform this identification in darkness. In some cases, skin incision above the central zone of inguinal lymph nodes has to be performed and fat tissue preparation is necessary to allow the identification of fluorescent nodes. The fluorescent technique also allows for lymphatic vessels identification during the biopsy procedure, allowing for their highly accurate identification and ligation. This clear, live view during the procedure offers the operating surgeon the ability to dissect lymphatic vessels carefully and close them accurately to avoid complications after the surgery such as lymphocoele and prolonged leakage of the lymph. Excision of the sentinel lymph node identified with the use of ICG and NIRF camera is presented in Video 24.3. Also, the intraoperatively use of Near-Infrared Fluorescent Camera system for fluorescent lymph nodes identification is shown in Video 24.4 (Fig. 24.4).

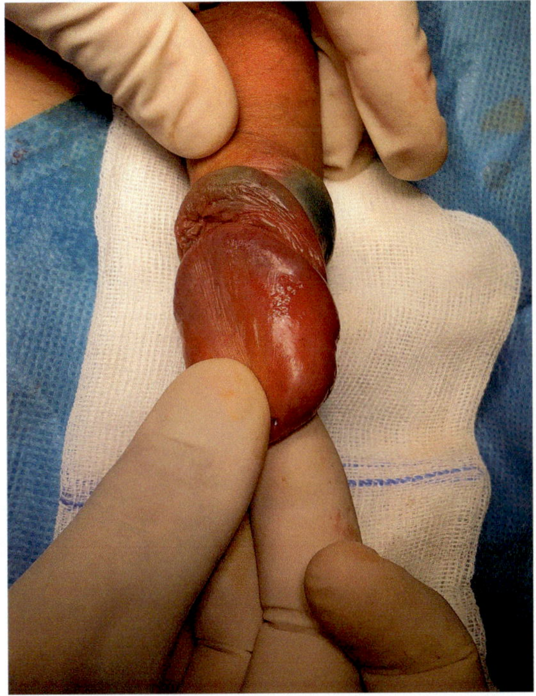

Fig. 24.2 Injection site of ICG proximally to the tumor site on the glans of the penis into the healthy tissue

Fig. 24.3 Identification of sentinel lymph node with the use of the fluorescent tracer ICG and a NIRF camera

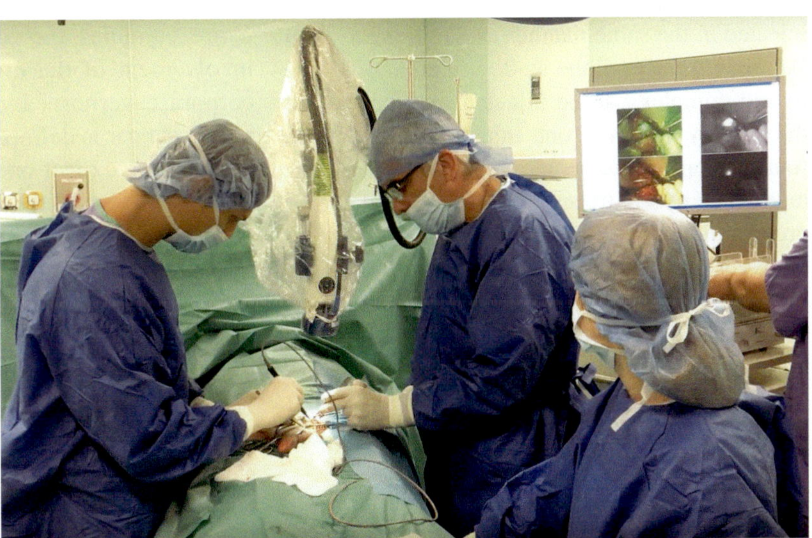

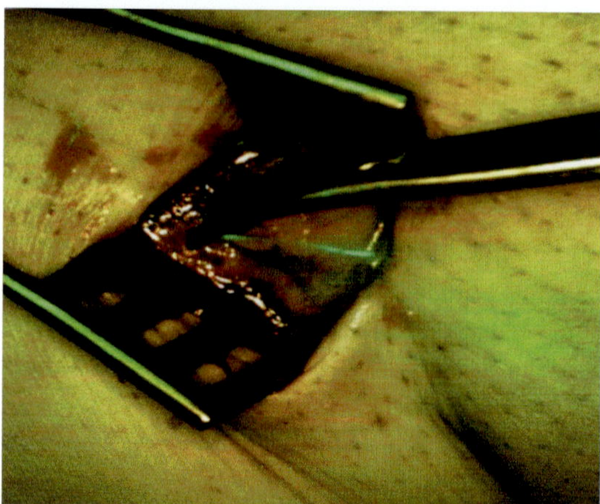

Fig. 24.4 Intraoperative identification of small lymphatic vessel draining the lymph from the tumor site to the first lymph node—sentinel lymph node

Hybrid Radio-Fluorescent Technique

A hybrid tracer 99mTc-nanocolloid—ICG is an innovative imaging tracer. It can provide additional information during sentinel lymph nodes detection and increase the accuracy of their excision [9]. With the use of the hybrid radio-fluorescent tracer (ICG-99mTch), both detecting systems have to be used during the surgery—hand-held gamma probe and a near-infrared camera (the hybrid tracer can be located with both systems in this manner). The hybrid tracer is injected in the same manner as a radiotracer or a fluorescent tracer alone as described above. The hybrid complex can be injected one day before the surgery and only one injection divided into four portions has to be administered. The advantage of the hybrid tracer is that it can be detected preoperatively in SPECT/CT scans and intraoperatively just before the skin incision, which in the case of the single fluorescent dye usage is in many cases difficult or impossible. What is more, this complex flows to the first lymph node and because of its big particle size it stays in the first lymph node and does not flow to secondary nodal stations (Fig. 24.5).

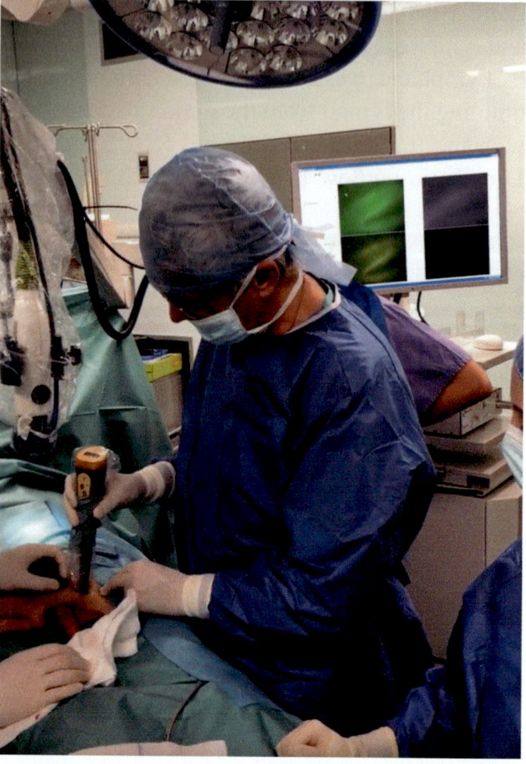

Fig. 24.5 Parallel sentinel lymph node identification during the DSLNB procedure with the use of a hand-held gamma probe and a near infrared fluorescent camera

Interpretation

Patients with penile cancer should be treated individually because of its rare incidence and many variables including the tumor position, involvement of the urethra, or invasion of the corpora cavernosa. Lymphatic drainage of the penile cancer is defined as simple, which means that we can expect one lymph node that drains the lymph from the penile cancer (primary lymph node) and secondary lymph nodes receiving the lymph from the primary node. This observation was made due to using radioactive tracers. In the case of a fluorescent agent such as ICG that has smaller particle size (1.2 nm) than nanocolloid (8 nm) means it can flow through lymphatic vessels to the secondary nodal stations more easily and mark higher number of lymph nodes than the radiotracer. It was proven that using both tracers (fluorescent and radioactive) independently in the same patient resulted in a different number of fluorescent-SLNs and radioactive-SLNs detected. In our experience, both methods of sentinel lymph nodes identification in the case of penile cancer offer comparable results [6, 10]. Video 24.5 presents intraoperative identification of sentinel lymph node with the use of NIRF system and hand-held gamma probe in the case of hybrid technique.

Pitfalls

Near-infrared fluorescence procedures in the case of penile cancer are a novelty. A dedicated team with previous experience in performing those procedures in a traditional way with the use of a radiotracer is recommended while performing the fluorescence technique because the learning curve has been described to achieve satisfactory results with the localization of sentinel lymph nodes [11]. We recommend performing the fluorescent procedure parallel to the radioactive one, which remains the standard technique. The most advanced technique with the use of a hybrid fluorescent-radioactive tracer and a hybrid image-guided surgery has been gaining much interest recently but their added value is yet to be proven. The procedures with the use of a hybrid tracer can be more accurate and independent of the use of other dyes such as methylene blue [12]. There are, however, some issues with fluorescent-guided surgery. Patients after previous surgical procedures on penis such as circumcision or other plastic surgeries should be evaluated with care; there are no data whether previous surgery on the penis may disturb the outflow of the lymph from the organ. Moreover, in patients after partial penectomy or laser treatment without lymph nodes estimation, the tracer injection can be difficult or even impossible to perform. In those cases, standard procedures of lymph nodes estimation should be applied. Also, patients after

previous procedures in the groin like hernia repair or orchidectomy should be considered for standard lymph nodes estimation since no data are available on this subject.

The fluorescent technique can be a challenge in patients with obesity since the dedicated cameras are capable of detecting the fluorescent dye at the depth up to 1–2 cm, which in such patients can provide false results of nodes detection. In some cases, simple small skin incision above the expected sentinel lymph node position and fat preparation should be enough for the fluorescence detection, yet it can cause problems during the image-guided surgery. Old NIRF systems required dimming the light in the operating room or even turning off the operating lamp and the light in the operating room to better see the fluorescence of the object of interest. New systems do not require such conditions and the whole visualization of the fluorescent object can be performed in normal operating conditions.

Different sentinel lymph nodes count with the use of parallel radio and fluorescent technique can cause unnecessary confusion during the DSLN biopsy procedure. This is because of the different particle sizes used for their identification and the different times of their administration. The ICG particle is much smaller than the 99m-technetium nanocolloid and can flow more easily through lymph nodes, thus making the identification of more ICG-stained lymph nodes possible. Different time of administration of both technetium and ICG is important. To have the best chance of visualization of only one—the first node that drains the lymph from the tumor—ICG should be administered during the surgical procedure. It is possible to visualize the lymphangiography live with the use of a near-infrared camera and assess the location of the first lymph node. As for now, we recommend to follow the standard recommendations and apply the radioactive method as the standard identification method unless proven otherwise. This problem should not appear in the case of hybrid tracer use.

Allergy to ICG is rare. Studies performed on large numbers of patients report serious adverse events after its administration as extremely rare—0.05% [13]. Other authors report only clinical cases of anaphylactic shock after the intravenous administration of ICG in the case of patients after partial nephrectomy [14].

Adverse effects and long-term morbidity after ICG usage for sentinel lymph node detection such as mild lymphedema or minor functional deficit have been observed. Moreover, persistent discoloration of the skin or a tattoo after subdermal ICG injection has been described by authors in one patient in whom it lasted for 11 months after the dye injection [15].

We can expect surgical field contamination after fluorescent agent injection into the penis. This can cause some problems with identifying healthy penile tissue and the tumor for resection (Fig. 24.6).

The fluorescent agent is injected superficially under the penile skin around the tumor. After penile skin incision the operating surgeon can identify colorful subcutaneous and lymphatic tissue making it hard to differentiate between healthy and cancerous tissue. We recommend not injecting the fluorescent agent into the glans of the penis and we recommend performing the injection proximal from the tumor site at least 2 cm into the healthy tissue. This allows the surgeon to maintain the surgical field uncontaminated (Fig. 24.7).

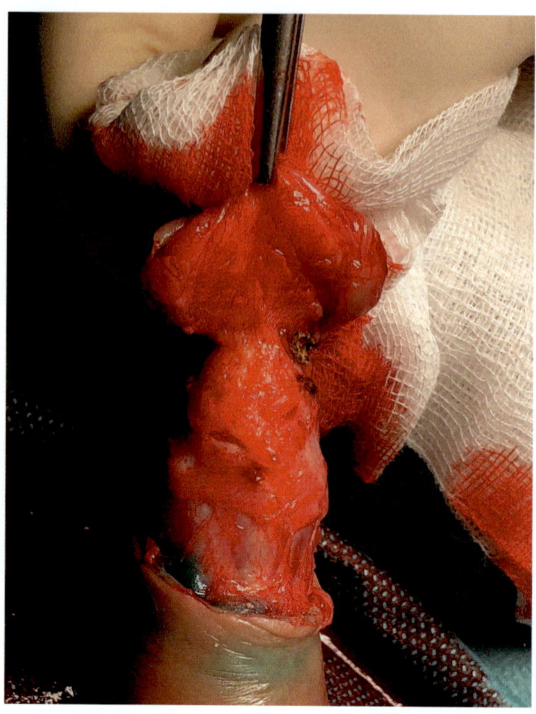

Fig. 24.7 Uncontaminated surgical field after the ICG injection around the tumor site during the glansectomy procedure, seen in white light with the naked eye. The injection site is preformed proximal to the tumor site

Near-infrared imaging systems have recently become more available clinically; indications for fluorescence image-guided surgery are expanding so we hope that this technique will find more approval in the case of penile cancer treatment. ICG offers a new and safe alternative or an addition to the standard DSLNB procedure with the use of radiotracers. Patients' benefit and clinical outcome still need to be proven.

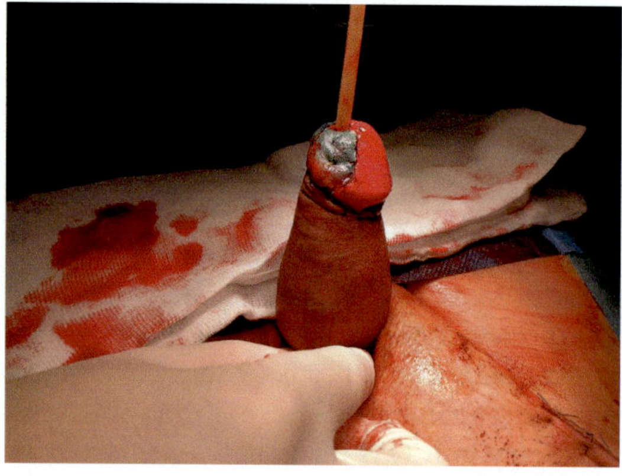

Fig. 24.6 Contamination of the skin flap used for partial glans reconstruction by fluorescent agent—the ICG injected too close to the tumor site

References

1. Windahl T, Andersson S-O. Combined laser treatment for penile carcinoma: results after long-term followup. J Urol. 2003;169(6):2118–21.
2. Colecchia M, Nicolai N, Secchi P, Bandieramonte G, Paganoni AM, Sangalli LM, et al. pT1 penile squamous cell carcinoma: a clinicopathologic study of 56 cases treated by C02 laser therapy. Anal Quant Cytol Histol. 2009;31(3):153–60.
3. Zou Z-J, Liu Z-H, Tang L-Y, Wang Y-J, Liang J-Y, Zhang R-C, et al. Radiocolloid-based dynamic sentinel lymph node biopsy in penile cancer with clini-

cally negative inguinal lymph node: an updated systematic review and meta-analysis. Int Urol Nephrol. 2016;48(12):2001–13.

4. van Bezooijen BP, Horenblas S, Meinhardt W, Newling DW. Laser therapy for carcinoma in situ of the penis. J Urol. 2001;166(5):1670–1.

5. Shindel AW, Mann MW, Lev RY, Sengelmann R, Petersen J, Hruza GJ, et al. Mohs micrographic surgery for penile cancer: management and long-term followup. J Urol. 2007;178(5):1980–5.

6. Markuszewski M, Polom W, Cytawa W, Czapiewski P, Lass P, Matuszewski M. Comparison of real-time fluorescent indocyanine green and99mTc-nanocolloid radiotracer navigation in sentinel lymph node biopsy of penile cancer. Clin Genitourin Cancer [Internet]. 2015;13(6):574–80. Available from: https://doi.org/10.1016/j.clgc.2015.06.005.

7. Bjurlin MA, Zhao LC, Kenigsberg AP, Mass AY, Taneja SS, Huang WC. Novel use of fluorescence lymphangiography during robotic groin dissection for penile cancer. Urology [Internet]. 2017;107:267. Available from: https://doi.org/10.1016/j.urology.2017.05.026.

8. Brouwer OR, Van Den Berg NS, Mathéron HM, Van Der Poel HG, Van Rhijn BW, Bex A, et al. A hybrid radioactive and fluorescent tracer for sentinel node biopsy in penile carcinoma as a potential replacement for blue dye. Eur Urol. 2014;65(3):600–9.

9. Stoffels I, Leyh J, Poppel T, Schadendorf D, Klode J. Evaluation of a radioactive and fluorescent hybrid tracer for sentinel lymph node biopsy in head and neck malignancies: prospective randomized clinical trial to compare ICG-(99m)Tc-nanocolloid hybrid tracer versus (99m)Tc-nanocolloid. Eur J Nucl Med Mol Imaging. 2015;42(11):1631–8.

10. Polom W, Markuszewski M, Cytawa W, Czapiewski P, Lass P, Matuszewski M. Fluorescent versus radioguided lymph node mapping in bladder cancer. Clin Genitourin Cancer [Internet]. 2017;15(3):e405–9. Available from: https://doi.org/10.1016/j.clgc.2016.11.007.

11. Ross GL, Shoaib T, Scott J, Soutar DS, Gray HW, MacKie R. The learning curve for sentinel node biopsy in malignant melanoma. Br J Plast Surg. 2002;55(4):298–301.

12. KleinJan GH, van Werkhoven E, van den Berg NS, Karakullukcu MB, Zijlmans HJMAA, van der Hage JA, et al. The best of both worlds: a hybrid approach for optimal pre- and intraoperative identification of sentinel lymph nodes. Eur J Nucl Med Mol Imaging. 2018;45(11):1915–25.

13. Hope-Ross M, Yannuzzi LA, Gragoudas ES, Guyer DR, Slakter JS, Sorenson JA, et al. Adverse reactions due to indocyanine green. Ophthalmology. 1994;101(3):529–33.

14. Chu W, Chennamsetty A, Toroussian R, Lau C. Anaphylactic shock after intravenous administration of indocyanine green during robotic partial nephrectomy. Urol Case Rep [Internet]. 2017;12:37–8. Available from: https://doi.org/10.1016/j.eucr.2017.02.006.

15. Murawa D, Polom K, Murawa P. One-year postoperative morbidity associated with near-infrared-guided indocyanine green (ICG) or ICG in conjugation with human serum albumin (ICG:HSA) sentinel lymph node biopsy. Surg Innov. 2014;21(3):240–3.

Part VIII

Applications in Breast Surgery

Masahiro Takada and Masakazu Toi

Introduction

Sentinel lymph node (SLN) biopsy is part of the standard of care for patients with primary clinically node-negative breast cancer [1]. Clinical trials and meta-analyses have shown that axillary node dissection for SLN-negative patients has no survival benefit [2–4]. Recent studies have shown that omission of axillary node dissection for patients with limited positive SLNs has no adverse impact on survival and decreases the incidence of lymphedema [5].

Both the radioisotope (RI) and blue dye methods are well-established techniques and are used worldwide. However, the RI method involves nuclear medicine, which limits its use to relatively high-volume centers, while the blue dye method requires special surgical skill to obtain sufficient accuracy and has a risk of anaphylactic reactions.

To overcome these problems, an indocyanine green (ICG) fluorescence method was developed in 2005 [6]. A near-infrared fluorescence imaging (NIR) system reveals subcutaneous lymphatic flow and enables the surgeon to navigate and perform sequential dissection of SLNs. Several clinical trials have shown that the ICG fluorescence method has an equal or higher SLN identification rate compared to conventional methods [7–9]. Meta-analyses have shown that there was no significant difference between ICG fluorescence and RI for SLN detection [10, 11].

In this chapter, we introduce the technical details and current data of SLN biopsy using the ICG fluorescence method, and describe the technical innovation of SLN mapping.

Indications

SLN biopsy using the ICG fluorescence method is indicated for patients with clinically node-negative breast cancer. However, ICG is contraindicated for patients with hypersensitivity or allergy to ICG or iodine, and the safety of ICG for pregnant or lactating women has not been established.

We recommend the combined use of RI with the ICG fluorescence method, especially for obese patients or patients undergoing preoperative systemic therapy (PST). Although only preliminary data have been obtained about the accuracy of the ICG fluorescence method after PST, our exploratory analysis showed that the

Electronic Supplementary Material The online version of this chapter (https://doi.org/10.1007/978-3-030-38092-2_25) contains supplementary material, which is available to authorized users.

M. Takada (✉) · M. Toi
Department of Breast Surgery, Kyoto University Hospital, Kyoto, Japan
e-mail: masahiro@kuhp.kyoto-u.ac.jp

identification rate was 100% among patients who underwent PST ($N = 70$) [7]. Although 42.8% of the sentinel lymphatic pathways changed owing to PST, the locations of the SLNs were not affected by PST [12]. The accuracy of the ICG fluorescence method after PST among patients with node-positive breast cancer has not yet been systematically evaluated.

Technical Description of the Procedure

ICG (5 mg in 1 mL; Diagnogreen®; Daiichi Sankyo Co., Tokyo, Japan) was injected intradermally at the edge of the areola. Fluorescent subcutaneous lymphatics were visualized using the NIR system and traced to the axilla where occasional nodes could be observed percutaneously (Fig. 25.1). SLNs detected by the NIR system were then excised. All these procedures were performed with the operating lights turned off, as per the manufacturer's recommendations. After SLN biopsy using the NIR system, residual SLNs were removed using RI, if used.

Interpretation

A previous meta-analysis showed that the identification rate of the ICG fluorescence method ranged from 88.6% to 100%, and there was no significant difference between the ICG fluorescence and RI methods for SLN detection [11]. There was no significant difference in the detection of positive SLNs between the ICG fluorescence and RI methods. Although SLNs identified using RI and ICG fluorescence generally overlapped, some of them are divergent [7]. Although the ICG fluorescence method may be an acceptable alternative to SLN detection using the RI method, ICG can function in a complementary manner to maximize the diagnostic performance of RI.

Currently, it is ethically difficult to evaluate the false-negative rate of the ICG fluorescence method. In addition, only few studies have investigated long-term survival after the application of ICG fluorescence method. Our retrospective study showed that axillary recurrence was observed in 6 of 1132 patients (0.53%) who underwent the ICG method between May 2007 and December 2015, and most of the patients with axillary recurrence were undertreated because of the patients' preference or age (data not shown). Long-term follow-up data regarding the survival or adverse events after the application of the ICG fluorescence method are required to confirm the clinical significance of this method.

Pitfalls

The detectable depth of the ICG fluorescence signal is limited. We usually use a plastic capsule to push and make the subcutaneous tissue thinner to help in the recognition of the fluorescence signals from SLNs percutaneously.

If the fluorescence signals from the SLNs cannot be detected percutaneously, surgeons should follow the lymphatic vessels and then reach the deeply located SLNs. Therefore, it is important not to disrupt the lymphatic vessels during procedures. If the lymphatic vessels get damaged, SLNs can still be recognized as green lymph nodes, as observed in the blue-dye method.

The number of SLNs identified using the ICG method is relatively higher than those identified using the conventional method (range 2.3–3.4) [7, 8]. In our study, skip metastasis to second or third metastasis was observed in 6 of 28 patients with positive SLNs [13]. Hence, we recommend that four-node resection could provide precise information on the nodal status, but the number of SLNs removed should be optimized based on individual patient and tumor characteristics.

Perspectives

Although the ICG fluorescence method is highly sensitive and easy to perform, current NIR systems have several technical issues that need to be improved. The current NIR systems display the fluorescence image on remote monitors, because the fluorescence signals are invisible under direct

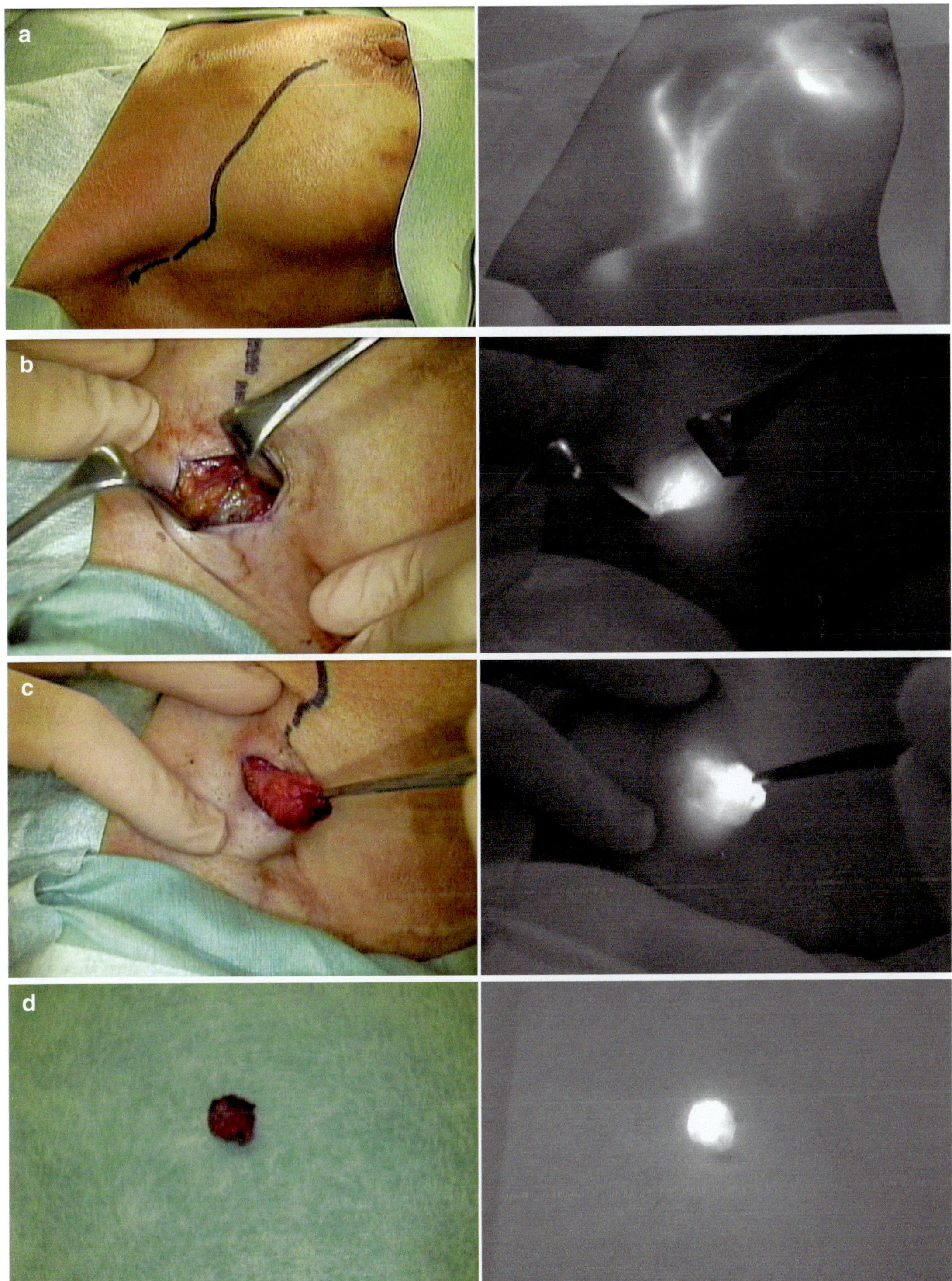

Fig. 25.1 The indocyanine green (ICG) fluorescence technique for sentinel lymph node (SLN) biopsy. (**a**) After intradermal injection of ICG at the edge of the areola, subcutaneous lymphatic vessels were visualized using the near-infrared fluorescence imaging (NIR) system (images on the right side). (**b**, **c**) Fluorescence signals from SLNs can be easily recognized, after skin incision. (**d**) All the excised SLNs were examined using the NIR system

observation of the surgical field. Therefore, surgeons have to look away from the surgical field to confirm the location of the fluorescence signals. These systems also require dimming of lights within the operative field to prevent white light contamination of images. These factors can disrupt surgical workflow and may increase the duration of surgery.

Hence, we developed a novel device, the medical imaging projection system (MIPS), to visualize fluorescence images directly on the surgical field using the projection mapping technique (Fig. 25.2; Video 25.1) [14]. The MIPS has a projection head that uses a half mirror to match the optical axis of the NIR camera and the projector.

The MIPS obtains the location of the fluorescence ICG emission and projects its image onto the location of the fluorescence emission in real time, irrespective of shifting and deformation of the organ. The projector of the MIPS can also illuminate the surgical field, allowing surgeons to perform the procedure without the need for operating lights. Our exploratory study showed that the identification rate of SLNs using this device was 100% (95% CI: 94–100%). This device could be useful in real-time navigation surgery for SLN biopsy.

Conclusions

SLN biopsy using the ICG fluorescence method is easy to perform and has an equal or higher SLN identification rate compared to conventional methods, making the ICG fluorescence method an acceptable alternative for SLN detection. Long-term follow-up data about survival or adverse events after the application of the ICG fluorescence method will confirm the clinical significance of this method. Nevertheless, recent technological innovation for SLN mapping enables us to perform real-time navigation surgery for SLN biopsy.

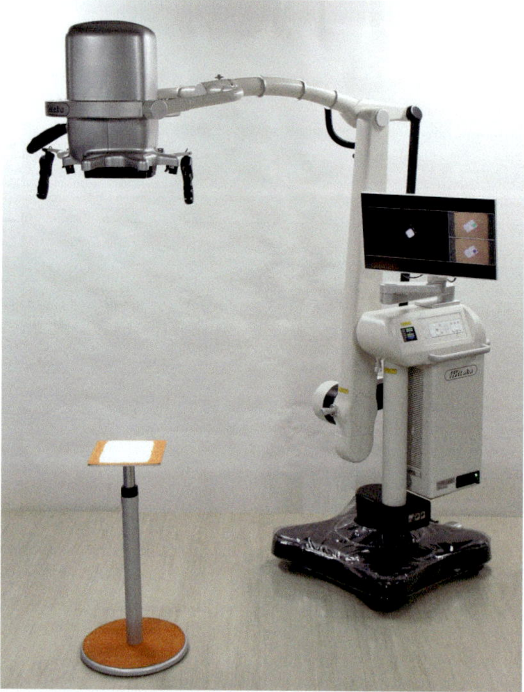

Fig. 25.2 The medical imaging projection system (MIPS). Photograph of the MIPS, showing the projection head and pole components. The MIPS has a projection head that uses a half mirror to match the optical axis of the near-infrared fluorescence imaging camera and the projector. The MIPS obtains the location of the fluorescence indocyanine green emission and projects its image onto the location of the fluorescence emission in real time, regardless of shifting and deformation of the organ. The projector of the MIPS can also illuminate the surgical field, allowing surgeons to perform the procedure without the need for operating lights

References

1. Lyman GH, Somerfield MR, Bosserman LD, Perkins CL, Weaver DL, Giuliano AE. Sentinel lymph node biopsy for patients with early-stage breast cancer: American Society of Clinical Oncology clinical practice guideline update. J Clin Oncol Off J Am Soc Clin Oncol. 2017;35(5):561–4.
2. Kim T, Giuliano AE, Lyman GH. Lymphatic mapping and sentinel lymph node biopsy in early-stage breast carcinoma: a metaanalysis. Cancer. 2006;106(1):4–16.
3. Krag DN, Anderson SJ, Julian TB, Brown AM, Harlow SP, Costantino JP, et al. Sentinel-lymph-node resection compared with conventional axillary-lymph-node dissection in clinically node-negative patients with breast cancer: overall survival findings from the NSABP B-32 randomised phase 3 trial. Lancet Oncol. 2010;11(10):927–33.
4. Veronesi U, Paganelli G, Viale G, Luini A, Zurrida S, Galimberti V, et al. A randomized comparison of sentinel-node biopsy with routine axillary dissection in breast cancer. N Engl J Med. 2003;349(6):546–53.

5. Giuliano AE, Hunt KK, Ballman KV, Beitsch PD, Whitworth PW, Blumencranz PW, et al. Axillary dissection vs no axillary dissection in women with invasive breast cancer and sentinel node metastasis: a randomized clinical trial. JAMA. 2011;305(6):569–75.

6. Kitai T, Inomoto T, Miwa M, Shikayama T. Fluorescence navigation with indocyanine green for detecting sentinel lymph nodes in breast cancer. Breast Cancer. 2005;12(3):211–5.

7. Sugie T, Kinoshita T, Masuda N, Sawada T, Yamauchi A, Kuroi K, et al. Evaluation of the clinical utility of the ICG fluorescence method compared with the radioisotope method for sentinel lymph node biopsy in breast cancer. Ann Surg Oncol. 2016;23(1):44–50.

8. Sugie T, Sawada T, Tagaya N, Kinoshita T, Yamagami K, Suwa H, et al. Comparison of the indocyanine green fluorescence and blue dye methods in detection of sentinel lymph nodes in early-stage breast cancer. Ann Surg Oncol. 2013;20(7):2213–8.

9. Wishart GC, Loh SW, Jones L, Benson JR. A feasibility study (ICG-10) of indocyanine green (ICG) fluorescence mapping for sentinel lymph node detection in early breast cancer. Eur J Surg Oncol. 2012;38(8):651–6.

10. Ahmed M, Purushotham AD, Douek M. Novel techniques for sentinel lymph node biopsy in breast cancer: a systematic review. Lancet Oncol. 2014;15(8):e351–e62.

11. Sugie T, Ikeda T, Kawaguchi A, Shimizu A, Toi M. Sentinel lymph node biopsy using indocyanine green fluorescence in early-stage breast cancer: a meta-analysis. Int J Clin Oncol. 2017;22(1):11–7.

12. Tsuyuki S, Yamaguchi A, Kawata Y, Kawaguchi K. Assessing the effects of neoadjuvant chemotherapy on lymphatic pathways to sentinel lymph nodes in cases of breast cancer: usefulness of the indocyanine green-fluorescence method. Breast. 2015;24(3):298–301.

13. Takeuchi M, Sugie T, Abdelazeem K, Kato H, Shinkura N, Takada M, et al. Lymphatic mapping with fluorescence navigation using indocyanine green and axillary surgery in patients with primary breast cancer. Breast J. 2012;18(6):535–41.

14. Takada M, Takeuchi M, Suzuki E, Sato F, Matsumoto Y, Torii M, et al. Real-time navigation system for sentinel lymph node biopsy in breast cancer patients using projection mapping with indocyanine green fluorescence. Breast Cancer. 2018;25:650.

Takashi Sakurai, Hirohito Seki, and Ken Shimizu

Introduction

Sentinel lymph node biopsy (SLNB) was introduced in the 1990s, and in the late 2010s, as a result of the ACOSOG-Z0011 and AMAROS trials, the proportion of axillary lymph node dissections (ALND) were gradually decreased [1–3]. However, there were still cases requiring ALND for tumor staging and local control in breast cancer treatment.

Secondary upper extremity lymphedema is nearly always the result of breast cancer treatment. With improved diagnostic accuracy and treatment, more patients are living longer, and there is an increased need for lymphedema management to maintain patients' quality of life.

Axillary reverse mapping (ARM) is a technique based on a hypothesis that there is a watershed of lymphatics and lymph nodes drainage from the upper extremity (ARM lymphatics, ARM lymph nodes) and lymphatics from the breast at the axillary lesion [4, 5]. If correct, preserving ARM lymphatics and ARM lymph nodes will reduce the risk of lymphedema after surgery.

Several studies have reported on the concordance of lymphatics from the ARM and breast, and the reduction of lymphedema with the ARM technique in ALND surgery.

In this chapter, we are going to explain our methods and the results of the ARM study, which compared the incidence of lymphedema in breast cancer patients after ALND and SLNB using ARM.

Electronic Supplementary Material The online version of this chapter (https://doi.org/10.1007/978-3-030-38092-2_26) contains supplementary material, which is available to authorized users.

T. Sakurai (✉) · H. Seki
Department of Breast Surgery, JCHO Saitama
Medical Center, Saitama, Japan
e-mail: sakurai-ssih@umin.org

K. Shimizu
Department of Pathology, JCHO Saitama Medical
Center, Saitama, Japan

Patients and Methods

Patients

From 2007 to December 2017, primary breast cancer patients who undergo SLNB and/or ALND were included. Updated data was used in patients with at least a one year observation period.

Indications

This technique was indicated for all patients undergoing SLNB and/or ALND.

E. M. Aleassa, K. M. El-Hayek (eds.), *Video Atlas of Intraoperative Applications of Near Infrared Fluorescence Imaging*, https://doi.org/10.1007/978-3-030-38092-2_26

Patients with allergies to indocyanine green (ICG) or iodine were excluded.

Technical Description of Procedures

Visualization Technique

Fluorescent dye technique was used because of the high visualization rate of ARM lymphatics and ARM lymph nodes [6, 7]. Our earlier study used blue dye and double tracer (blue dye and fluorescent dye) techniques, but we found that many cases were visualized only by fluorescent dye, while no cases were visualized only by blue dye. Hence, we stopped using blue dye technique.

Fluorescent dye is also preferred for our SLNB method. We use triple mapping technique (preoperative lymphoscintigraphy, Tc99m-RI tracer, and blue dye), and fluorescent dye can be clearly identified from the other tracers.

Injection of Indocyanine Green (ICG)

At least 2 hours before surgery, we injected 0.1 ml of ICG (25 mg of ICG with 10 ml of 5% glucose) in the second and third web space of the ipsilateral hand of the affected breast (Fig. 26.1).

Observation of ARM Lymphatics Before Incision

Before incision in the operating room, we examined the number and location of ARM lymphatics running from the upper limb to the axillary site through the skin using an ICG camera (Fig. 26.2). We hypothesized that the probability of preserving the lymphatics would be higher and the risk of developing lymphedema would be lower with a larger number of lymphatics at the axillary site.

Anatomical Classification

Many studies use the anatomical classification made by Clough [8]. However, we think the most important anatomical landmark in ARM lymphatics is the second intercostobrachial nerve (2ICBN), so we divided the axilla into three parts for classification: the area surrounding the 2ICBN, and the cranial and caudal sides of the 2ICBN (Fig. 26.3).

SLNB Maneuvers

When the sentinel lymph node (SLN) was identified and extracted, it was observed for fluorescence using an ICG camera. Fluorescence (shine) indicates that the SLN is also an ARM lymph node, and ARM lymphatics will be disrupted. Conversely, when the SLN is dark, it is not an ARM node and ARM lymphatics will probably be saved. The fatty tissue around the SLN was divided as precisely as possible, and only the targeted lymph node was resected.

ALND Maneuvers

After cutting the deep fascia on the ventral side of the axillary vein, ICG cameras were used to

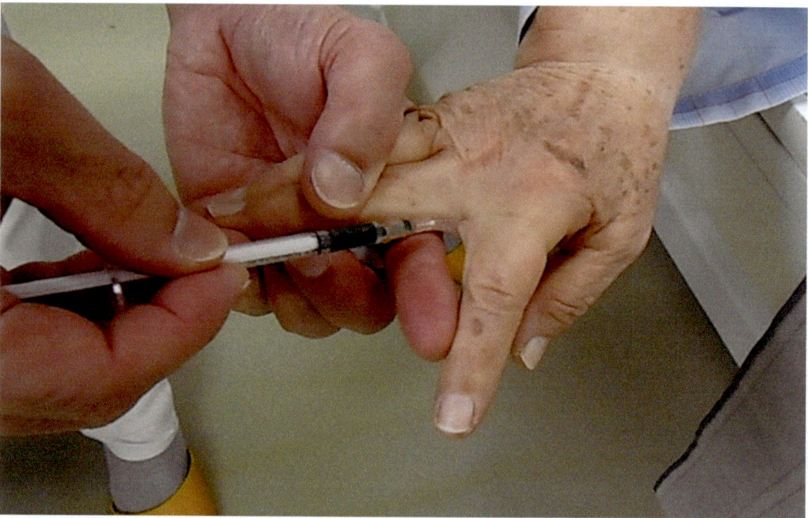

Fig. 26.1 Injection of ICG. 0.1 ml of ICG was injected into the ipsilateral hand (second and third web space)

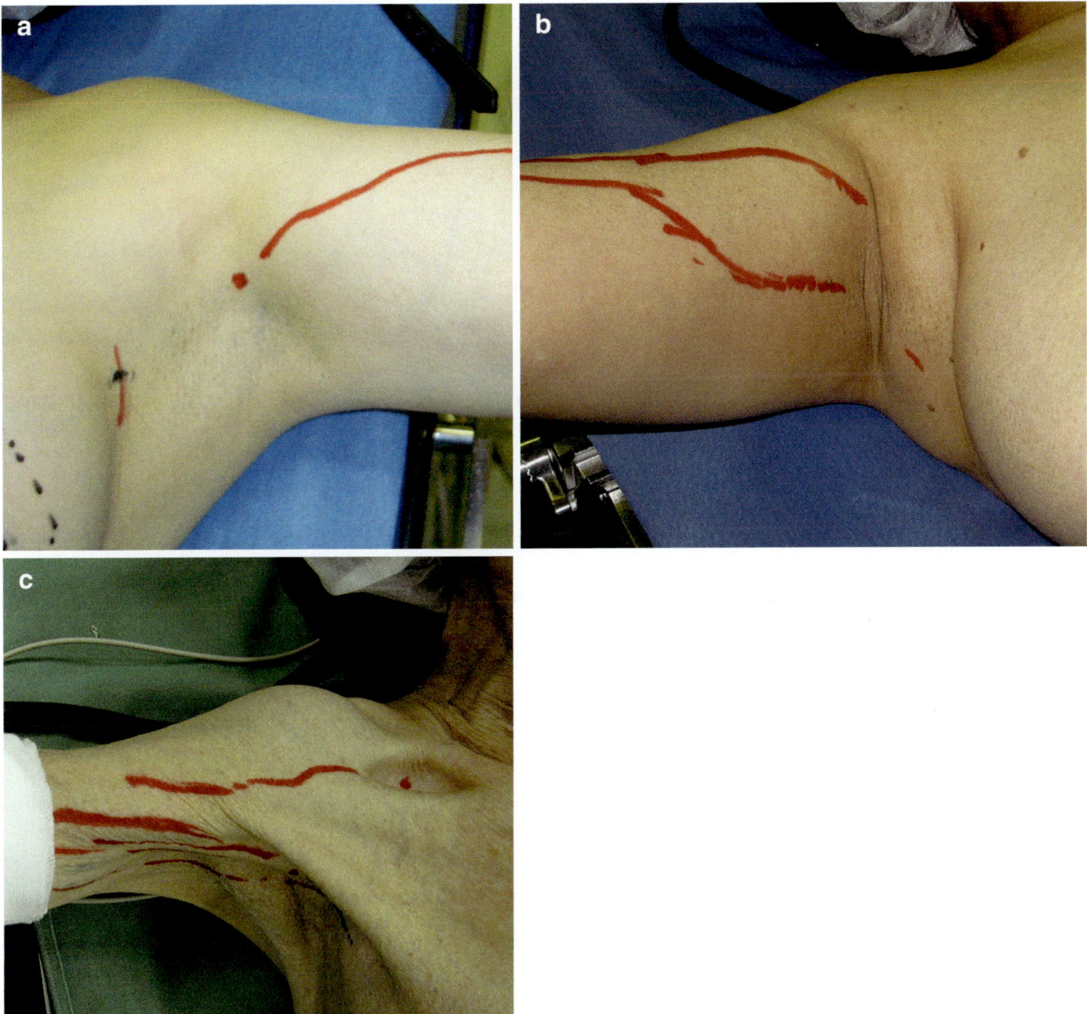

Fig. 26.2 Pattern of upper extremity lymphatics at axilla. (**a**) Single lymphatics, (**b**) two or more lymphatics, (**c**) two or more lymphatics and one lymphatics near the phrenic vein (shine lymphatics were marked in red ink)

search for fluorescent lymphatics and lymph nodes. Any fluorescent lymphatics and/or lymph nodes existing outside the ordinary dissection field (e.g., cranial side of axillary vein) were divided and preserved. Fluorescent lymphatics inside the dissection field were ligated and cut for the purpose of shortening the period of axillar drainage.

During the operation, the room was darkened to detect fluorescent images. Head-mounted LED lights were used to perform axillary dissection, and the ICG camera monitor and operating field were viewed alternately (Video 26.1).

Interpretation (Results)

Observation of ARM Lymphatics Before Incision

Single ARM lymphatic was observed at the axilla in 740 patients (53%), two or more were observed in 551 patients (40%), and lymphatics running in the axilla plus other parts of body (e.g., near the phrenic vein) were observed in 101 patients (7%).

Anatomical Classification

ARM lymphatics in ALND cases were primarily located around the 2ICBN (53%), with 18% on

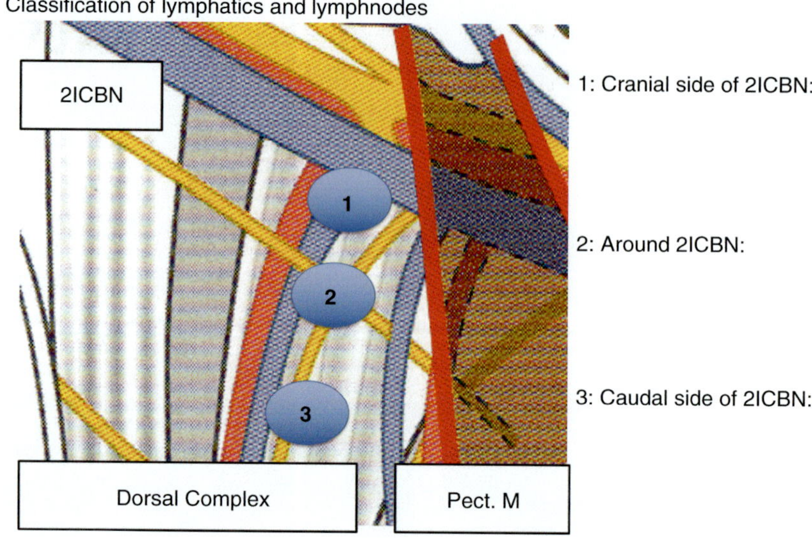

Fig. 26.3 Classification of lymphatics and lymph nodes. Location of lymphatics and lymph nodes were classified into three parts anatomically (position of numbered blue node)

the cranial side and 29% along the periaxillary vein (Fig. 26.3).

SLNB Maneuvers

The concordance of ARM lymphatics and lymph nodes with the SLN is the most important factor in predicting postoperative lymphedema [7, 9]. When the SLN is also an ARM node, resecting the SLN will disrupt ARM lymphatics. When the SLN is distinct from the ARM lymph node, a precise maneuver can preserve ARM lymphatics.

In 1310 patients, the concordance rate of the ARM lymph node and the SLN was 24.7% (323 patients), and the concordance rate of the ARM lymph node and the dissected non-SLN, immediately adjacent to the SLN, was 10.5% (137 patients). Almost all ARM lymphatics were either surrounding or on the cranial side of 2ICBN. If the SLN was located on the caudal side of 2ICBN, there was no concern of developing lymphedema (Fig. 26.4). There were eight patients who developed lymphedema in the 45-month mean follow-up period. All patients who developed lymphedema were in the ARM lymph nodes dissected group ($p = 0.0001$).

ALND Maneuvers

Lymphedemas of more than 2 cm in arm circumference developed in 71 of 339 patients (20.9%) who underwent ALND in the 55-month mean follow-up period. ARM lymphatics were totally or partially preserved in 37 patients (10.9%). Lymphedema was observed in considerably fewer patients in the preserved group than in the not-preserved group, although the difference was not statistically significant (13.5% vs. 21.9%, $p = 0.29$). In addition, the severity of lymphedema was considerably mild in the group for whom ARM lymphatics were totally or partially preserved.

There are several reports of the clinical use of the ARM procedure. Yue et al. reported that lymphedema occurred in 6% of patients in the ARM lymphatics-preservation group compared to 33% in the control group [10]. Pasko et al. reported that 27% of patients that underwent ARM developed lymphedema, while 50% of patients in the non-ARM group developed lymphedema, based on the results of a patient-based questionnaire [11].

Challenges

We think there are some problems to be solved.

First, observation through the skin was difficult in obese patients. In addition, lymphatics could not be detected in about 1% of our patient population in Japan.

Second, in 10.5% of the SLNB cases, a non-sentinel node immediately adjacent to the SLN was the ARM lymph node. It is rare but possible

Fig. 26.4 Location of SLN and concordance rate of ARM lymphatics and nodes. Almost all ARM lymphatics and lymph nodes were located around 2ICBN (37.6%) or at the cranial side of 2ICBN (40.6%)

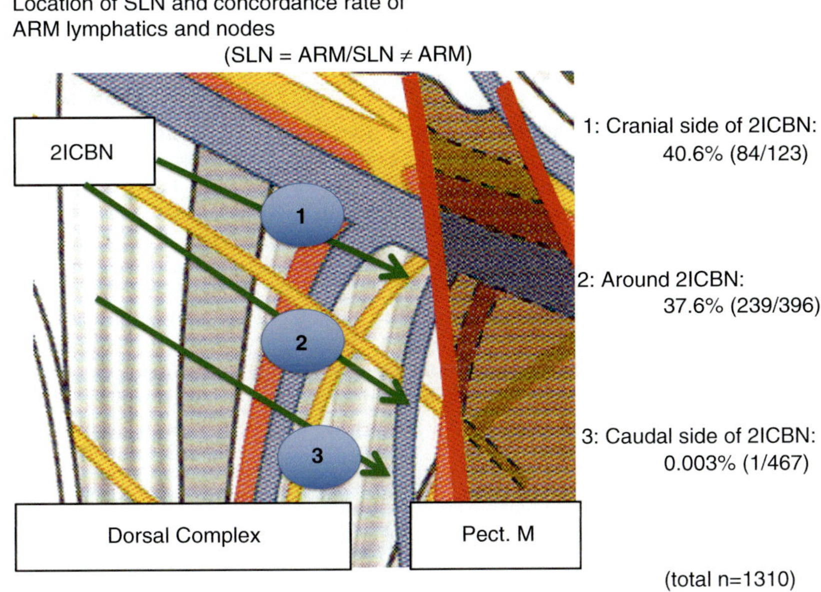

that only the non-sentinel node had metastasis, in which case extensive dissection will increase the risk of lymphedema.

Third, several studies have reported on the oncologic safety of preserving ARM lymphatics and lymph nodes in the ordinary anatomical dissection field during ALND. Especially for the clinical node-negative but pathologically SLN-positive patients, they found no metastatic involvement in the ARM lymphatics. Conversely, we found that 24.4% of the clinical node-negative, SLN-positive patients had metastases to more than four lymph nodes. In these 30 cases, only 10 were in the ARM and SLN concordance group. Since many ARM lymph node involvements were revealed pathologically in the group with metastases to more than four lymph nodes, reduction surgery should be carefully considered.

In our study, we did not improve the rate of lymphedema occurrence with ALND. We assumed the preserving maneuver itself could have contributed to the lymphedema rate, as lymphatics might be narrowed or obstructed by adhesions and/or inflammation after surgery, without enough fatty tissue attached to the lymphatics.

Conclusions

During SLNB, the ARM procedure is useful for identifying those at risk of developing lymphedema. Further review is necessary to determine if the ARM procedure is useful for reducing the risk of developing lymphedema during ALND.

References

1. Giuliano AE, Hawes D, Ballman KV, Whitworth PW, Blumencranz PW, Reintgen DS, et al. Association of occult metastases in sentinel lymph nodes and bone marrow with survival among women with early-stage invasive breast cancer. JAMA. 2011;306:385–93.
2. Giuliano AE, Ballman KV, McCall L, Beitsch PD, Brennan MB, Kelemen PR, et al. Effect of axillary dissection vs no axillary dissection on 10-year overall survival among women with invasive breast cancer and sentinel node metastasis: the ACOSOG Z0011 (Alliance) Randomized Clinical Trial. JAMA. 2017;318:918–26.
3. Donker M, van Tienhoven G, Straver ME, Meijnen P, van de Velde CJ, Mansel RE, et al. Radiotherapy or surgery of the axilla after a positive sentinel node in breast cancer (EORTC 10981–22023 AMAROS): a randomized, multicentre, open-label, phase 3 non-inferiority trial. Lancet Oncol. 2014;15:1303–10.

4. Thompson M, Korourian S, Henry-Tillman R, Adkins L, Mumford S, Westbrook KC, et al. Axillary reverse mapping (ARM); a new concept to identify and enhance lymphatic preservation. Ann Surg Oncol. 2007;14:1890–5.
5. Nos C, Lesieur B, Clough KB, Lecuru F. Blue dye injection in the arm in order to conserve the lymphatic drainage of the arm in breast cancer patients requiring an axillary dissection. Ann Surg Oncol. 2007;14:2490–6.
6. Noguchi M, Yokoi M, Nakano Y. Axillary reverse mapping with indocyanine fluorescence imaging in patients with breast cancer. J Surg Oncol. 2010;101:217–21.
7. Noguchi M, Noguchi M, Nakano Y, Ohno Y, Kosaka T. Axillary reverse mapping using a fluorescence imaging system in breast cancer. J Surg Oncol. 2012;105:229–34.
8. Clough KB, Nasr R, Nos C, Vieira M, Inguenault C, Poulet B. New anatomical classification of the axilla with implications for sentinel node biopsy. Br J Surg. 2010;97:1659–65.
9. Sakurai T, Endo M, Shimizu K, Yoshimizu N, Nakajima K, Nosaka K, et al. Axillary reverse mapping using fluorescence imaging is useful for identifying the risk group of postoperative lymphedema in breast cancer patients undergoing sentinel node biopsies. J Surg Oncol. 2014;109:612–5.
10. Yue T, Zhuang D, Zhou P, Zheng L, Fan Z, Zhu J, et al. A prospective study to assess the feasibility of axillary reverse mapping and evaluate its effect on preventing lymphedema in breast cancer patients. Clin Breast Cancer. 2015;15:301–6.
11. Pasko JL, Garreau J, Carl A, Ansteth M, Glissmeyer M, Johnson N. Axillary reverse lymphatic mapping reduces patient perceived incidence of lymphedema after axillary dissection in breast cancer. Am J Surg. 2015;209:890–5.

Vahe Fahradyan, Michael J. Annunziata, Risal S. Djohan, and Graham S. Schwarz

Introduction

Pedicled flap transposition and free flap transfer have become an integral part of plastic surgery in providing the means for reconstruction of complex defects that can present with missing bone structure and soft tissue coverage. Therefore, composite free flaps that include bone, muscle, subcutaneous tissue, and skin are often needed. The complexity of the design of these kinds of composite free flap requires planning and detail in designing the extent and reliability of the free flap. Advanced microsurgical techniques increased free flap survival rate 94–99%, however up to 14% of cases still require re-exploration [1]. Clinical signs such as flap color, capillary refill time and flap temperature and Doppler ultrasound assessment of vascular pedicle still remain the "gold standard" for free flap evaluation; however, clinical evaluation is subjective and largely depends on experience. Indocyanine green (ICG) fluorescence angiography can be utilized as an additional imaging method to identify pedicle location, evaluate tissue perfusion, visualize anastomotic patency, detect arterial insufficiency or venous congestion helping to design flaps and avoid postoperative complications [2, 3]. ICG angiography can help guide decision making in pedicled or free flap surgery intra- and perioperatively.

Application of ICG for Perforator Mapping

Perforator flaps became very popular in the last two decades as they cause less donor site morbidity and allow harvesting of thinner flaps. However, harvesting the flap can take a longer time and perforators can be easily damaged intraoperatively. Normal anatomical variations of the perforator vessels further complicate flap dissection. Preoperative identification of the perforators can help with flap design, significantly ease the dissection, and shorten the operative time [4]. By evaluating the perforators of anterolateral thigh flap (ALT), deep inferior epigastric perforator flap (DIEP), and fibular osteocutaneous flap,

Electronic Supplementary Material The online version of this chapter (https://doi.org/10.1007/978-3-030-38092-2_27) contains supplementary material, which is available to authorized users.

V. Fahradyan · R. S. Djohan · G. S. Schwarz (✉)
Department of Plastic Surgery, Dermatology and Plastic Surgery Institute, Cleveland Clinic, Cleveland, OH, USA
e-mail: schwarg@ccf.org

M. J. Annunziata
Case Western Reserve University School of Medicine, Cleveland, OH, USA

© Springer Nature Switzerland AG 2020
E. M. Aleassa, K. M. El-Hayek (eds.), *Video Atlas of Intraoperative Applications of Near Infrared Fluorescence Imaging*, https://doi.org/10.1007/978-3-030-38092-2_27

Onoda et al. have shown that ICG angiography has a 84% positive predictive value and 76% sensitivity in detecting perforators [5]. They concluded that the identification of perforators is difficult in patients with a flap thickness greater than 20 mm [5]. In a series of 24 breast reconstructions, Pestana and Zenn showed that CT angiography successfully identified the actual largest perforators in 78% of cases [6]. However, they were unable to demonstrate significant correlation between computed CT angiography identified perforator location and ICG angiography skin blush location, size, or intensity [6]. Contrary, Wu et al. found an 85% correlation between ICG angiography and preoperative CT angiography identified perforators [7].

Application of ICG for Evaluation of Flap Perfusion After Raising the Flap

Detection of poorly perfused areas after raising the flap can significantly decrease the area of partial flap necrosis and improve surgical outcomes. ICG angiography can be used to verify adequate perfusion of pedicled or free flaps before their transposition or transfer to the recipient region. Still et al. were the first to use ICG angiography for the evaluation of perfusion immediately after flap elevation. In their clinical trial of 21 flaps, they describe one case where ICG angiography successfully detected diminished perfusion of the distal three-fourths of the flap, which was subsequently treated in a delayed fashion [8]. Mothes et al. evaluated perfusion before transposition in 11 flaps. In their study, none of the flaps displayed insufficient perfusion at an early stage [9]. Buchrer et al. presented a case report of a planned anterolateral thigh (ALT) flap used to reconstruct a large lower leg defect in which intraoperative ICG monitoring had a significant impact on the surgical plan. After dissection of the two main ALT perforators, ICG angiography revealed perforasome coverage that was inadequate for the size of flap required. Addition of an adjacent tensor fascia lata perforator and intraoperative conversion from ALT to a conjoined fabricated flap

allowed complete coverage of the extensive defect [10]. In evaluating DIEP flaps harvested after abdominal liposuction, Casey et al. found no difference in the rate of anastomotic complications or total flap loss in those assessed on clinical grounds alone compared to those visualized with ICG angiography [11]. However, they demonstrated statistically significant decrease in the rate of partial flap loss and fat necrosis (from 71.4% to 0%) in those flaps in which ICG angiography was used to monitor flap perfusion. There was a decrease of postoperative flap volume reduction from 24.3% to 0% [11].

Application of ICG for Intraoperative Evaluation of Vascular Anastomosis

Patency and sufficiency of vascular anastomosis is integral to the success of free autologous tissue transfers. Conventional methods of evaluating the need for repair or revision of anastomosis (vessel filling, flap color and bleeding, milking tests) can be supplemented with ICG-angiography. In a series of 50 free flaps, Holm et al. compared clinical and ICG-angiographic assessments of anastomotic patency. After initial clinical determination of patency, ICG angiography was performed. Anastomoses deemed occluded after angiography were revised intraoperatively. In 11 cases of clinically determined patency, luminal occlusion or altered venous flow velocity was observed with ICG. Of these cases, six flaps experienced failure and three in total underwent intraoperative revision [12]. Pestana et al. presented a series of cases that highlight another notable example of ICG-angiography as used to evaluate vascular anastomosis. In one facial reanimation case, the absence of a Doppler signal after completion of anastomosis was consistent with both a low-flow state and absent venous flow. ICG angiography allowed direct visualization of positive venous outflow and reassurance that revision was not indicated—the postoperative course was uneventful and there were no flap complications [13]. Holm et al. further outline one case where intraoperative arterial spasm at the microvascular anastomotic site was directly visualized by ICG-videography. Repeat images of the site 2 minutes later showed resolution and continued arterial flow with no further complication [3]. While clinical tests remain the most accessible method of evaluating anastomotic quality, ICG angiography can prove to be a valuable aid in the decision process.

Application of ICG for Intraoperative Evaluation of Flap Perfusion During Flap Inset

In 2002, Holm et al. first monitored free flaps using ICG intraoperatively, immediately after inset. They found that intraoperative indicators of arterial spasm, venous congestion, and regional hypoperfusion on ICG-videography had a strong correlation with clinical outcome [3]. Duggal et al. evaluated the clinical outcomes of ICG angiography-guided excision in 71 pedicled or free transverse rectus abdominis muscle (TRAM) or DIEP flaps and 59 historical control flaps. They found a trend in the reduction of the rate of fat and partial flap necrosis from 22% to 14% ($p = 0.237$) [14]. Probability of flap edge necrosis is increased when wounds are closed under high tension. ICG angiography allows assessment of tissue-border perfusion and can direct intraoperative interventions aimed at reducing closure tension and preventing skin/soft tissue necrosis, such as modification on initial suture placement or selective removal of constricting sutures [15].

Application of ICG for Postoperative Monitoring of Flap Perfusion

Traditional postoperative evaluation of free and pedicled flaps is accomplished clinically, through prick tests, flap color, turgor, capillary refill, temperature, and Doppler assessment of the vascular pedicle. ICG angiography may be used to complement these techniques. Clinical detection of complications such as vessel thrombosis may be hindered by examiner inexperience, difficulty in examining buried tissues, and other factors. Mothes et al. have shown that postoperative ICG angiography predicted free flap failure in 77.8% of cases, in contrast to clinical signs turgor 33.3%, reperfusion 22.2%, tissue temperature 55.6%, and puncture bleeding test 11.1% [9]. Adelsberger et al. report that after 7 years of experience using routine postoperative ICG angiography flap monitoring alongside clinical assessment, their detection rates of vascular thrombosis have reached 85%. Furthermore, they found that postoperative monitoring using ICG angiography alone had a thrombosis detection rate of 64%, while clinical tests were only able to identify 29% of thromboses [16]. They propose a 5-day monitoring schedule beginning with an immediate postoperative clinical assessment, supplemented with ICG angiography. For the first 72 hours, clinical assessments occur every 2 hours and ICG angiography is applied every 4 hours. In the final two days, clinical assessments without ICG angiography are performed every 4 hours [16]. In a series of 20 free flap cases reported by Hitier et al., the time course of flap fluorescence and recovery to baseline at day 1 was found to have 100% sensitivity and 100% specificity in detecting postoperative complications requiring flap revision [17]. They also report that in two cases where postoperative clinical assessment was inconclusive, reassurance was provided by ICG angiography data that appeared normal—in those cases no complications were observed [17].

Technical Description of the Procedure

After reconstitution of 25 mg indocyanine green with 10 mL of sterile water (concentration 2.5 mg/mL), ICG is administered via intravenous bolus. ICG has a short half-life (3–5 minutes in tissue) that allows repetitive intraoperative reassessments. Raw ICG videography images are obtained in grayscale. With low latency, image processing is overlaid in color (green is conventional, though other colors may be used) on a white light image of the surgical field. At our institution, for skin blush imaging and identification of cutaneous perforators, 10 mg (4 cc) ICG is utilized, and 5 mg (2 cc) of ICG is given for pedicle and microsurgical anastomosis imaging.

Mapping of Arterial Perforators

After final positioning of patient on the operative table, 10 mg (4 cc) ICG is given intravenously. Next, the proposed flap area is imaged, and real-time video fluorescent angiography is recorded. The aim of this technique is to identify fluorescent skin blushes that correspond to the location of arterial perforators supplying blood to the skin of the proposed flap. Within 15–30 seconds of ICG bolus delivery, the origin of all skin blushes within the flap area are identified with real-time ICG videography and marked with sterile surgical ink (see Video 27.1). Standard dissection in preparation for perforator-based free-tissue transfer is then performed.

Assessing Flap Perfusion

Following flap elevation, 10 mg (4 cc) ICG is delivered intravenously in order to determine flap perfusion. ICG videography is performed as described above. Flap perfusion quality is assessed based on fluorescent signal intensity, with the highest intensity indicating most perfusion and lowest intensity least perfusion. Areas of flap tissue that still appear dark and hypoperfused

are marked according to videography results and excised in a lit environment, ensuring that only tissue that is well-perfused will be included in the final flap (see Video 27.2 and Fig. 27.1).

Assessing Arterial and Venous Anastomoses and Vascular Pedicle of the Flap

The patency and quality of arterial and venous anastomoses are assessed using 5 mg (2 cc) ICG intravenously. Immediately following injection of ICG, videography is examined for the presence of any suture gaps, kinked vessels, or other flow disturbances (see Video 27.3). When assessing anastomoses, it is also important to begin recording ICG videography before bolus injection, otherwise movement of fluorescent signal through the anastomotic site may be overlooked. Video 27.4 demonstrates assessment of the vascular pedicle of a pedicled flap.

Assessing Perfusion During Flap Inset and Wound Closure

Finally, ICG angiography is performed following flap inset and final wound closure, as well as postoperatively (see Fig. 27.2, Video 27.5). ICG videography is performed as described earlier. Flap position may be adjusted accordingly to ensure minimal tension. Additional tissue trimming and

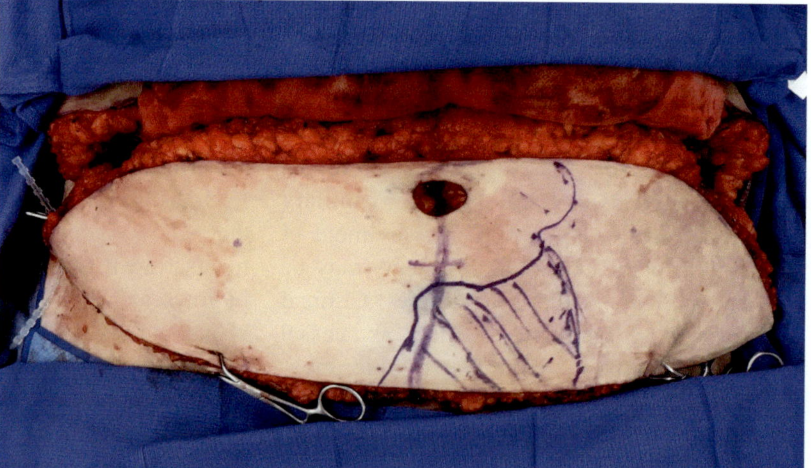

Fig. 27.1 ICG angiography-guided marking of hypoperfused DIEP flap

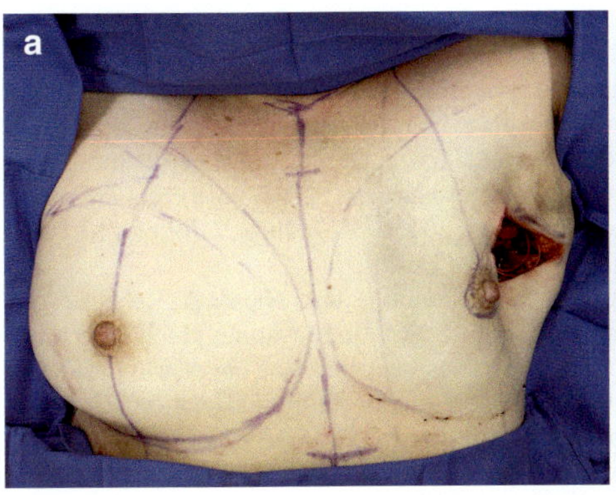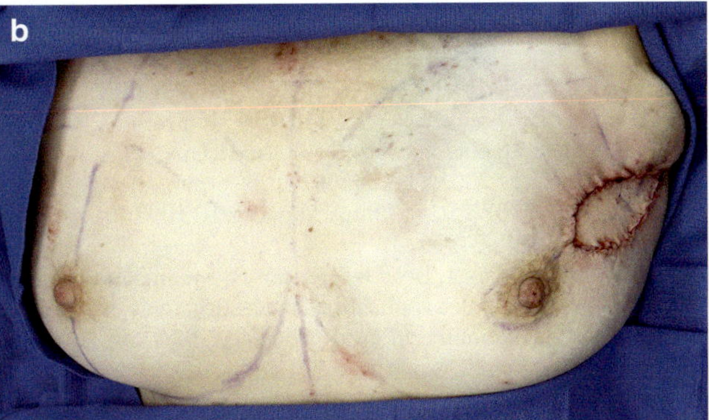

Fig. 27.2 (**a**) Tissue defect following left breast mastectomy. (**b**) Left breast following final DIEP flap inset

suture replacement is performed to ensure optimal flap perfusion.

Interpretation

Although the principles of ICG angiography used in free and pedicled flaps appear straightforward, there is not yet a standard set of guidelines to inform interpretation. Additionally, a diversity of qualitative and quantitative methods is represented within the literature. In general, tissue is defined as well-perfused or hypoperfused based on either relative or absolute fluorescence intensity levels. The earliest phases of dye uptake from the arterial system into the tissues generally reveal the most well-perfused tissue. However, late uptake does not always indicate poor perfusion as there is transit time for dye flowing through the tissues. The tissue distribution of larger pedicles may be mapped spatially using confinement patterns of fluorescence and used to guide flap design, but signal becomes more difficult to distinguish at tissue depths greater than 1–2 cm. Cutaneous perforators can be identified by monitoring the initial phases of fluorescent skin blush as dye moves into the microcirculation. When the anatomy of a vascular bed is reasonably well-known, suspected areas of hypoperfusion are identified as tissue where fluorescence intensity is closer to background. The patency of arterial anastomosis can be visualized either directly as uninterrupted fluorescence across suture lines, or indirectly based on fluorescence patterns within distal tissue. Similarly, venous anastomosis can be assessed based on dye movement from tissues and veins more proximal. For example, anastomotic occlusion from any source is strongly suggested by impaired dye flow across suture lines. Flap congestion may be suspected when there is good dye uptake and slow removal, or sometimes when there is poor flap uptake alone.

Pitfalls

- Frequent injections of ICG over short intervals (<3–5 minutes apart) can increase background fluorescence within the tissue, making areas of relative hypoperfusion less distinct [18].
- Boundaries of perfused areas may be overpredicted using ICG angiography, complicating the decision to excise or preserve hypoperfused tissue.
- Venous congestion can be difficult to judge because the venous phase fluorescence of the dye is not as precise as the initial arterial uptake phase [18].
- External factors that affect tissue perfusion (tumescent solutions with epinephrine, vasopressor administration, blood pressure, oxygen saturation, FiO2, temperature, hematocrit) can alter dye uptake, tissue distribution, and outflow [18–20].
- Fluorescence intensity is not correlated in a standardized fashion with a specific relative or absolute level of perfusion [18]. Clinical experience and judgment are still required to interpret ICG angiography results.

References

1. Bui DT, Cordeiro PG, Hu QY, Disa JJ, Pusic A, Mehrara BJ. Free flap reexploration: indications, treatment, and outcomes in 1193 free flaps. Plast Reconstr Surg. 2007;119(7):2092–100. e-pub ahead of print 2007/05/24; https://doi.org/10.1097/01.prs.0000260598.24376.e1.

2. Burnier P, Niddam J, Bosc R, Hersant B, Meningaud JP. Indocyanine green applications in plastic surgery: a review of the literature. J Plast Reconstr Aesthet Surg. 2017;70(6):814–27. e-pub ahead of print 2017/03/16; https://doi.org/10.1016/j.bjps.2017.01.020.

3. Holm C, Tegeler J, Mayr M, Becker A, Pfeiffer UJ, Muhlbauer W. Monitoring free flaps using laser-induced fluorescence of indocyanine green: a preliminary experience. Microsurgery. 2002;22(7):278–87. e-pub ahead of print 2002/10/31; https://doi.org/10.1002/micr.10052.

4. Ayhan S, Oktar SO, Tuncer S, Yucel C, Kandal S, Demirtas Y. Correlation between vessel diameters of superficial and deep inferior epigastric systems: Doppler ultrasound assessment. J Plast Reconstr Aesthet Surg. 2009;62(9):1140–7. e-pub ahead of print 2008/06/24; https://doi.org/10.1016/j.bjps.2008.02.012.

5. Onoda S, Azumi S, Hasegawa K, Kimata Y. Preoperative identification of perforator vessels by combining MDCT, doppler flowmetry, and ICG fluorescent angiography. Microsurgery. 2013;33(4):265–9. e-pub ahead of print 2013/01/25; https://doi.org/10.1002/micr.22079.

6. Pestana IA, Zenn MR. Correlation between abdominal perforator vessels identified with preoperative CT angiography and intraoperative fluorescent angiography in the microsurgical breast reconstruction patient. Ann Plast Surg. 2014;72(6):S144–9. e-pub ahead of print 2014/05/20; https://doi.org/10.1097/SAP.0000000000000104.

7. Wu C, Kim S, Halvorson EG. Laser-assisted indocyanine green angiography: a critical appraisal. Ann Plast Surg. 2013;70(5):613–9. e-pub ahead of print 2013/04/13; https://doi.org/10.1097/SAP.0b013e31827565f3.

8. Still J, Law E, Dawson J, Bracci S, Island T, Holtz J. Evaluation of the circulation of reconstructive flaps using laser-induced fluorescence of indocyanine green. Ann Plast Surg. 1999;42(3):266–74. e-pub ahead of print 1999/03/30; https://doi.org/10.1097/00000637-199903000-00007.

9. Mothes H, Donicke T, Friedel R, Simon M, Markgraf E, Bach O. Indocyanine-green fluorescence video angiography used clinically to evaluate tissue perfusion in microsurgery. J Trauma. 2004;57(5):1018–24. e-pub ahead of print 2004/12/08; https://doi.org/10.1097/01.ta.0000123041.47008.70.

10. Buehrer G, Taeger CD, Ludolph I, Horch RE, Beier JP. Intraoperative flap design using ICG monitoring of a conjoined fabricated anterolateral thigh/tensor fasciae latae perforator flap in a case of extensive soft tissue reconstruction at the lower extremity. Microsurgery. 2016;36(8):684–8. e-pub ahead of print 2015/05/27; https://doi.org/10.1002/micr.22424.

11. Casey WJ 3rd, Connolly KA, Nanda A, Rebecca AM, Perdikis G, Smith AA. Indocyanine green laser angiography improves deep inferior epigastric perforator flap outcomes following abdominal suction lipectomy. Plast Reconstr Surg. 2015;135(3):491e–7e. e-pub ahead of print 2015/02/27; https://doi.org/10.1097/PRS.0000000000000964.

12. Holm C, Mayr M, Hofter E, Dornseifer U, Ninkovic M. Assessment of the patency of microvascular anastomoses using microscope-integrated near-infrared angiography: a preliminary study. Microsurgery. 2009;29(7):509–14. e-pub ahead of print 2009/03/24; https://doi.org/10.1002/micr.20645.

13. Pestana IA, Coan B, Erdmann D, Marcus J, Levin LS, Zenn MR. Early experience with fluorescent angiography in free-tissue transfer reconstruction. Plast Reconstr Surg. 2009;123(4):1239–44. e-pub ahead of print 2009/04/02; https://doi.org/10.1097/PRS.0b013e31819e67c1.

14. Duggal CS, Madni T, Losken A. An outcome analysis of intraoperative angiography for postmastectomy breast reconstruction. Aesthet Surg J. 2014;34(1):61–5. e-pub ahead of print 2014/01/08; https://doi.org/10.1177/1090820X13514995.

15. Wyles CC, Taunton MJ, Jacobson SR, Tran NV, Sierra RJ, Trousdale RT. Intraoperative angiography provides objective assessment of skin perfusion in complex knee reconstruction. Clin Orthop Relat Res. 2015;473(1):82–9. e-pub ahead of print 2014/07/10; https://doi.org/10.1007/s11999-014-3612-z.

16. Adelsberger R, Fakin R, Mirtschink S, Forster N, Giovanoli P, Lindenblatt N. Bedside monitoring of free flaps using ICG-fluorescence angiography significantly improves detection of postoperative perfusion impairment(#)(). J Plast Surg Hand Surg. 2019;53(3):149–54. e-pub ahead of print 2019/01/25; https://doi.org/10.1080/2000656x.2018.1562457.

17. Hitier M, Cracowski JL, Hamou C, Righini C, Bettega G. Indocyanine green fluorescence angiography for free flap monitoring: a pilot study. J Craniomaxillofac Surg. 2016;44(11):1833–41. e-pub ahead of print 2016/10/18; https://doi.org/10.1016/j.jcms.2016.09.001.

18. Ludolph I, Horch RE, Arkudas A, Schmitz M. Enhancing safety in reconstructive microsurgery using intraoperative indocyanine green angiography. Front Surg. 2019;6:39. e-pub ahead

of print 2019/07/25; https://doi.org/10.3389/fsurg.2019.00039.

19. Xue EY, Schultz JJ, Therattil PJ, Keith JD, Granick MS. Indocyanine green laser angiography in the setting of tumescence. Eplasty. 2019;19:e1. e-pub ahead of print 2019/01/27.

20. Munabi NC, Olorunnipa OB, Goltsman D, Rohde CH, Ascherman JA. The ability of intra-operative perfusion mapping with laser-assisted indocyanine green angiography to predict mastectomy flap necrosis in breast reconstruction: a prospective trial. J Plast Reconstr Aesthet Surg. 2014;67(4):449–55. e-pub ahead of print 2014/02/11; https://doi.org/10.1016/j.bjps.2013.12.040.

Implant-Based Breast Reconstruction

Cagri Cakmakoglu, Thomas Y. Xia, Risal S. Djohan, and Graham S. Schwarz

Introduction

Surgical management of breast cancer has evolved in the last decade, and with more treatment options available, patients face more choices than ever before. Implant-based breast reconstruction is the most frequently employed breast reconstruction approach due to its relative technical ease and short postoperative recovery. Efforts to abbreviate the traditionally staged reconstruction process, improve aesthetic outcomes and reduce long-term chest wall morbidity have led to innovations in techniques. In particular, increasing usage of both direct-to-permanent implant placement and pre-pectoral positioning

Electronic Supplementary Material The online version of this chapter (https://doi.org/10.1007/978-3-030-38092-2_28) contains supplementary material, which is available to authorized users.

C. Cakmakoglu · R. S. Djohan · G. S. Schwarz (✉)
Department of Plastic Surgery, Cleveland Clinic, Cleveland, OH, USA
e-mail: schwarg@ccf.org

T. Y. Xia
School of Medicine, Case Western Reserve University, Cleveland, OH, USA

of breast implants necessitate a trustworthy test for mastectomy skin flap perfusion.

Nipple-sparing mastectomy incurs a higher risk of mastectomy skin flap loss postoperatively, especially in patients with risk factors such as high BMI and smoking [1]. Therefore, removal of the poorly perfused mastectomy skin flap and coverage of the implant or tissue expander with well-perfused soft tissue is important for preventing wound healing complications, implant exposure and infection.

Widespread adoption of biologic and synthetic mesh materials to support and cover the implant device has reduced the need to disrupt the soft tissue of the chest wall. Whereas vascularized chest wall tissues (e.g., muscle and fascia) have the advantage of protecting an implant from exposure and contamination, biologic implants (e.g. acellular dermal matrix) require a period of vascular and cellular in-growth, during which time they cannot provide effective immunologic protection to an implant in the case of mastectomy flap ischemic change or wound dehiscence.

Proper assessment and intraoperative removal of inadequately perfused mastectomy skin can prevent complications, reoperation, reconstructive failure and their associated economic impacts [2].

Near infrared fluorescence imaging for implant-based breast reconstruction is generally used for:

- Evaluation of the nipple areolar complex and mastectomy skin flap viability to select the ideal breast reconstruction technique after mastectomy.

- Determination of the resection boundaries of mastectomy skin flap after reconstruction.
- Evaluation of mastectomy skin flap tension and perfusion after expander/implant insertion.

Technical Description of the Procedure

After constitution of indocyanine green (ICG) with 10 cc of sterile water, ICG is injected intravenously. For mastectomy skin flap evaluation 7.5–10 mg (3–4 cc) is injected. ICG's short half-life (4–5 minutes) allows for quick, supplementary reassessments intraoperatively, with appropriate redosing as required.

ICG angiographic video images are obtained in grayscale. With low latency, a processed image is overlaid in color (green in this case) on a white light image of the surgical field.

Furthermore, gradient on-lay software technology shows skin perfusion assessment based on the signal intensity, with red indicating the highest intensity and blue, the lowest. Mastectomy skin flap areas seen as black or dark blue on the gradient on-lay scale are excised before the reconstruction.

Summary of the Technical Steps

1. Pre-reconstruction assessment of the mastectomy skin flaps after mastectomy
2. Determination of the resection margin, preparation of dermal flap (sling) via de-epithelization for additional coverage of the implant if needed
3. Selection of expander or implant-based breast reconstruction technique based on mastectomy skin flap perfusion
4. Reconstruction of the breast with either expander or implant
5. Evaluation of the mastectomy skin after insertion of either the expander of implant
6. Inflation, deflation or selection of differently sized prosthetic device (expander or implant) after mastectomy skin flap assessment with ICG angiography

Interpretation

Evaluation of the Mastectomy Skin Flap Viability

Mastectomy skin flap necrosis and wound dehiscence are associated with impending loss of the implanted device due to exposure and subsequent contamination or infection. Intraoperative identification of potentially ill-perfused mastectomy skin flap allows for preventative excision of inadequately perfused skin. In cases of implant-based breast reconstruction, the reconstruction technique will include placement of a full-sized, heavier, permanent implant, or a partially deflated expander, which can be securely inflated to its full volume over time as satisfactory mastectomy incisional healing and skin envelope viability are demonstrated. If a wide area of skin has low perfusion, pre-pectoral or partial, sub-pectoral device placement can be changed to complete, submuscular expander breast reconstruction with minimal volume fill. In this instance, highly vascularized muscle will provide well-vascularized soft tissue coverage for the device. Less commonly, device placement may be abandoned altogether should perfusion be severely impaired over a large area of the skin flap (Fig. 28.1).

Cases Examples

Case I: Breast Reconstruction Stage I with Tissue Expander

This is a case presentation of a 66-year-old non-smoker female with a history of oncoplastic reduction for breast cancer (Fig. 28.2). Patient could not tolerate post-mastectomy radiation therapy; therefore, right nipple-sparing mastectomy was planned. This patient had a BMI of 30 kg/m², D breast size, and grade 2, ptotic breast before the mastectomy.

Four months elapsed between the oncoplastic surgery and the planned nipple-sparing mastectomy.

Intravenously, 3 cc of ICG was injected. Mastectomy skin perfusion was analyzed with grayscale, green, and gradient on-lay technology. The poorly perfused nipple-areolar complex is marked. After analyzing its perfusion through the different image onlays, the nipple-areolar complex was preserved as decided by the surgeon, despite its poor perfusion as shown by ICG angiography.

The pre-operative plan of pre-pectoral implant reconstruction was changed to placement of an expander. The expander was partially filled for the purpose of preventing tension on the mastectomy skin flap and 3 cc ICG was reinjected to assess perfusion of the skin flap. Again, the nipple-areolar complex showed poor perfusion, but it was not excised by the surgeon. Patient was sent to hyperbaric oxygen therapy after surgery.

Figure 28.3a was taken immediately after the surgery, which shows ischemic, poorly perfused NAC and mastectomy skin flap.

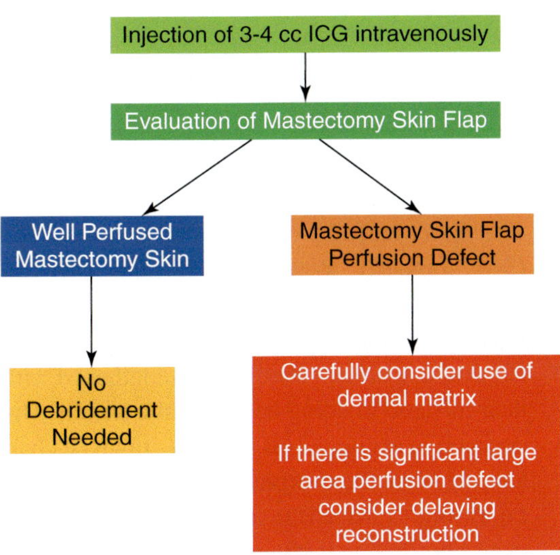

Fig. 28.1 Decision making in indocyanine green guided implant-based breast reconstruction

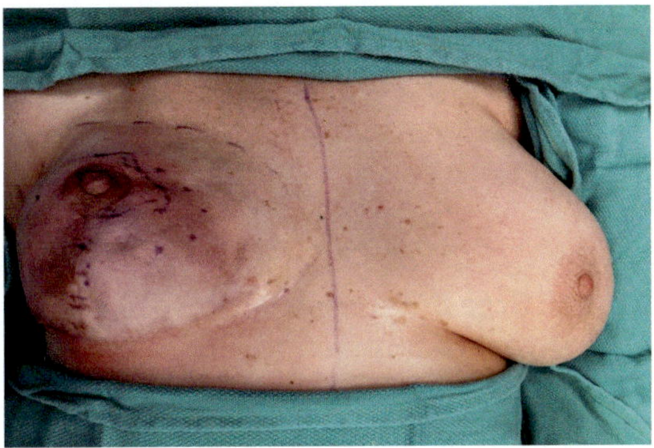

Fig. 28.3 Postoperative photograph, immediately after surgery

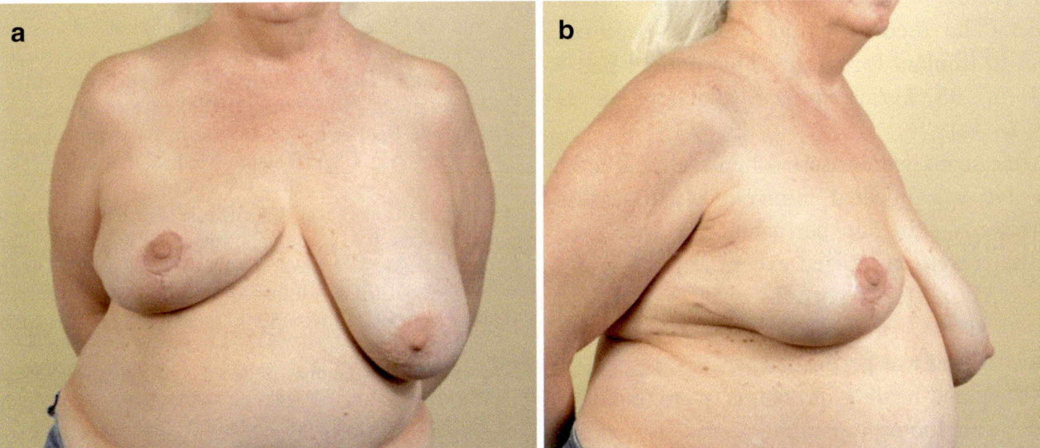

Fig. 28.2 Preoperative photographs. (**a**) Frontal view. (**b**) Lateral View

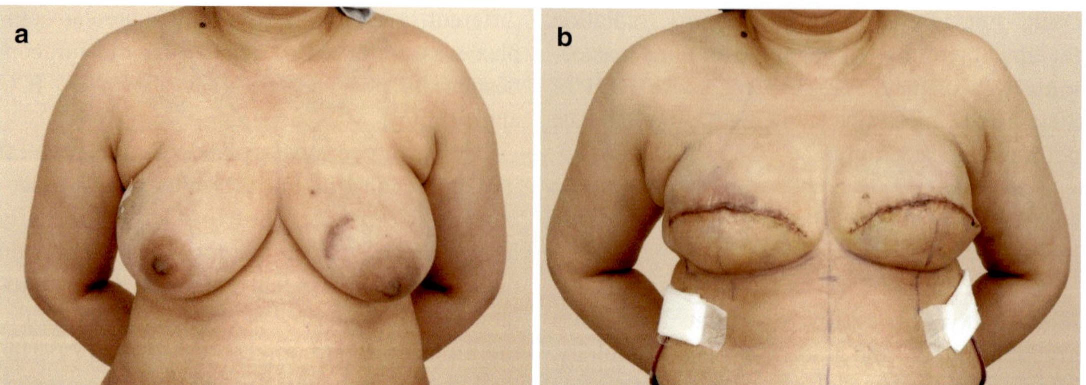

Fig. 28.4 Preoperative (**a**) and postoperative (**b**) photographs of a 41-year-old patient

At postoperative week 2, there was partial nipple necrosis despite hyperbaric oxygen therapy. This demonstrates that ICG is a reliable technique since it showed poor nipple perfusion during the surgery. The surgeon decided to preserve the NAC despite ICG angiography showing poor perfusion (Fig. 28.3b) (Video 28.1). Partial nipple re-excision and closure were performed during follow-up.

Case II: Breast Reconstruction with Direct to Implant

This is a 41-year-old nonsmoker, diabetic female patient with a history of left partial mastectomy and sentinel lymph node biopsy at an outside institution. She underwent bilateral skin-sparing mastectomy for recurrent breast cancer. The reconstruction was pre-pectoral, direct-to-implant technique. This patient had a BMI of 33 kg/m^2, breast size of 38 D (Fig. 28.4a).

After sizers were inserted bilaterally, 3 cc of ICG dye was injected intravenously to assess mastectomy skin flap perfusion. Well-perfused skin flaps were visualized except at the margin. The poorly perfused portions were marked and excised. Next, pre-pectoral, direct-to-implant reconstruction was performed.

No wound-healing problems were encountered during the postoperative period, as demonstrated in this photo that was taken 2 weeks after surgery (Fig. 28.4b) (Video 28.2).

Pitfalls

- The short half-life of indocyanine green dye (3–4 minutes) incurs a wait-time between sequential monitoring of skin perfusion between injections, which might cause delays in surgery.
- Clinical assessment should be strengthened with near-infrared imaging before skin excision. The decision to excise versus preserve might be challenging since the overprediction of ICG angiography might mislead the surgeon to overzealously excise borderline perfused areas [3, 4].

References

1. Sue GR, Long C, Lee GK. Management of mastectomy skin necrosis in implant based breast reconstruction. Ann Plast Surg. 2017;78(5 Suppl 4):S208–11. https://doi.org/10.1097/SAP.0000000000001045.
2. Jones G. Bostwick's plastic and reconstructive breast surgery. NY, USA: Thieme Medical Publisher Inc.; 2009.
3. Jeon FHK, Varghese J, Griffin M, Butler PE, Ghosh D, Mosahebi A. Systematic review of methodologies used to assess mastectomy flap viability. BJS Open. 2018;2(4):175–84. https://doi.org/10.1002/bjs5.61.
4. Mattison GL, Lewis PG, Gupta SC, Kim HY. SPY imaging use in postmastectomy breast reconstruction patients: preventative or overly conservative? Plast Reconstr Surg. 2016;138(1):15e–21e. https://doi.org/10.1097/PRS.0000000000002266.

Rebecca Knackstedt, Cagri Cakmakoglu,
Graham S. Schwarz, and Risal S. Djohan

Indication

A successful breast reduction requires ample postoperative blood supply to the nipple and remaining tissue. However, this must be performed while resecting adequate volume and providing an aesthetic postoperative shape. While this may be relatively easy to achieve in smaller breasts, larger, ptotic breasts can provide a surgical challenge. For extremely large or ptotic breasts, the surgeon must decide if a free nipple graft is required. With numerous breast pedicles to choose from, each patient must be evaluated individually to determine the best operative plan. However, sometimes these surgical decisions are not clear and vascular compromise in the perioperative period can often be difficult to assess. To that end, indocyanine green (ICG) can be utilized to assess blood supply and help guide clinical decision-making pre-, intra-, and perioperatively.

The vascular pedicle in a breast reduction is comprised of breast parenchyma that is isolated and preserved and serves as the source of blood supply to the nipple and areola following tissue rearrangement. Various pedicles for breast reductions have been described and can be combined with any skin resection [1–3]. While each pedicle may receive blood supply from more than one named vessel, there is typically a dominant blood source that must be preserved for ample nipple vascularity. A superior pedicle relies on the descending branch of the artery coming from the second interspace of the internal mammary system. This lies in the subcutaneous tissue and can be easily visualized and located with a Doppler. The arterial supply for a medial breast reduction curves around the periphery of the breast from the second and third interspace and runs in the subcutaneous tissue toward the nipple. Inferior and central pedicles receive their blood supply from the deep system from the fourth interspace. While arteries from the fifth interspace can provide additional blood supply to an inferior pedicle, they cannot be utilized for a central pedicle. When a free nipple graft is utilized, it functions like a skin graft and relies on the same stages of healing, imbibition, inosculation, and neovascularization, as a skin graft.

Technical Description

At the desired time, 3 cc of ICG can be introduced intravascularly by the anesthesia team. This is then flushed with 10 cc of normal saline.

Electronic Supplementary Material The online version of this chapter (https://doi.org/10.1007/978-3-030-38092-2_29) contains supplementary material, which is available to authorized users.

R. Knackstedt (✉) · C. Cakmakoglu
G. S. Schwarz · R. S. Djohan
Department of Plastic Surgery, Cleveland Clinic, Cleveland, OH, USA
e-mail: knacksr@ccf.org

© Springer Nature Switzerland AG 2020

E. M. Aleassa, K. M. El-Hayek (eds.), *Video Atlas of Intraoperative Applications of Near Infrared Fluorescence Imaging*, https://doi.org/10.1007/978-3-030-38092-2_29

The surgeon must be prepared to visualize the results as fluorescence appears almost immediately and is transient. The ICG perfusion pattern can be viewed in grayscale or with color onlay to determine overall vascularity of the nipple areolar complex, dermal-parenchymal pedicle and skin flap (see Video 29.1).

Interpretation

There are multiple times pre-, intra-, and perioperatively that ICG can help guide decision-making in breast reduction surgery. The first would be preoperatively prior to skin incision. ICG utilized at this time point allows for evaluation of the blood supply to the skin and nipple and may demonstrate a robust superficial superior blood supply to the nipple. If there is poor blood flow demonstrated preoperatively, this could suggest the necessity of a free nipple graft. If large superficial, superior blood vessels are observed, they can be marked on the skin and preserved, especially if they supply the pedicle of choice or remaining breast tissue. This can be especially useful in superior and superomedial pedicles where the blood supply is mainly superficial.

Once the pedicle has been isolated, ICG can be utilized to assess the viability of the nipple, to evaluate blood flow to the flap edges and to determine if more tissue can be safely resected from the pedicle, if desired. If poor blood flow to the nipple is observed, a free nipple graft should be considered. If there is not ample blood supply to skin flap edges, they should be resected until healthy tissue is observed. If blood supply to the nipple is clinically questionable, the pedicle can be thinned out and the perfusion can be reassessed with repeat ICG dosing.

Once the incisions are tacked together or closed, ICG can be utilized to assess the viability of the nipple and to determine if skin flap edges are receiving good blood flow. Once again, if poor blood flow to the nipple is observed, a free nipple graft should be considered or the pedicle should be interrogated, and if there is not ample blood supply to skin flap edges, they should be resected as required.

Postoperatively, nipple and areolar vascular compromise can result from injury or kinking of the pedicle or may occur secondary to tissue edema. If there is concern in the perioperative period, ICG can be utilized to assess nipple viability or determine if tissue ecchymosis is superficial or potentially indicative of tissue compromise. If poor flow to the nipple is observed, sutures can be released and perfusion can be reassessed. If there is still poor flow, return to the operating room should be considered for pedicle exploration and possible conversion to free nipple graft. If skin edges appear ischemic, expectant wound management, hyperbaric oxygen, or operative exploration and debridement should be considered.

In conclusion, while breast reduction surgery is a procedure that many plastic surgeons perform routinely, demanding surgical cases can present a challenge. ICG can be utilized in planning, execution, and postoperative assessments to help guide clinical decision-making and ensure the safety, efficacy, and outcomes of this surgery.

References

1. Hall-Findlay EJ. Pedicles in vertical breast reduction and mastopexy. Clin Plast Surg. 2002;29(3):379–91. PubMed PMID: 12365638.
2. van Deventer PV, Page BJ, Graewe FR. The safety of pedicles in breast reduction and mastopexy procedures. Aesthet Plast Surg. 2008;32(2):307–12. PubMed PMID: 18064510.
3. Hall-Findlay EJ, Shestak KC. Breast reduction. Plast Reconstr Surg. 2015;136(4):531e–44e. PubMed PMID: 26397273.

Junkichi Yokoyama and Shinich Ohba

Parapharyngeal Space and Parapharyngeal Space Tumors

The parapharyngeal space (the lateral pharyngeal space) is a narrow area of clinical importance for head and neck cancer due to it being the point at which a variety of original parapharyngeal space tumors and metastatic tumors develop.

The parapharyngeal space is shaped like an inverted pyramid with its superior aspect at the skull and its inferior apex at the hyoid bone. The superior pharyngeal constrictor muscle forms the medical boundary and the parotid gland, mandible, and lateral pterygoid muscle bound it laterally. The parapharyngeal space contains significant organs such as internal carotid artery, internal jugular vein, sympathetic chain, and cranial nerves IX, X, XI, and XII. The parapharyngeal space is known as the danger space. As a result, it is exceedingly difficult to resect tumors without complications such as dysphagia and carotid artery rupture in the narrow-complicated space [1]. In order to minimize surgical complications and preserve organs, endoscopic, or robotic surgery is often executed when performing head and neck surgery [2]. While highly effective, a disadvantage of these procedures is that it is not possible for the surgeon to physically touch tumors or to directly observe diffusely invaded deep organs. As a result, we have proposed using ICG florescence imaging method for navigation surgery and have demonstrated the advantage and effectiveness of ICG fluorescent image-guided surgery for the safe resection of parapharyngeal space tumors [3].

Indications

There are many kinds of malignant parapharyngeal tumors including salivary gland tumors, pharyngeal tumors, metastatic tumors and paragangliomas. Metastatic tumors from head and neck cancers are the highest occurring among malignant parapharyngeal tumors.

Electronic Supplementary Material The online version of this chapter (https://doi.org/10.1007/978-3-030-38092-2_30) contains supplementary material, which is available to authorized users.

J. Yokoyama (✉)
Department of Otolaryngology, Head and Neck Surgery, Kyorin University, Mitaka, Tokyo, Japan

Department of Otolaryngology, Head and Neck Surgery, Edogawa Hospital, Tokyo, Japan
e-mail: jyokoya@juntendo.ac.jp

S. Ohba
Department of Otolaryngology, Head and Neck Surgery, Juntendo University, Tokyo, Japan

Technical Description of the Procedure(s)

Initially, 0.5 mg/kg of ICG is injected via the cephalic vein. Observation of the fluorescent image is conducted with HEMS (Hyper Eye Medical System, Mizuho Medical Co. Ltd., Tokyo, Japan) between 5 and 30 min after the initial injection (Video 30.1) [4]. Firstly, the position of the tumor is marked over pharyngeal mucosa through the use of ICG fluorescence imaging with HEMS (Fig. 30.1). The pharyngeal mucosa is then incised transorally (Fig. 30.2a). The submucosal tumor cannot initially be visualized as it is obscured by fascia under natural light. However, the submucosal tumor obscured is seen under the fascia clearly after application of the HEMS color imaging (Fig. 30.2b). The submucosal tumor under the fascia is then clearly seen under HEMS imaging by observing conventional image (Fig. 30.2c). The position of the tumor obscured by fascia is then detected and seen following removal of the fascia. Owing to clear visualization, the proximity of the tumor is confirmed in relation to the carotid artery and lower cranial nerves, thus aiding in avoidance of stretching and injuring these vital structures. As a result, the tumors are able to be safely separated from the carotid artery and lower cranial nerves while protecting organs (Video 30.1).

In addition, by using this technology, parapharyngeal tumors can be resected by a transparotid approach. Tumors located behind the carotid sheath in parapharyngeal space are challenging to manipulate and locate in relation to deep organs. In order to visualize and safely resect these tumors in such cases, ICG can be used for navigation surgery. ICG fluorescence imaging with HEMS facilitates this procedure by revealing the tumor behind the carotid sheath even in cases where they are obscured (Fig. 30.3). Consequently, parapharyngeal tumors can be completely and safely resected by ICG navigation surgery without complications.

Tumors display bright fluorescence emissions that clearly contrast them with surrounding normal structures. When the submucosal tumor is

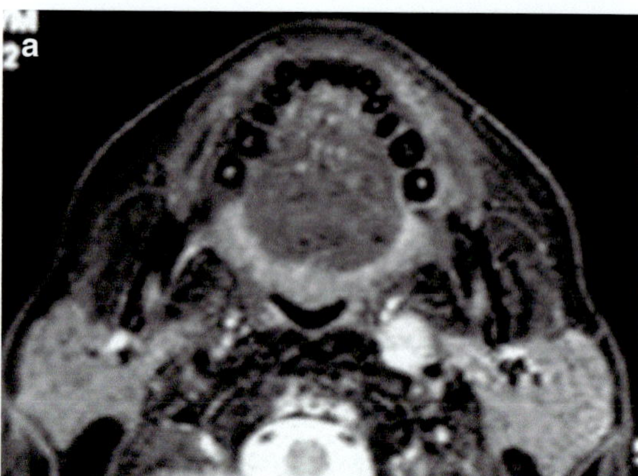
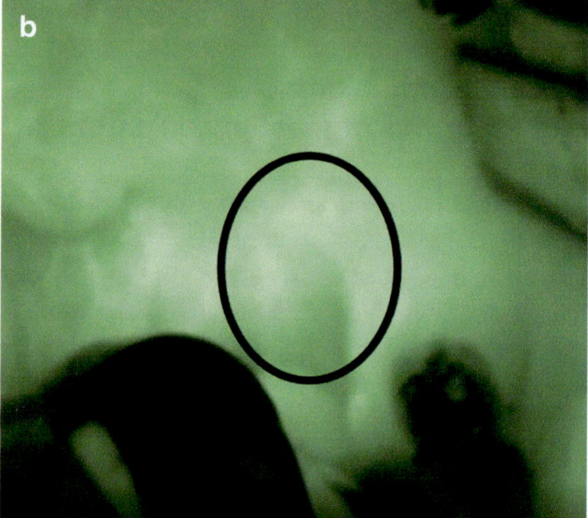
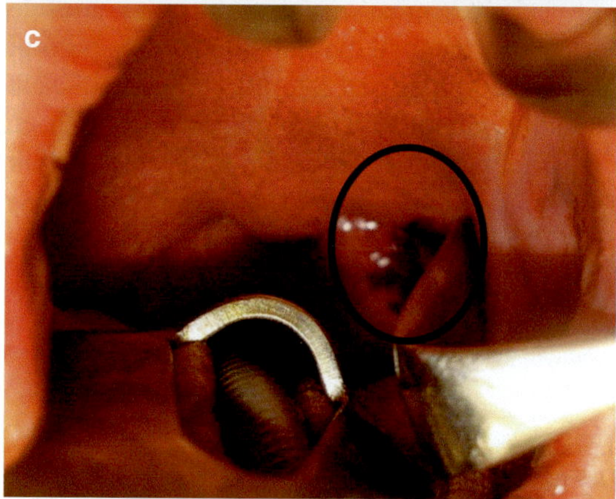

Fig. 30.1 *Case 1* Transoral resection by guiding ICG imaging. Recurrent parapharyngeal metastasis was resected transorally, guiding ICG imaging. (**a**) MRI (Magnetic Resonance Imaging). (**b**) ICG image. Tumor location was marked based on ICG image (circle). (**c**) Tumor location based on ICG image. Tumor location was marked on the pharyngeal mucosa based on ICG image (circle)

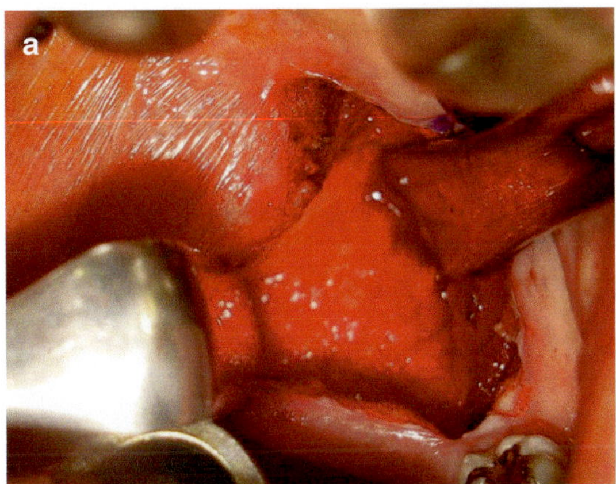

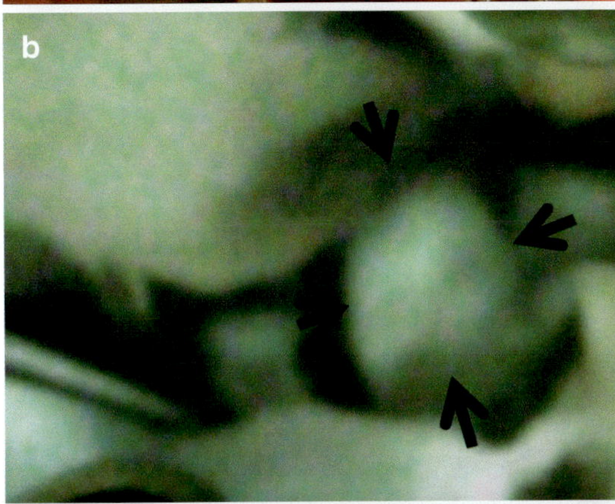

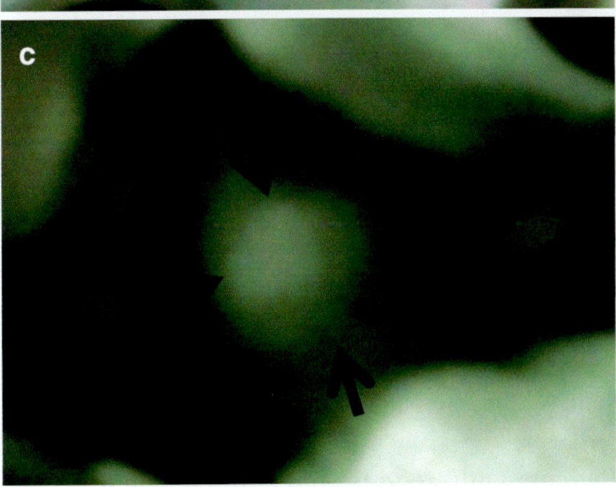

Fig. 30.2 *Case 1 Operative findings by ICG navigation surgery.* (**a**) Submucosal tumor. Submucosal tumor was visually obscured by fascia. (**b**) ICG color image. ICG color image clearly indicated the obscured tumor in pharynx (arrows). (**c**) Conventional ICG image. Conventional ICG image indicated the obscured tumor (arrows). The tumor was removed while preserving function

covered with and obscured by fascia, or vascular bundles such as carotid artery and internal jugular vein, it can be clearly seen under HEMS imaging. Near-infrared (NIR) Fluorescence

Imaging Visibility Score by Poellinger [5] exhibited no difference between squamous cell carcinoma and other malignant tumors. In the case example, the tumor was completely resected pathologically including the entire tumor capsule. Furthermore, the tumor was safely and noninvasively resected in order to preserve pharyngeal functions. These findings are particularly useful for detection and safe resection of tumors invading the parapharyngeal space [6].

Interpretation

Optical imaging using ICG is a new technique for visualizing tumors real-time during surgery. Some reports have indicated that ICG fluorescence imaging guided surgery is efficient in liver cancer surgery to detect not only large cancers, but also when detecting micro-cancers [7]. We have also reported the usefulness of ICG fluorescence imaging not only in liver cancer surgery, but also in head and neck cancer surgery [3, 8].

The handheld HEMS can significantly aid in the detection and visual confirmation of pharyngeal tumors located behind the oral cavity or nasal cavity by ICG-enhanced imaging with vivid color. Of note is that it can be freely operated intraoperatively by surgeons. Because of the high sensitivity of ICG fluorescence imaging, ICG fluorescence imaging under HEMS can assist surgeons in the identification and resection of tumors that have invaded the parapharyngeal space behind the internal carotid artery, internal jugular vein, and lower cranial nerves.

We have demonstrated a successful method for distinguishing cancerous tissue from healthy tissue and the optimum surgical time with HEMS in animal models [4]. Application of endoscopic and robotic surgery for the parapharyngeal space lesions enables surgeons to perform minimally invasive surgery with superior results [2]. However, we need to be able to detect parapharyngeal tumors in deeper and invisible areas when palpation is not possible. This is required in order to resect tumors safely and can be aided through effective tumor detection carried out with ICG fluorescent imaging.

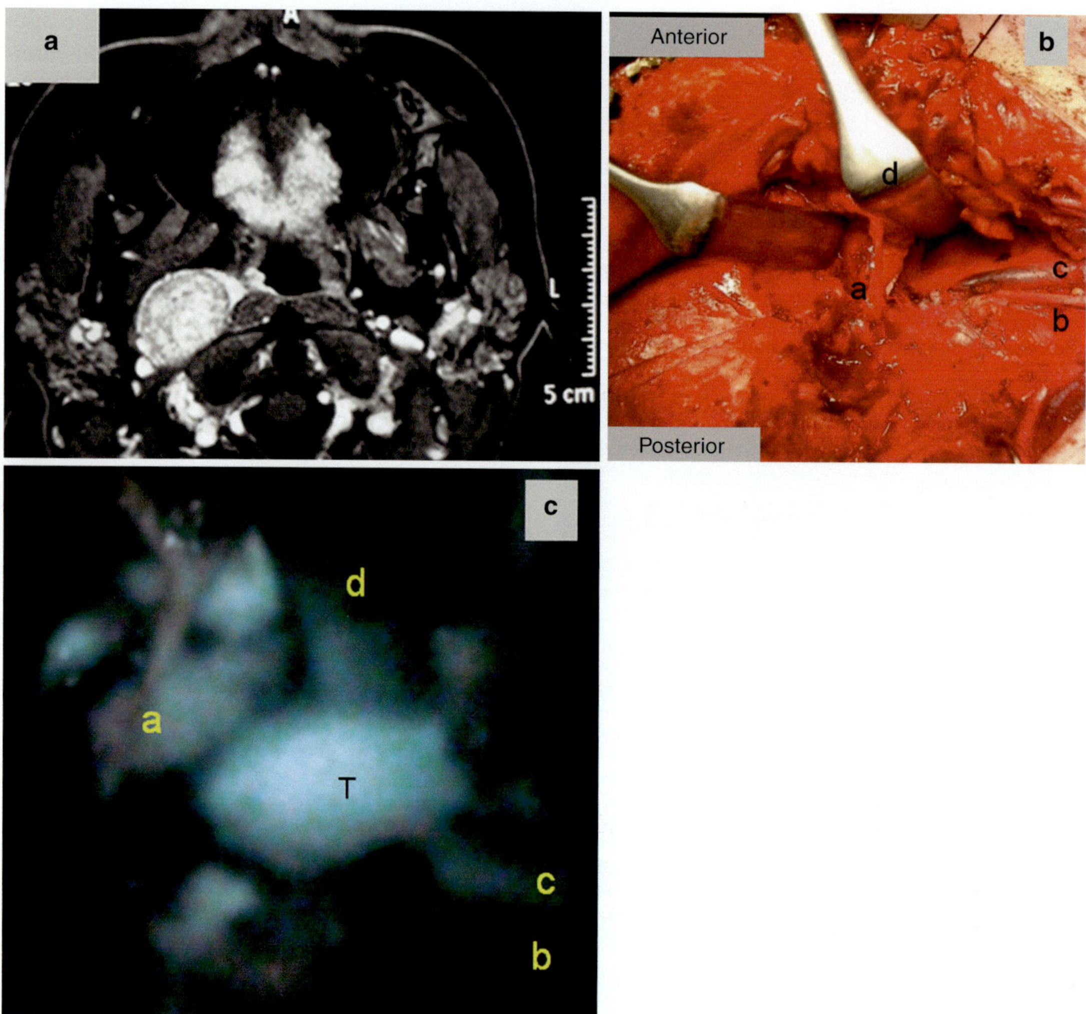

Fig. 30.3 *Case 2* Transparotid resection by guiding ICG imaging. Parapharyngeal space tumor (malignant paraganglioma). (**a**) MRI (magnetic resonance imaging); (**b**) intraoperative findings. The tumors located behind the carotid sheath in parapharyngeal space cannot be detected and physically touched. (a) Facial nerve, (b) accessory nerve, (c) internal jugular vein, (d) retractor, (**c**) ICG navigation surgery for parapharyngeal space tumor. ICG florescence imaging with HEMS clearly reveals the tumor behind the carotid sheath. (a) Facial nerve, (b) accessory nerve, (c) internal jugular vein, (d) retractor

We conclude that ICG fluorescence imaging is effective for the detection and resection of the parapharyngeal space tumors that enables greater preservation of functions.

Pitfalls

There are two approaches to parapharyngeal space tumors, the transoral approach and the approach from the neck (transparotid procedure).

Patients with trismus are contraindicated for the transoral approach. This is because the handheld HEMS is too large to eradicate enough excitation light to target cancers or detect enough fluorescent emissions in patients with trismus. Parapharygeal space tumors without invasion into the carotid artery are indicated for an intra oral and neck approach.

As fluorescence emitted by ICG is scattered through fat tissue, it is sometimes difficult to detect enough ICG fluorescence deeper than

1 cm. In cases of neck approach (transparotid procedure), there is the possibility that ICG fluorescence imaging may not be able to detect parapharyngeal tumors behind the internal carotid artery, internal jugular vein, and lower cranial nerves in patients with fatty tissue. It is therefore necessary to carefully remove fatty tissue around parapharyngeal tumors in order to clearly detect tumors by ICG fluorescence imaging.

References

1. Carrau RL, Myers E, Johnson J. Management of tumors arising in the parapharyngeal space. Laryngoscope. 1990;100:583–9.
2. Desai SC, Sung CK, Genden EM. Transoral robotic surgery using an image guidance system. Laryngoscope. 2008;118:2187–9.
3. Yokoyama J, Ooba S, Fujimaki M, et al. Impact of indocyanine green fluorescent image-guided surgery for parapharyngeal space tumors. J craniomaxillofacial Surg. 2014;42:835–8.
4. Fujimaki M, Yokoyama J, Ohba S, et al. Dynamic imaging in determining the optimum surgical time for NIR fluorescent image-guided surgery. Head Neck Oncol. 2012;4:50.
5. Poellinger A, Burock S, Grosenick D, et al. Breast Cancer: early- and late-fluorescence near-infrared imaging with indocyanine green-a preliminary study. Radiology. 2011;258:409–16.
6. Yokoyama J, Ohba S. ICG fluorescent image-guided surgery in head and neck cancer. In: Kusano M, Kokudo N, Toi M, Kaibori M, editors. ICG fluorescence imaging and navigation surgery. Tokyo: Springer; 2016. p. 49–62.
7. Ishizawa T, Fukushima N, Shibahara J, Masuda K, Tamura S, Aoki T, Hasegawa K, Beck Y, Fukayama M, Kokudo N. Real-time identification of liver cancers by using indocyanine green fluorescent imaging. Cancer. 2009;115:2491–504.
8. Yokoyama J, Ito S, Ohba S, Fujimaki M, Ikeda K. A novel approach to translymphatic chemotherapy targeting sentinel lymph nodes of patients with oral cancer using intra-arterial chemotherapy. Head Neck Oncol. 2011;3:42.

Andrea Papadia, Junjie Wang,
Maria Luisa Gasparri, Anda Petronela Radan,
Jarmila Anna Zdanowicz, and Michael D. Mueller

Indications

Background of Indocyanine Green (ICG)/Near Infrared (NIR)

Indocyanine green (ICG) is a fluorescent dye developed during World War II by Kodak. Initially meant to be employed in photography, it was granted FDA approval in 1959, after being tested in the United States at Mayo Clinic.

Ever since, its use via intravenous injection has found application in ophthalmology, but also in internal medicine and cardiology. In the last decades, ICG has been successfully employed in oncological surgery [1, 2].

The main advantages, which led to a rapid acceptance of the compound, are the low rate of adverse effects and the rapid excretion, the presence of peak absorption around 800 nm, close to the isobestic point of hemoglobin. This allows the employment of ICG with near infrared light (NIR) for in vivo detection of tissue, with virtually no interference from background autofluorescence caused by water and blood, and excellent applicability in minimally invasive surgery [2, 3]. Indocyanine green has a half-life of around 3 min and is excreted almost exclusively through the bile [4].

Electronic Supplementary Material The online version of this chapter (https://doi.org/10.1007/978-3-030-38092-2_31) contains supplementary material, which is available to authorized users.

A. Papadia (✉)
Department of Obstetrics and Gynecology, Ospedale Regionale di Lugano, Ente Ospedaliero Cantonale, Svizzera Italiana, Lugano, Switzerland
e-mail: andrea.papadia@eoc.chJunjie

J. Wang
Department of Gynaecological Oncology,
KK Women's & Children's Hospital,
Singapore, Singapore

M. L. Gasparri
Department of Gynecology and Obstetrics,
"Sapienza" University of Rome, Rome, Italy

A. P. Radan · J. A. Zdanowicz · M. D. Mueller
Department of Obstetrics and Gynecology,
University Hospital of Bern and University of Bern,
Bern, Switzerland

Application in Sentinel Lymph Node (SLN) Mapping

The first approach in sentinel lymph node (SLN) mapping was made in 1977 by the American urologist Cabanas [5]. Ever since, the method has been adopted in the surgical treatment of melanoma and vulvar and breast cancer [6].

The assessment of lymph node status in gynecological oncology is of great importance for the prognosis of the patient. Regional lymph nodes are, however, often negative for tumor involvement. In the last decades, efforts have been made in avoiding a routine systematic lymphadenectomy in

E. M. Aleassa, K. M. El-Hayek (eds.), *Video Atlas of Intraoperative Applications of Near Infrared Fluorescence Imaging*, https://doi.org/10.1007/978-3-030-38092-2_31

patients with negative nodal status. Analogue to breast cancer, where the method of SLN biopsy is well established, SLN mapping in genital cancers could lead to an improvement in quality of life after surgery, to better surgical results, a faster recovery, reduced blood loss, and a shorter hospital stay. It has been shown that long-term complications such as lymphedema of the lower extremities and sensory loss were more common when routine systematic lymphadenectomy was performed [7, 8].

Technetium-99 radiocolloid (Tc-99 m) and blue dyes (methylene, isosulfan or patent blue) are other commonly used tracers in the surgery of genital cancers. Blue dyes are relatively often associated with severe allergic reactions (0.7–1.9%), as well as with discoloration of the urine, tegument necrosis, and interference with pulsoxymetry readings [6]. ICG has an outstanding toxicity profile, with a low rate of allergic reactions (0.05% after intravenous application) [9].

The manufacturers recommend caution in patients allergic to iodide, as ICG contains sodium iodide, as well as in patients with severe liver disease [6]. Indocyanine green has also been employed during pregnancy [10].

Tc-99 m is also described as safe; however, it leads to low patient satisfaction when employed, due to the fact that its employment requires additional hospital appointments and it is not injected under general anesthesia [6, 11].

After submucosal injection of ICG (off-label), this distributes in lymph pathways and lymph nodes, making it a suitable tracer for these structures. Its small particles exhibit fluorescence when using NIR technology, which makes it excellent for employment in minimal invasive surgery, but also in open surgery [6].

SLN Mapping in Gynecologic Oncology

Endometrial Cancer

The diagnosis of endometrial cancer occurs in most cases at an early stage. One important prognostic factor is the nodal status, as 5-year survival drops from 95% to 70% in case of nodal involvement. Nodal involvement in endometrial cancer

is not uncommon; however, the risk for lymph node metastasis is low in small, well-differentiated tumors [12].

The lymphatic drainage of the uterus is known to be complex. Anatomic studies describe four lymphatic pathways: the upper and the lower cervical pathway, an infundibulo-pelvic pathway, and a pathway that runs around the round ligament to the inguino-femoral and to Cloquet's lymph nodes. The upper cervical pathway drains the lymph nodes situated in the obturator fossa as well as those of the iliac vessels; the lower cervical pathway is responsible of draining the presacral lymph nodes. The latter are not included in a systematic pelvic lymphadenectomy.

Since 1988, following the GOG#33 trial, FIGO recommends a surgical rather than a clinical staging in endometrial cancer. The adherence to this recommendation worldwide is however low, assumingly due to the complexity of the procedure and patients' characteristics (often presence of comorbidities, mostly patients with obesity). Identifying patients who benefit most from a surgical staging is of great importance. A widespread approach is the intraoperative identification of risk factors by analyzing the uterus at frozen section. However, the method has intrinsic limitations and reports regarding its accuracy vary among different series [12].

In the past years, identification of SLNs has been proposed as an alternative to this method, respectively, as a solution between performing a systematic lymphadenectomy or no lymphadenectomy at all. The procedure has, however, only been accepted by a part of the international guidelines so far.

Whereas the National Comprehensive Cancer Center (NCCN) guidelines consider SLN mapping in endometrial cancer as acceptable when employed in selected cases, the ESMO-ESGO-ESTRO consensus conference recommends only offering it in the setting of clinical trials [13, 14].

Two large prospective trials to SLN mapping in endometrial cancer are available: the SENTI-ENDO trial and the FIRES trial [8, 15]. In the SENTI-ENDO trial, the detection was performed by employing Tc-99 m combined with blue dye. The authors report a false negative rate of 18%

(3 out of 20 patients with lymph node involvement). It is worth mentioning that all false negative events occurred in cases of type II endometrial cancer, which raises concern with employing the method in these patients [15].

However, recent trials report promising results for SLN mapping in high-risk constellations, with false negative rates comparable to those found in low-risk patients [8]. One of those is the FIRES trial, where sentinel lymph node detection was performed by using ICG, which has been injected directly in the cervix. The trial reports an excellent false negative rate of only 3%. Rossi et al. reportedly adopted the mapping algorithm proposed by Barlin et al. from the Memorial Sloan Kettering Center (MSKCC). This algorithm suggests beyond unilateral mapping in case of SLN positivity the removal of all clinically suspicious lymph nodes. Barlin et al. also describe a low false negative rate of only 2%, as opposed to 15% before introducing their algorithm [8, 16]. The NCCN guidelines also recommend adopting the MSKCC algorithm [12, 13].

Although false negative rates play a great role in analyzing the accuracy of a method, it is the disease-free survival of the patient that is of most interest in oncology. How et al. found that SLN mapping prior to pelvic lymphadenectomy led to less pelvic side recurrences, which suggests that lymph node harvesting by mapping is more accurate. By performing a systematic lymphadenectomy, one risks omitting relevant lymph nodes [11].

After 30 years of controversy on lymphadenectomy in endometrial cancer, SLN mapping seems to be an equitable alternative to take into consideration.

Cervical Cancer

Early-stage cervical cancer is routinely treated by radical hysterectomy. In selected cases, patients can be offered fertility-sparing surgery, meaning performing wide conization or trachelectomy. Similar to endometrial cancer, nodal involvement plays a great prognostic role in cervical cancer. For this reason, a systematic pelvic lymphadenectomy should be performed in early stages [17].

Analogue to endometrial cancer, the method of SLN mapping was proposed in the management of cervical cancer. The considerations are similar: reducing morbidity by reducing surgical trauma. Although the method is not yet established, it is progressively being adopted in clinical practice. The first trials show promising results, with good detection rates (Cormier et al. unilateral detection rate 93% [18], bilateral detection rate 75%; Diaz et al. unilateral detection rate 95% [19]). Moreover, ultrastaging allows better detection of micro-metastasis [18, 19].

Vulvar Cancer

Squamous cell cancer of the vulva is rare, with an incidence of 3/100,000 women per year. The 5-year survival rates reach 90% without lymph node involvement, and rapidly drop at 50% when positive lymph nodes are present. Until 10 years ago, radical excision of the tumor and radical inguino-femoral lymphadenectomy was considered standard of care for the affected patients, although lymph node metastasis was ultimately present in only 25–35% of the cases [20]. Around 50% of the women who underwent surgery suffer a wound complication [21]. While local complications such as wound dehiscence or infection are temporary, lymphedema can accompany the patient throughout her lifetime.

Meanwhile, based on the results of two big trials, SLN mapping in the treatment of vulvar cancer is considered standard of care. Detection of SLNs is standardly performed by using Tc-99 m and blue dye; however, employment of ICG has increasingly gained acceptance in the past years [20, 21].

Ovarian Cancer

Although SLN mapping is rapidly gaining popularity in most types of female genital cancer, its applicability in the treatment of ovarian cancer has been so far limited. Its limitations arise from the fact that in most cases, disease is diagnosed at an advanced stage. The method has only been employed in experimental pilot cases so far. In most cases, lymph node detection was performed by using Tc-99 m and blue dye. Multiple questions are still open, beginning with adequate selection of the patients to proper site of tracer injection, as the literature on this topic is still scarce [22].

Technical Description of the Procedure

LSC

Typically, the surgery for cervical and endometrial cancer using ICG has been performed laparoscopically. To date, there are two main protocols for injecting ICG, directly into the cervix and using hysteroscopic guidance, respectively [1, 23–27]. Other possible injection sites will be also discussed in this section.

One important difference between Tc-99m and ICG is that ICG is injected at the beginning of surgery under general anesthesia [11, 23]. A more detailed comparison of ICG with other dyes will be presented in the following section.

In general, ICG powder is suspended in sterile water to yield a green solution. The dosage and concentration used vary in literature. Once ICG is injected, it travels via lymphatic vessels to the SLNs where it persists for some time. However, ICG also spreads not only to echelon but also to second-echelon lymph nodes, potentially leading to removal of additional, non-SLNs (NSLNs) (Video 31.1) [6].

Algorithms have been established with regard to SLNs as well as to the removal of suspicious looking lymph nodes, such as the MSKCC algorithm [16]. According to this algorithm, all the SLNs along with clinically suspicious lymph nodes have to be removed. Additionally, in case of unilateral mapping, a side-specific lymphadenectomy has to be performed. A para-aortic lymphadenectomy is performed at physician's discretion.

In endometrial cancer, four lymphatic systems that drain the uterus have been identified [28]: a lower paracervical pathway draining into the internal iliac and/or presacral lymph nodes [29]; an upper paracervical pathway that drains to lymph nodes in the obturator fossa as well as external iliac vessels; in addition, para-aortic lymphatic drainage occurs at the aortic infra-mesenteric level, as well as the aortic infrarenal level [30].

After performing the SLN mapping, the removed lymph nodes are further analyzed according to an ultrastaging protocol. Here, an in-depth pathological examination allows for an even more thorough investigation of nodal disease, which is then classified according to tumor size [31]. The steps of the laparoscopic ICG SLN mapping for uterine malignancies are depicted in Figs. 31.1, 31.2, 31.3, 31.4, 31.5, and 31.6.

However, some open questions remain, such as defining the optimal time between tracer injection and detection as well as finding the optimal dose of ICG, including for bilateral detection [3]. It is important that lymph nodes on both sides of the pelvis are detected, bilateral detection is

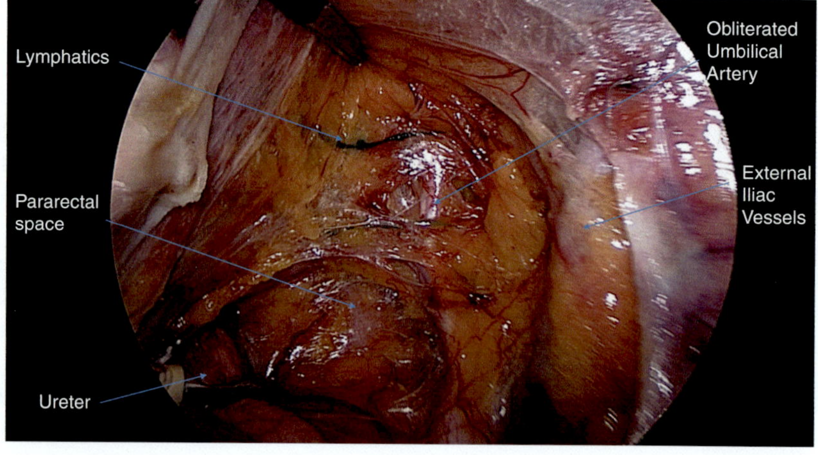

Fig. 31.1 Left retroperitoneal space after administration of ICG. Lymphatics could often be visible under white light

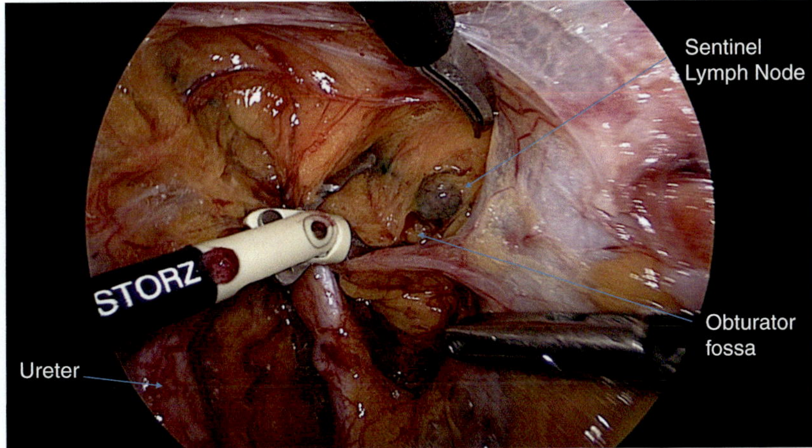

Fig. 31.2 Sentinel lymph node (under white light) found in left obturator fossa—the most common location

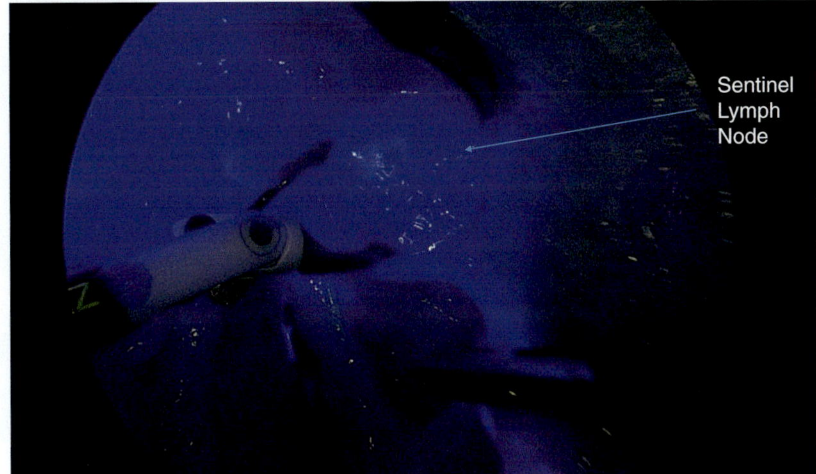

Fig. 31.3 Visualization of sentinel lymph node under near-infrared fluorescence imaging. We can see the lymphatics leading toward the sentinel lymph node

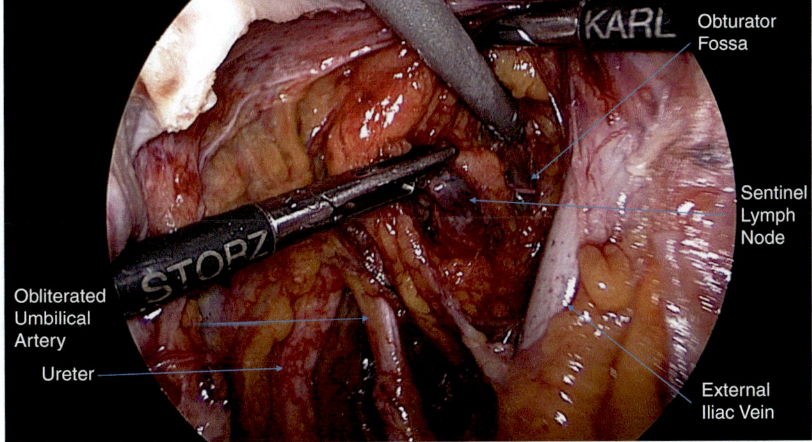

Fig. 31.4 Dissection and removal of sentinel lymph node from the left obturator fossa

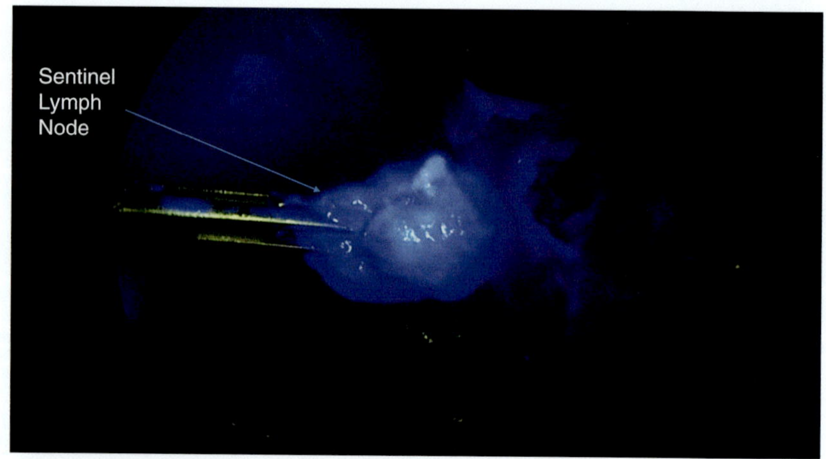

Fig. 31.5 Confirmation of sentinel lymph node under near-infrared fluorescence imaging after dissection

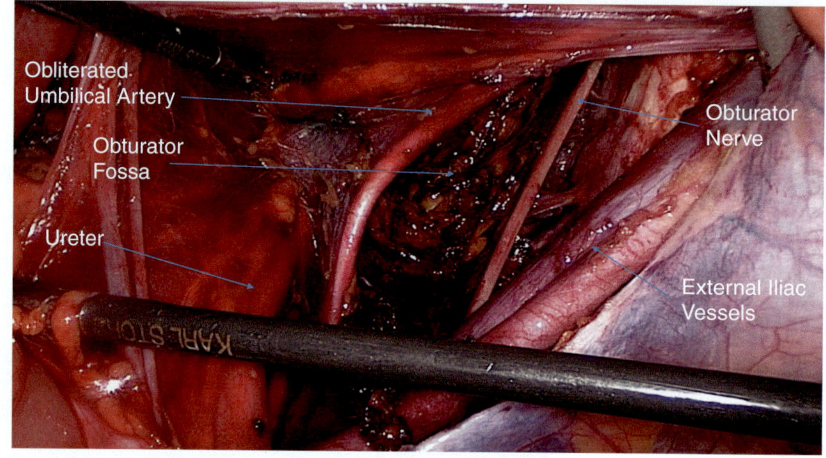

Fig. 31.6 Left retroperitoneal space after pelvic lymph node dissection, showing important structures like the ureter, external illiac vessels, obturator nerve, and obliterated umbilical artery

therefore crucial in ICG SLN mapping [16]. Here, ICG has also shown to be superior when compared to other dyes [6, 11, 23, 32–35]. A larger dose of ICG does seem to yield a higher number of marked SLN, however, not a higher bilateral detection rate [36].

Cervical Injection

For cervical as well as endometrial cancer, the injection of ICG can be performed intracervically. In this case, the dye is usually injected submucosally as well as inside the cervical stroma.

After the standard laparoscopic setup, a diagnostic laparoscopy is performed to ascertain operability. The ICG injections are then performed with a 21–23-gauge needle, typically into the four quadrants of the cervix at 2, 4, 8, and 10 o'clock, although injections at 3, 6, 9, and 12 o'clock have been described as well [6, 27–28, 36]. Alternatively, only two injection sites have been used, namely, at 3 and 9 o'clock [8, 11, 32]. The injection occurs usually at a deep as well as superficial level of the cervix.

Usually, 25 mg of ICG powder is diluted in sterile water to achieve a concentration between 0.5 mg/ml and 2.5 mg/ml [8, 11, 27–28, 32, 37], although a concentration of 5 mg/ml has been used as well [36]. Using a laparoscopic NIR setup, the fluorescent signal is then identified and the SLNs are removed for further examination. A higher ICG concentration has been shown to remove more SLNs; however, if too much dye is applied, there is a greater risk of labeling NSLNs as well [36]. The total dose of ICG injected varies from 1 mg up to 40 mg [1, 8, 32, 36].

The advantages of intracervical injection are quite obvious: the technique is easy to reproduce and it provides an easier accessibility for the surgeon. However, in endometrial cancer, it has been argued that the injection site is remote to the actual tumor location.

Hysteroscopic Peritumoral Injection for Endometrial Cancer

Several studies have also described a hysteroscopic peritumoral injection of tracer for endometrical cancer [25, 26]. Using this protocol, after a standard laparoscopic setup and diagnostic laparoscopy, a hysteroscopy is performed. Tracer injection occurs with an 18–23-gauge needle subendometrially around the lesion, or, in cases where the tumor fills the entire uterine cavity, injection occurs at 3, 6, 9, and 12 o'clock peritumorally [25–27, 37]. As in the cervical injection, ICG powder is diluted in sterile water to achieve a concentration between 0.5 mg/ml and 1.25 mg/ml [25–27]. A laparoscopic NIR setup is used to detect the fluorescent signal and, consequently, the SLN are removed. In some studies, a tubal occlusion has been performed prior to tracer injection to prevent peritoneal spilling of dye [25, 27].

When comparing the two possible injection protocols, cervical tracer injection is easier to perform, while a hysteroscopic injection is more invasive and requires an additional surgical procedure [27]. In addition, the learning curve for hysteroscopic tracer injection may be longer and require a more skilled surgeon, while the tumor itself might be a visual impediment during hysteroscopic injection [12]. Overall, a combination of hysteroscopic and intracervical might lead to the most effective detection of the SLNs [25].

Infundibulo-Pelvic Ligament Injection

As described above, the lymphatic drainage of the uterus is quite complex. In addition to the pelvic drainage, there is a non-pelvic pathway along the infundibulo-pelvic ligament to the para-aortic lymph nodes [31]. In high-risk endometrial carcinoma, the removal of para-aortic lymph nodes is recommended [38]. An algorithm has been proposed for management of lymphadenectomy in high-risk patients [39].

No study to date has evaluated the direct tracer injection into the infundibulo-pelvic ligament as a possible additional site for enhanced SLN mapping. However, transabdominal fundal injection seems to result in visualization of lymphatic vessels that run along the IP ligament, but also to cause greater leakage of ICG into the abdomen [28].

Open Surgery (VITOM®)

Laparotomy

To date, there have been relatively few data on the SLN mapping in gynecology and open surgery. In open gynecological cancer surgery for vulvar carcinoma, ICG tracking for SLN mapping has been conducted using the Karl Storz VITOM® Fluorescence Camera (VITOM® II ICG). The VITOM® II exoscope consists of a telescope connected to an NIR camera for detection of fluorescent light.

As previously described, ICG powder is diluted in sterile water to a concentration of 1.25 mg/ml and is injected intracervically at 3 and 9 o'clock in case of cervical and endometrial cancer, respectively [40]. In vulvar cancer, peritumoral injection with the same ICG concentration was performed with 28-gauge needle after a preoperative lymphoscintigraphy [40].

Inguino-Femoral SLN Mapping

Lymphatic drainage of vulvar cancer occurs along the labia majora from dorsal to ventral, further implicating the inguinal as well as pelvic lymph nodes. In early-stage vulvar cancer, a complete lymphadenectomy may be unnecessary, hence SLN mapping via ICG could provide a useful alternative here [41].

Interpretation

False Negative Rate

The false negative rate of an SLN mapping is defined as the number of false negative SLNs divided by the number of cases with lymph nodal metastases and represents the most important characteristic of the procedure. In order for the procedure to be safe and reliable, the false negative rate has to be low so that the chance of missing an affected lymph node is low. The SLN mapping algorithm was described by MSKCC and adopted by Barlin et al. in their study in 2012 [16]. The algorithm recommends removing all the clinically suspicious NSLNs other than the SLNs, performing a side-specific lymphadenectomy in case of unilateral mapping and performing a para-aortic lymphadenectomy based on surgeon's indication. Barlin et al. found that with the application of this algorithm, they were able to reduce the false negative rate of SLN mapping in endometrial cancer from 15% to 2%. In a retrospective series of fully staged endometrial cancer patients, Papadia et al. recorded a false negative rate of 8.3% for the ICG sentinel lymph node mapping [10]. This result correlates well with those reported by Barlin et al. [16]. The FIRES trial is a prospective multicenter validation trial that was performed in the United States, following the SLN mapping algorithm. In the FIRES trial, the SLN mapping was performed via intracervical injection of ICG followed by robotic-assisted systematic pelvic lymphadenectomy in every patient and para-aortic lymphadenectomy in approximately half of the patients [8]. In this trial, Rossi et al. recorded one false negative SLN and 35 true positive SLNs accounting for an excellent false negative rate of approximately 3%.

Detection Rate

Another characteristic that defines a successful SLN node mapping is a high detection rate. In order to have a complete and successful mapping, SLNs need to be detected on both sides of the pelvis. A high bilateral detection rate will additionally help in reducing the number of side-specific pelvic lymphadenectomies when the MSKCC SLN mapping algorithm is adopted [16].

In 2015, Imboden et al. showed, in a retrospective study, that ICG has higher bilateral detection rates as compared to a combination of Tc-99 m and blue dye in cervical cancer patients [37]. Papadia et al. also showed that in patients with endometrial cancer who underwent an ICG laparoscopic sentinel lymph node mapping, the overall and bilateral detection rates were 96% and 88%, respectively [23]. Both studies were performed with the tracer injected intracervically.

In 2016, a meta-analysis on endometrial cancers, performed on the data available at that time, demonstrated that the SLN mapping had higher overall and bilateral detection rates when the procedures were performed with ICG, as compared to blue dyes (OR 0.27 95% CI 0.15–0.50; $p < 0.0001$; OR 0.27; 95% CI 0.19–0.40; $p < 0.00001$, respectively). However, ICG SLN was not significantly superior to the combination of blue dyes and Tc-99 m, in terms of overall and bilateral detection rates and false negative rate [42]. In a multicenter cohort study, involving five European centers, the bilateral detection rate for ICG was 84.1%, as compared to the 73.5% obtained with Tc-99 m in association with blue dye ($p = 0.007$) [23]. Recently, the FILM trial, a randomized, phase III multicenter study, confirmed that ICG with near-infrared fluorescence imaging is able to identify more SLNs than blue dye in women with endometrial and cervical cancers, defining the NIR-ICG SLN mapping technique as the current standard of care [32].

Comparison Between Dyes

ICG has an excellent toxicity profile, has higher overall and bilateral detection rates as compared to blue dyes and higher bilateral detection rates as compared to a combination of Tc-99 m and blue dye [6]. As compared to Tc-99 m, ICG is not radioactive and can be injected after induction of anesthesia in the operating room at the time of the surgery. Tc-99 m is injected the day prior to surgery in a radio-protected outpatient setting and is followed by a lymphoscintigraphy or SPECT–CT to determine number and anatomic location of the SLNs. A significant delay in the surgical schedule may compromise the identification of a radioactive signal with the gamma probe. ICG is also overall more cost-effective than Tc-99 m and blue dye. As compared to the other tracer, ICG is associated with a lower incidence of allergic reactions.

Role of SLN Mapping in Endometrial Cancer

Pathological lymph node assessment is a controversial issue in low-risk endometrial cancer. However, in these preoperatively low-risk patients, some may turn out to have high-risk endometrial carcinoma after the final pathology. This group of patients has a 40% risk of nodal involvement [43]. If lymph node assessment was not performed, then there will be an indication for adjuvant radiotherapy.

In a group of patients with preoperative diagnosis of complex atypical hyperplasia or grade 1 or 2 endometrial cancer, Papadia et al. showed that a strategy based on SLN mapping is more accurate in detecting patients with lymph nodal metastases as compared to a strategy based on triage to a systematic lymphadenectomy based on intraoperative frozen section analysis of the uterus [44]. SLN mapping identified all lymph nodal metastases, whereas one out of six patients with nodal metastases was missed with the strategy that relies on a full lymphadenectomy when uterine risk factors are identified at frozen section. The latter strategy has a false negative rate of 16.7% at the cost of performing a systematic lymphadenectomy in approximately one-third of patients considered to be at low risk preoperatively. Sinno et al. recommend performing an SLN mapping in patients who are preoperatively considered to be at low risk [45]. A frozen section of the uterus is performed in cases wherein the SLN mapping fails, and a bilateral or side-specific pelvic lymphadenectomy is performed when the frozen section analysis of the uterus defines the endometrial cancer as a high-risk one.

In a large retrospective study involving over 1000 patients with endometrial cancer and limited myometrial invasion from the Mayo Clinic and from the MSKCC, a comparable 3-year disease-free survival was recorded for patients undergoing a systematic lymphadenectomy versus an SLN mapping according to the MSKCC algorithm [46]. In an Italian multicenter retrospective study comparing 145 patients undergoing an SLN mapping according to the MSKCC algorithm versus 657 patients undergoing a full lymphadenectomy for an early-stage endometrial cancer, the recorded disease-free survival was comparable [47].

In 2014, the NCCN guidelines first recognized the SLN mapping as an acceptable alternative to a systematic lymphadenectomy in selected case of endometrial cancer. Since then, the NCCN guidelines have extended the indication to an SLN mapping algorithm even in high-risk endometrial cancer patients [13]. On the other hand, the ESMO-ESGO-ESTRO guidelines recommend the adoption of the SLN mapping in endometrial cancer patients only within controlled trials [14].

Role of SLN Mapping in Cervical Cancer

In cervical cancer, lymph node metastasis is the most important prognostic factor influencing prognosis and treatment. Concomitant chemoradiotherapy is indicated in nodal involvement. The combination of radical surgery and adjuvant radiotherapy is not associated with a better oncologic outcome but is associated with a higher incidence of treatment-related toxicity than radiotherapy alone. If metastatic nodal disease could be identified prior to radical surgery, an unnecessary and potentially toxic multimodality treatment could be avoided. SLN mapping may be useful for decreasing the need for full pelvic lymphadenectomy in patients with early-stage cervical cancer [18].

Tax et al. in a meta-analysis of 44 studies comprising 3931 patients found an overall sensitivity of the SLN biopsy and ultrastaging to be 94% [48]. Similarly, a retrospective review of 188 patients with early-stage cervical cancer performed showed a sensitivity of 96.4% and negative predictive value of 99.3% [49].

SLN mapping is considered in the surgical management of selected stage I cervical cancer as mentioned in the NCCN guidelines for cervical cancer (NCCN). The sensitivity of SLN mapping coupled with ultrastaging seems to be better in patients with tumors of 2 cm or smaller [18, 51]. NCCN recommends that the best detection and mapping results are in tumors of less than 2 cm in diameter. Surgeons should also remove all suspicious or grossly enlarged nodes regardless of SLN mapping and perform side-specific nodal dissection in the event of failed mapping [13].

Role of SLN Mapping in Vulvar Cancer

Lymph node metastasis is the most significant prognostic factor in vulvar carcinoma. Up to 35% of patients with early-stage vulvar cancer have lymph node metastases. Therefore, 65% of these patients do not benefit from elective inguino-femoral lymphadenectomy but may suffer from its complications like lymphedema and wound infection. Sentinel lymph node mapping allows assessment of the inguinal lymph nodes without the need to remove all nodes, and provides an opportunity to reduce the morbidity associated with full lymphadenectomy.

Technetium-99 m with or without blue dye has been used in SLN mapping of vulvar cancer with very high detection rates of the SLN ranging up to 100% [50, 51]. A more recently introduced technique involves near-infrared fluorescence-guided SLN mapping using ICG.

NCCN guideline for vulvar cancer recommends SLN mapping for vulvar cancer patients with negative clinical groin examination and imaging, a primary unifocal vulvar tumor size of <4 cm, and no previous vulvar surgery that may have impacted lymphatic flow to the inguinal region [52–54].

SLN mapping is used in patients with depth of invasion greater than 1 mm (FIGO stage IB or worse) or when the maximum diameter of the tumor is greater than 2 cm but less than 4 cm. If the SLN is negative, there is no need for full lymphadenectomy. This protocol is associated with a groin recurrence rate of 2.3% in unifocal vulvar disease and 3% in multifocal disease [55]. A complete inguino-femoral lymphadenectomy is recommended if an ipsilateral SLN is not detected.

Pitfalls

The excellent integration between near-infrared platforms and minimally invasive surgery has significantly accelerated the development and the clinical acceptance of the sentinel lymph node mapping in uterine malignancies. However, various pitfalls that physicians adopting this technique need to be aware of, still exist.

First, as of now ICG has been FDA approved for intravenous use only. Consequently, the patients need to be informed and consented about the off-label use of this compound that needs to be injected interstitially for the SLN mapping. Despite its favorable toxicity profile, severe allergic reactions to ICG have been reported [6, 55]. The recent publication of a prospective randomized controlled trial comparing the performance of ICG and blue dye in endometrial and cervical cancer patients may help to get the FDA for the interstitial injection of ICG [32].

Second, the dose of ICG employed for the SLN mapping has been empirically set. Various institutions have adopted different doses and concentrations of the dose [6, 12, 29, 36]. Regardless of the dose adopted, the reported results in terms of detection rates and false negative rates have been consistently superior to those reported with other tracers, suggesting that the adopted dose probably only plays a minor role in the performance of the mapping. However, higher doses of ICG have been shown to lead to an increase of the number of detected lymph nodes and to an increase of the bilateral detection of all the upper and lower paracervical lymphatic pathways [29, 36]. On the other hand, the removal of a larger number of SLNs does not seem to translate into a lower false negative rate [56]. As compared to the blue dyes, the visual signal of ICG is more persistent. After having traveled to the SLNs it moves cephalad to the non-SLN located downstream of the SLN. Both the SLN and the non-SLNs remain stained and it may become difficult to differentiate between the two. This may lead to an oversampling of lymph nodes that are erroneously labeled as SLNs.

Third, the site of tracer injection for the SLN mapping in endometrial cancer remains debatable. Some authors suggest that a hysteroscopic peritumoral injection is more "anatomically correct" as compared to a pericervical injection leading to a different distribution of the SLNs [24–26, 37].

Finally, fluorescence surgery in gynecologic oncology remains an experimental procedure both for the adoption of the SLN mapping, at least for endometrial and cervical cancer, and for the adoption of ICG as a tracer. The diffusion of fluorescence surgery and of the SLN mapping in this setting did not strictly follow the IDEAL recommendations to evaluate surgical interventions [57].

References

1. Papadia A, Imboden S, Siegenthaler F, et al. Laparoscopic indocyanine green sentinel lymph node mapping in endometrial cancer. Ann Surg Oncol. 2016;23:2206–11.
2. Alander JT, Kaartinen IL, Laakso A, et al. A review of indocyanine green fluorescent imaging in surgery. Int J Biomed Imaging. 2012;2012:940585.
3. Gasparri ML, Mueller MD, Papadia A. Instead of feeling blue, go green! Lancet Oncol. 2018; 19:1273–4.
4. Scott P, Optical absorption of Indocyanine green. Oregon Medical Laser Center. https://omlc.org/spectra/icg/.
5. Cabanas RM. An approach for the treatment of penile carcinoma. Cancer. 1977 Feb;39(2):456–66.
6. Papadia A, Gasparri ML, Buda A, Mueller MD. Sentinel lymph node mapping in endometrial cancer: comparison of fluorescence dye with traditional radiocolloid and blue. J Cancer Res Clin Oncol. 2017;143:2039–48. https://doi.org/10.1007/s00432–017–2501–8. PubMed PMID: 28828528.
7. Papadia A, Remorgida V, Salom EM, et al. Laparoscopic pelvic and paraaortic lymphadenectomy in gynecologic oncology. J Am Assoc Gynecol Laparosc. 2004;11:297–306.
8. Rossi EC, Kowalski LD, Scalici J, et al. A comparison of sentinel lymph node biopsy to lymphadenectomy for endometrial cancer staging (FIRES trial): a multicentre, prospective, cohort study Lancet Oncol. 2017;18:384–92.
9. Hope-Ross M, Yannuzzi LA, Gragoudas ES, et al. Adverse reactions due to indocyanine green. Ophthalmology. 1994;101:529–33.
10. Papadia A, Mohr S, Imboden S, et al. Laparoscopic indocyanine green sentinel lymph node mapping in pregnant cervical cancer patients. J Minim Invasive Gynecol. 2016;1:270–3.
11. Buda A, Elisei F, Palazzi S, et al. Quality of care for cervical and endometrial cancer patients: the impact of different techniques of sentinel lymph node mapping on patient satisfaction. Ann Surg Oncol. 2016;23:2975–81.
12. Papadia A, Gasparri ML, Wang J, et al. Sentinel Node biopsy for treatment of endometrial cancer. State of the art. Minerva Ginecol. 2019;71:25–35. https://doi.org/10.23736/S0026–4784.18.04337-X. PMID: 30318882.
13. NCCN Clinical Practice Guidelines in Oncology. Uterine neoplasms. Version 2. 2018. http://www.nccn.org/professionals/physician_gls/pdf/uterine.pdf. Accessed 7 Aug 2018).
14. Colombo N, Creutzberg C, Amant F, et al. ESMO-ESGO-ESTRO consensus conference on endometrial cancer: diagnosis, treatment and follow-up. Ann Oncol. 2016;27:16–41.
15. Daraï E, Dubernard G, Bats AS, et al. Sentinel node biopsy for the management of early stage endometrial cancer: long-term results of the SENTI-ENDO study. Gynecol Oncol. 2015;136:54–9.
16. Barlin JN, Khoury-Collado F, Kim CH, et al. The importance of applying a sentinel lymph node mapping algorithm in endometrial cancer staging: beyond removal of blue nodes. Gynecol Oncol. 2012;125:531–5.
17. Buda A, Papadia A, et al. From conventional radiotracer Tc-99(m) with blue dye to indocyanine green fluorescence: a comparison of methods towards optimization of sentinel lymph node mapping in early stage cervical cancer for a laparoscopic approach. Ann Surg Oncol. 2016;23:1959–65.
18. Cormier B, Diaz JP, Shih K, et al. Establishing a sentinel lymph node mapping algorithm for the treatment of early cervical cancer. Gynecol Oncol. 2011;122:275–80.
19. Diaz JP, et al. Sentinel lymph node biopsy in the management of early-stage cervical carcinoma. Gynecol Oncol. 2011;120:347–52.
20. Van der Zee AG, Oonk MH, De Hullu JA, et al. Sentinel node dissection is safe in the treatment of early-stage vulvar cancer. J Clin Oncol. 2008;26:884–9.
21. Levenback CF, Ali S, Coleman RL, et al. Lymphatic mapping and sentinel lymph node biopsy in women with squamous cell carcinoma of the vulva: a gynecologic oncology group study. J Clin Oncol. 2008;26:884–9.
22. Uccella S, Gisone B, Stevenazzi G, et al. Laparoscopic sentinel node detection with ICG for early ovarian cancer: Description of a technique and literature review. Eur J Obstet Gynecol Reprod Biol. 2018;221:193–4.
23. Papadia A, Zapardiel I, Bussi B, Ghezzi F, Ceccaroni M, De Ponti E, Elisei F, Imboden S, de la Noval BD, Gasparri ML, Di Martino G, De Santiago J, Mueller M, Vecchione F, Dell'Orto F, Buda A. Sentinel lymph node mapping in patients with stage I endometrial carcinoma: a focus on bilateral mapping identification by comparing radiotracer Tc99$_m$ with blue dye versus

indocyanine green fluorescent dye. J Cancer Res Clin Oncol. 2017;143:475–80.

24. Martinelli F, Ditto A, Signorelli M, Bogani G, Chiappa V, Lorusso D, Scaffa C, Recalcati D, Perotto S, Haeusler E, Raspagliesi F. Sentinel node mapping in endometrial cancer following Hysteroscopic injection of tracers: a single center evaluation over 200 cases. Gynecol Oncol. 2017;146:525–30.

25. Martinelli F, Ditto A, Bogani G, Signorelli M, Chiappa V, Lorusso D, Haeusler E, Raspagliesi F. Laparoscopic sentinel node mapping in endometrial cancer after hysteroscopic injection of indocyanine green. J Minim Invasive Gynecol. 2017;24: 89–93.

26. Ditto A, Martinelli F, Bogani G, Papadia A, Lorusso D, Raspagliesi F. Sentinel node mapping using hysteroscopic injection of indocyanine green and laparoscopic near-infrared fluorescence imaging in endometrial cancer staging. J Minim Invasive Gynecol. 2015;22:132–3.

27. Rossi EC, Jackson A, Ivanova A, Boggess JF. Detection of sentinel nodes for endometrial cancer with robotic assisted fluorescence imaging: cervical versus hysteroscopic injection. Int J Gynecol Cancer. 2013;23:1704–11.

28. Geppert B, Lönnerfors C, Bollino M, Arechvo A, Persson J. A study on uterine lymphatic anatomy for standardization of pelvic sentinel lymph node detection in endometrial cancer. Gynecol Oncol. 2017;145:256–61.

29. Persson J, Geppert B, Lönnerfors C, Bollino M, Måsbäck A. Description of a reproducible anatomically based surgical algorithm for detection of pelvic sentinel lymph nodes in endometrial cancer. Gynecol Oncol. 2017;147:120–5.

30. Querleu D, Morrow CP. Classification of radical hysterectomy. Lancet Oncol. 2008;9:297–303.

31. Greene FL, Page DL, Irvin D, et al. AJCC cancer staging manual. 6th ed. New York: Springer-Verlag; 2003. p. 223–40.

32. Frumovitz M, Plante M, Lee PS, Sandadi S, Lilja JF, Escobar PF, Gien LT, Urbauer DL, Abu-Rustum NR. Near-infrared fluorescence for detection of sentinel lymph nodes in women with cervical and uterine cancers (FILM): a randomised, phase 3, multicentre, non-inferiority trial. Lancet Oncol. 2018;19:1394–403.

33. Buda A, Papadia A, Di Martino G, Imboden S, Bussi B, Guerra L, De Ponti E, Reato C, Gasparri ML, Crivellaro C, Mueller M. Real-time fluorescent sentinel lymph node mapping with indocyanine green in women with previous conization undergoing laparoscopic surgery for early invasive cervical cancer: comparison with radiotracer±blue dye. J Minim Invasive Gynecol. 2018;25:455–60.

34. Di Martino G, Crivellaro C, De Ponti E, Bussi B, Papadia A, Zapardiel I, Vizza E, Elisei F, Diestro MD, Locatelli L, Gasparri ML, Di Lorenzo P, Mueller M, Buda A. Indocyanine green versus radiotracer with or without blue dye for sentinel lymph node mapping in

stage >IB1 cervical cancer (>2 cm). J Minim Invasive Gynecol. 2017;24:954–9.

35. Holloway RW, Bravo RA, Rakowski JA, James JA, Jeppson CN, Ingersoll SB, Ahmad S. Detection of sentinel lymph nodes in patients with endometrial cancer undergoing robotic-assisted staging: a comparison of colorimetric and fluorescence imaging. Gynecol Oncol. 2012;126:25–9.

36. Papadia A, Buda A, Gasparri ML, Di Martino G, Bussi B, Verri D, Mueller MD. The impact of different doses of indocyanine green on the sentinel lymph-node mapping in early stage endometrial cancer. J Cancer Res Clin Oncol. 2018;144:2187–91.

37. Imboden S, Papadia A, Nauwerk M, McKinnon B, Kollmann Z, Mohr S, Lanz S, Mueller MD. A comparison of radiocolloid and indocyanine green fluorescence imaging, sentinel lymph node mapping in patients with cervical cancer undergoing laparoscopic surgery. Ann Surg Oncol. 2015;22:4198–203.

38. Mariani A, Dowdy SC, Cliby WA, Gostout BS, Jones MB, Wilson TO, Podratz KC. Prospective assessment of lymphatic dissemination in endometrial cancer: a paradigm shift in surgical staging. Gynecol Oncol. 2008;109:11–8.

39. Kumar S, Podratz KC, Bakkum-Gamez JN, Dowdy SC, Weaver AL, McGree ME, Cliby WA, Keeney GL, Thomas G, Mariani A. Prospective assessment of the prevalence of pelvic, paraaortic and high paraaortic lymph node metastasis in endometrial cancer. Gynecol Oncol. 2014;132:38–43.

40. Buda A, Dell'Anna T, Vecchione F, Verri D, Di Martino G, Milani R. Near-infrared sentinel lymph node mapping with indocyanine green using the VITOM II ICG exoscope for open surgery for gynecologic malignancies. J Minim Invasive Gynecol. 2016;23:628–32.

41. Martínez-Palones JM, Pérez-Benavente MA, Gil-Moreno A, Díaz-Feijoo B, Roca I, García-Jiménez A, Aguilar-Martínez I, Xercavins J. Comparison of recurrence after vulvectomy and lymphadenectomy with and without sentinel node biopsy in early stage vulvar cancer. Gynecol Oncol. 2006;103:865–70.

42. Ruscito I, Gasparri ML, Braicu EI, Bellati F, Raio L, Sehouli J, Mueller MD, Panici PB, Papadia A. Sentinel node mapping in cervical and endometrial cancer: indocyanine green versus other conventional dyes-a meta-analysis. Ann Surg Oncol. 2016;23:3749–56.

43. Ouldamer L, Bendifallah S, Body G, et al. Call for surgical nodal staging in women with ESMO/ESGO/ESTRO high-intermediate risk endometrial cancer: a multicentre cohort analysis from the FRANCOGYN Study Group. Ann Surg Oncol. 2017;24:1660–6.

44. Papadia A, Gasparri ML, Siegenthaler F, et al. FIGO stage IIIC endometrial cancer identification among patients with complex atypical hyperplasia, grade 1 and 2 endometrioid endometrial cancer: laparoscopic indocyanine green sentinel lymph node mapping versus frozen section of the uterus, why get around the problem? J Cancer Res Clin Oncol. 2017;143:491–7.

45. Sinno AK, Peijnenburg E, Fader AN, et al. Reducing overtreatment: a comparison of lymph node assessment strategies for endometrial cancer. Gynecol Oncol. 2016;143:281–6.

46. Eriksson AG, Ducie J, Ali N, et al. Comparison of a sentinel lymph node and a selective lymphadenectomy algorithm in patients with endometrioid endometrial carcinoma and limited myometrial invasion. Gynecol Oncol. 2016;140:394–9.

47. Buda A, Di Martino G, Restaino S, De Ponti E, Monterossi G, Giuliani D, Ercoli A, Dell'Orto F, Dinoi G, Grassi T, Scambia G, Fanfani F. The impact on survival of two different staging strategies in apparent early stage endometrial cancer comparing sentinel lymph nodes mapping algorithm and selective lymphadenectomy: an Italian retrospective analysis of two reference centers. Gynecol Oncol. 2017;147:528–34.

48. Tax C, Rovers MM, de Graaf C, Zusterzeel PLM, Bekkers RLM. The sentinel node procedure in early stage cervical cancer, taking the next step; a diagnostic review. Gynecol Oncol. 2015;139:559–67.

49. Salvo G, Ramirez PT, Levenback CF, Munsell MF, Euscher ED, Soliman PT, Frumovitz M. Sensitivity and negative predictive value for sentinel lymph node biopsy in women with early-stage cervical cancer. Gynecol Oncol. 2017;145:96–101.

50. Bats AS, Mathevet P, Buenerd A, Orliaguet I, Mery E, Zerdoud S, Le Frère-Belda MA, Froissart M, Querleu D, Martinez A, Leblanc E, Morice P, Daraï E, Marret H, Gillaizeau F, Lécuru F. The sentinel node technique detects unexpected drainage pathways and allows nodal ultrastaging in early cervical cancer: insights from the multicenter prospective SENTICOL study. Ann Surg Oncol. 2013;20:413–22.

51. De Cicco C, Sideri M, Bartolomei M, Grana C, Cremonesi M, Fiorenza M, Maggioni A, Bocciolone L, Mangioni C, Colombo N, Paganelli G. Sentinel node biopsy in early vulvar cancer. Br J Cancer 2000;82:295–9.

52. Levenback CF, Ali S, Coleman RL, Gold MA, Fowler JM, Judson PL, Bell MC, De Geest K, Spirtos NM, Potkul RK, Leitao MM Jr, Bakkum-Gamez JN, Rossi EC, Lentz SS, Burke JJ 2nd, Van Le L, Trimble CL. Lymphatic mapping and sentinel lymph node biopsy in women with squamous cell carcinoma of the vulva: a gynecologic oncology group study. J Clin Oncol. 2012;30:3786–91.

53. Covens A, Vella ET, Kennedy EB, Reade CJ, Jimenez W, Le T. Sentinel lymph node biopsy in vulvar cancer: systematic review, meta-analysis and guideline recommendations. Gynecol Oncol. 2015;137:351–61.

54. Van der Zee AG, Oonk MH, De Hullu JA, Ansink AC, Vergote I, Verheijen RH, Maggioni A, Gaarenstroom KN, Baldwin PJ, Van Dorst EB, Van der Velden J, Hermans RH, van der Putten H, Drouin P, Schneider A, Sluiter WJ. Sentinel node dissection is safe in the treatment of early-stage vulvar cancer. J Clin Oncol. 2008;26:884–9.

55. Papadia A, Gasparri ML, Mueller MD. Are allergic reactions to indocyanine green really that uncommon? A single institution experience. Obstet Gynecol Rep. 2017;1:1–2.

56. Papadia A, Imboden S, Gasparri ML, et al. Endometrial and cervical cancer patients with multiple sentinel lymph nodes at laparoscopic ICG mapping: How many are enough? J Cancer Res Clin Oncol. 2016;142:1831–6.

57. McCulloch P, Altman DG, Campbell WB, Flum DR, Glasziou P, Marshall JC, Nicholl J, Balliol Collaboration, Aronson JK, Barkun JS, Blazeby JM, Boutron IC, Campbell WB, Clavien PA, Cook JA, Ergina PL, Feldman LS, Flum DR, Maddern GJ, Nicholl J, Reeves BC, Seiler CM, Strasberg SM, Meakins JL, Ashby D, Black N, Bunker J, Burton M, Campbell M, Chalkidou K, Chalmers I, de Leval M, Deeks J, Ergina PL, Grant A, Gray M, Greenhalgh R, Jenicek M, Kehoe S, Lilford R, Littlejohns P, Loke Y, Madhock R, McPherson K, Meakins J, Rothwell P, Summerskill B, Taggart D, Tekkis P, Thompson M, Treasure T, Trohler U, Vandenbroucke J. No surgical innovation without evaluation: the IDEAL recommendations. Lancet. 2009;374:1105–12.

Fluorescent Lymphangiography: Sentinel Node Navigation Surgery in Melanoma

Rene Aleman, Fernando Dip, Emanuele Lo Menzo, and Raul J. Rosenthal

Introduction

Melanoma is the most serious and most common form of skin cancer in the United States. According to the Centers for Disease Control and Prevention (CDC), melanoma is the sixth most prevalent form of cancer in men and women, with an incremental age-related incidence [1]. The 5-year survival rates for patients diagnosed with melanoma is dependent on the stage of the disease at the time of diagnosis. Ever since Morton et al.'s description of the sentinel lymph node (SLN) concept in cutaneous malignant melanoma, preoperative lymphatic mapping and lymphadenectomy of SLN biopsy has been widely developed and proven to be a minimally invasive approach that conveys relevant information for outstanding outcomes [2]. Recently, indocyanine green (ICG) fluorescence-guided surgery (FGS) has been developed to detect SLN and it has been successfully applied to the treatment of various types of skin cancers, with reports of accurate SLN detection in both cutaneous melanomas as well as non-melanoma skin cancers [3–5]. Herein, we present current applications, essential techniques, and novel intraoperative tools.

Melanoma

Overview of Surgical Approach

Due to the physiological behavior of melanoma, early diagnosis plays a significant role in patients' overall course of the disease. There are five stages: stage 0 is in situ (intraepithelial)

Electronic Supplementary Material The online version of this chapter (https://doi.org/10.1007/978-3-030-38092-2_32) contains supplementary material, which is available to authorized users.

R. Aleman
Bariatric and Metabolic Institute, Cleveland Clinic Florida, Weston, FL, USA

F. Dip
Hospital de Clinicas Jose de San Martin, Buenos Aires, Argentina

E. Lo Menzo · R. J. Rosenthal (✉)
Department of General Surgery, The Bariatric and Metabolic Institute, Cleveland Clinic Florida, Weston, FL, USA
e-mail: ROSENTR@CCF.ORG

melanoma; stages I and II are considered localized invasive cutaneous; stage III is regional nodal disease; and stage IV implies distant metastatic disease. Commonly, stage I melanoma is associated to prolonged survival rates and likely cure following treatment, whereas the more advanced stages have a tendency to develop metastatic disease [6, 7]. In terms of prognosis, tumor thickness is the determinant factor, followed by histologic ulceration and mitotic rate, in accordance with the American Joint Committee on Cancer (AJCC) [8]. Considering that survival rates rapidly decline as tumor thickness increases, early detection of melanoma is hence imperative in leading the improvement of patient outcome and survival.

Adequate surgical management is critical for the diagnosis, staging, and optimal therapeutic treatment of melanoma. Thus, surgery surrounding the management of melanoma should aim for four main endpoints:

1. Histology: Pathologic confirmation of the diagnosis with appropriate planned biopsy
2. Staging: Achievement of complete and accurate microstaging of the primary tumor to guide therapy
3. Oncologic surgery: Proper excision of margins around primary site to minimize risks of local recurrence, allowing additional potential surgical interventions
4. Quality of life: Optimal functional outcome and cosmetics

Prior to any surgery, biopsy is required for the initial diagnosis of melanoma. Following staging and surgical planning—if deemed necessary or adequate—proper surgical resection can be achieved for the initial management of melanomas in order to maximize the chances of long-term survival. Conversely, the decision of SLN biopsy (SLNB) will be based upon the risk of recurrence:

- For patients with clinically negative regional lymph nodes (LN) and a low risk of recurrence primary melanoma (stage IA without ulceration), lymphatic omission is viable.

- For patients with clinically negative nodes and a primary melanoma with intermediate or high risk of LN metastasis, mapping and SLNB is recommended [9, 10].
- SLNB is standard of care for staging regional LN in stage IB-IIC melanoma [8].

The dual localization with the aid of radiolabeled colloids and blue dyes provides optimal accuracy for identification. However, the patient is exposed to cumulative radiation. Current available probes, like ICG, can be used as a visual enhancer for fluorescence-guided surgery via near infrared imaging to detect SLN in melanoma. Sentinel node navigational surgery (SNNS) involves both preoperative and intraoperative detection of SLN. Therefore, the availability of fluorescence guidance can potentially lead to earlier risk-free detection of SLN, and increase success rates after treatment.

Near Infrared (NIR) Imaging

To better understand the applicability and limits of NIR imaging for fluorescence in melanoma SNNS, it is important to recognize the mechanism of infrared-navigated SNNS using ICG. Indocyanine green is a dye with great tropism for plasma protein binding. Once bonded, ICG can emit fluorescence of maximum wavelength around 845 nm when excited by NIR light at a wavelength range of 750–810 nm. The fluorescence of ICG can be detected at least 10 mm beneath the skin surface by an infrared camera unit. The aforementioned mechanisms and functional characteristics are the most important factors when considering melanoma SNNS.

Administration of ICG

Although SLNB is a widely accepted diagnostic staging procedure in melanoma patients, there are still controversies in regard to the technical aspects of the procedure, especially on the time of administration, delivery method, dosage, and replicability of SNNS [11]. SLNB using ICG was recently introduced to clinical practice, and various studies have reported successful fluorescence-guided surgery for noninvasive detection of fluorescent SLN with high accuracy and sensitivity [4, 12–15]. However, there are no guidelines that have standardized the optimum fluorescence contrast ratio with a definitive time of administration, delivery method, and dosage. Table 32.1 summarizes current case reports and prospective and retrospective studies regarding the reported techniques [13, 16–40].

As per usual standard of other fluorescence-guided procedures, 25 mg of ICG vials are diluted into 5 mL of sterile distilled water prior to administration. As presented in Table 32.1, the current clinical practice for SNNS is to administer ICG through an intradermal injection in patients with melanoma. It is well known that fluorescence of ICG can be detected at least 10 mm beneath the skin surface by an infrared camera unit; hence, intradermal administration should be directed anatomically toward the

Table 32.1 Studies on fluorescence-guided melanoma SNNS: Applied methods

Study	Dose	Cases (#)	Preop. LSN	Concomitant tracer/dye	Time of administration	Type of administration
Lo et al.	N/A	62	Yes	Yes: Tc^{99} radiolabeled nanocolloid and patent blue dye	Intraoperatively	Intradermal
Knackstedt et al.	0.2–0.3 mL	61	Yes	No	Intraoperatively	Intradermal
Vahabzadeh-Hagh et al.	0.25 mL	14	Yes	No	Intraoperatively	Intradermal
McGregor et al.	N/A	14	No	No	Intraoperatively	Around tumor bed
KleinJan et al.	N/A	8	Yes	Yes: Tc^{99} radiolabeled nanocolloid	Intraoperatively	Intradermal
Goppner et al.	0.25–2.5 mg	10	Yes	Yes: Blue dye	Preoperatively and escalating scheme	Intradermal
Stoffels et al.	0.25 mg	40	Yes	Yes: Tc^{99} radiolabeled nanocolloid	Preoperatively	Intradermal
Stoffels et al.	N/A	80	Yes	Yes: Tc^{99} radiolabeled nanocolloid	Preoperatively	Intradermal
van den Berg et al.	N/A	104	Yes	Yes: Tc^{99} radiolabeled nanocolloid	Preoperatively (24 h prior or on the morning of operation)	Intradermal
Cloyd et al.	2 mL (2.5 mg/mL)	52	Yes	Yes: Blue dye	After induction of anesthesia	Intradermal
Korn et al.	0.5–1.5 mL	90	Yes	No	Intraoperatively	Intradermal
Jain et al.	0.9 mL (2.25 mg)	15	Yes	Yes: Blue dye	Intraoperatively	Intradermal
Murawa et al.	2.5 mg	10	N/A	Yes: Human serum albumin	Intraoperatively	Intradermal
Gilmore et al.	1 mL	25	Yes	Yes: Human serum albumin	After intubation	Intradermal
Namikawa et al.	0.4–1.0 mL (2–5 mg)	86	Yes	Yes: Blue dye	Preoperatively	Intradermal
van der Vorst et al.	1.6 mL	15	Yes	Yes: Human serum albumin	Intraoperatively	Intradermal
Brouwer et al.	0.25 mg	25	Yes	Yes: Tc^{99} radiolabeled nanocolloid	Preoperatively	Intradermal
Fujisawa et al.	0.5%	34	Yes	Yes: Blue dye	After intubation	Intradermal

(continued)

Table 32.1 (continued)

Study	Dose	Cases (#)	Preop. LSN	Concomitant tracer/dye	Time of administration	Type of administration
Brouwer et al.	0.25 mg	11	Yes	Yes: Tc⁹⁹ radiolabeled nanocolloid	5 h preoperatively	Intradermal
Stoffels et al.	1 mL (0.2 mg)	22	Yes	No	Intraoperatively	Intradermal
Uhara et al.	0.5%	562	Yes	Yes: Tc⁹⁹ radiolabeled nanocolloid and blue dye	Intraoperatively	Intradermal
Polom et al.	2–2.4 mL	10	Yes	Yes: Human serum albumin	Preoperatively prior to incision	Intradermal
Fujisawa et al.	0.5%	16	Yes	Yes: Blue dye	After induction of anesthesia	Intradermal
Hayashi et al.	0.4 mL (2 mg)	1	Yes	No	Intraoperatively	Intradermal
Fujiwara et al.	0.1 mL (0.5 mg)	7	Yes	No	Intraoperatively	Intradermal

LSN lymphoscintigraphy, *N/A* information not available in original article, *Tc* technetium, *mL* milliliters, *mg* milligrams

location of relevant lymphatics (Video 32.1). The points of interest for tracing administration in melanoma are in contiguity of the tumor or the scar following excisional diagnostic biopsy, roughly 1 mm from the tumoral borders of potential excision. Table 32.2 summarizes the suggested sites for injection of ICG.

The time of administration will depend on the surgeon's preference and protocols followed during SLN harvesting in patients with melanoma. Most of the reported literature on SNNS in melanoma suggest an intraoperative and intradermal administration of ICG. Similarly, applied doses range from 0.2 to 12 mg, implying numerous variables that may bias visual feedback from the emitted fluorescence [13, 16–40]. Based on the lack of standardization and definitive evidence of ICG-mediated SNNS in melanoma, the standard of care remains to concomitantly inject radiocolloids and/or dyes to confirm and optimize of localization of SLN. Different type of dyes and probes—technetium-99, 0.4% indigo carmine, 2% isosulfan blue—can be administered prior to ICG injection to provide an evident mapping of the evaluated lymphatic tracts [5]. Overall, the time of administration, delivery method, and dosage require further evaluation in order to achieve consensus and standardization regarding the most suitable technique during SNNS in melanoma.

Table 32.2 Administration of ICG according to type and size of lesion

Type of lesion	Diameter extent (cm)	Site of injection
Flattened small	≤5	Around lesion
Large plaques	≥5	In the proximity of the most elevated or eroded lesions

Fluorescent Lymphatic Visualization

A recent systematic review and meta-analyses of SLN identification in breast cancer and melanoma reported an average time for detection of fluorescent SLN between 5 and 15 mins following peritumoral injection with ICG [41]. Hence, following ICG administration, fluorescence of the lymphatic channels to the SLNs is nearly immediately visible from the skin surface with the use of an infrared camera system. The availability of handheld devices, such as VITOM® (KARL STORZ (KARL STORZ SE & Co. KG—Tuttlingen, Germany) and IC-Flow™ Imaging System (Diagnostic Green Munich, Germany), allows for the visualization of fluorescent images in real-time, without the need of turning the operating room lights off, allowing an uninterrupted surgical approach [42, 43]. Other infrared camera systems like the Photodynamic

Table 32.3 Dermal fluorescence interpretation

Dermal finding	Cause	Feedback
Diffuse fluorescence and pooling of tracer, known as *dermal backflow*	Lymphatic obstruction	Probable regional node metastasis
Opaque fluorescence	Deeper location of the SLN covered by thicker adiposity	Overlying skin and subcutaneous tissue should be pressed to reduce distance from skin surface-to-SLN
Linear tracing	Lymphatic tract	Tracts often rather than not, lead to location of relevant SLN

SLN sentinel lymph node

Eye (pde-neo, Hamamatsu Photonics, Hamamatsu, Japan) or the Hamamatsu Photonics (Hamamatsu Photonics K.K, Shizuoka, Japan) require the operating room lamps to be switched off for the ICG-INR guided observation. The time required for detecting SLN fluorescence is within 5 min for inguinal nodes. Conversely, nodes located in the trunk, head, neck, and upper limbs require approximately 10 more minutes [41]. An extensive anatomical understanding of the lymphatic tracts and SNL of interest is helpful when interpreting dermal fluorescence. To further elaborate on this, Table 32.3 summarizes suggestable interpretations of the superficial imagery conveyed by fluorescence through infrared image filtering.

Surgical Resection

Fluorescence Implications

Historically, surgery has represented the optimal treatment for patients with cutaneous melanoma. Various solid tumors require neoadjuvant therapy as a multidisciplinary approach, either prior to surgical resection or without definitive suggestibility for surgery [44]. Contemporary effective therapies have expanded the potential of therapeutic approaches for patients with unresectable and regionally advanced melanoma. The development of said techniques has increased positive outcomes and prognosis for patients who have melanoma with locally advanced or metastatic disease [41].

Many studies have reported noninvasive detection of SLN with high accuracy and sensitivity [4, 12–15]. This principle is supported by ICG's physical properties. After subcutaneous administration, ICG flows through the lymphae and accumulates in the SLN within minutes, which allows for the detection of fluorescence through NIR imaging. So far, there are no reported adverse reactions in any of the conducted studies regarding SNNS [41]. Moreover, ICG-enhanced fluorescence-guided surgery enables high, real-time imagery feedback, is relatively cheap, lacks radiation exposure, and offers high sensitivity and specificity rates [45].

Limitations

Despite the many benefits of this technique, ICG-guided SNNS presents several limitations.

Fluorescence emission is limited to a 10 mm depth perception, mainly due to absorption and scattering of photons when propagating through tissue [46]. Albeit, a meta-analysis conducted for SLN identification demonstrated that the number of identified SLN per patient using ICG was considerably higher compared to solely blue dye, solely radiocolloid, or a combination of the two [41]. A potential issue with this technique is that non-sentinel LN can be mistaken for SLN, leading to overtreatment and associated comorbidity. The drawback associated with "over diagnosis" can be virtually eliminated with the concomitant administration of human serum albumin, so as to reduce ICG diffusion speed and increase sensitivity and specificity [47].

Also, the lack of reliable quantifiable data on the intensity of the fluorescent emission limits the interpretation of the images.

Local allergic reactions to ICG, although rare, have been reported.

Identification

Overall, the identification of SLN through standard methods like blue dye has been estimated to be around 8% [48]. Radiolabeled colloid tracers have played a significant role as well in the identification of SLN through lymphoscintigraphy; nevertheless, this method is expensive, exposes the patient to radioactivity, and has limited availability. More so, both methods require an unequivocal learning curve that implies high costs, and the dual approach of said techniques does not further increase the SLN identification rate [49, 50]. Additionally, the use of blue dye as a guidance probe in SNNS may lead to increasing tissue damage when tracing lymphatics toward the SLN of interest, and the allergic reactions have been reported in 0.14–3% of patients [51, 52].

ICG-mediated fluorescence for melanoma SNNS has influenced SLN identification rates. In melanoma, the volume of injection (in milliliters) was associated with an improved SLN identification rate for ICG. No significant association has yet been found between identification rate and age, tumor size, number of SLN removed, injection site, timing of injection, or the type and concentration of ICG [41]. Although these findings suggest that identification rates and SNNS should focus solely on the technique rather than methodology, the photodynamics associated with ICG-mediated fluorescence are yet to be extensively investigated to draw conclusive statements. Furthermore, ICG-mediated fluorescence has proven to be safe, effective, and feasible, and remains to be an exploitable technique for accurate SLN identification.

Pitfalls

As previously mentioned, the major limitation of this technique is the limited penetration of the fluorescence emission (10 mm depth). In fact, beyond this depth the absorption and scattering of photons may lead to inaccurate identification. Also the presence of local inflammation or scarring might alter the identification of fluorescent light. Additionally an over sensitivity of this technique might identify a superior number of LN, including the non-sentinel ones, leading to unnecessary more extensive procedures. As mentioned, this "over diagnosis" can be virtually eliminated with the concomitant administration of human serum albumin, so as to reduce ICG diffusion speed and increase sensitivity and specificity.

Conclusions

There is a long-withstanding controversy on the role of applicability of fluorescence-guided surgery in SLN resection. ICG-mediated fluorescence is a novel technique that continues to thrive in providing real-time and noninvasive clear image feedback to the surgeon. Its applicability in melanoma SNNS has been widely accepted and continues to be explored. The use of this dye seems a promising technique for oncologic surgery due to safety and feasibility. The identification rate via this method resulted in outstanding outcomes in correlation to current clinical practice and gold standard methods. As with every other interventional approach, this technique carries certain limitations. The lack of dosage, timing, administration method, and location of administration is yet to be standardized. The lack of objective and quantifiable data limits the interpretation of the images. Nonetheless, with the development of novel probes like ICG-human serum albumin hybrid and the development of infrared filtering imaging devices, ICG promises to surpass expectations.

References

1. USCS Data visualizations. Available at: https://gis.cdc.gov/grasp/USCS/DataViz.html. Accessed: 12 Mar 2019.
2. Morton DL. Technical details of intraoperative lymphatic mapping for early stage melanoma. Arch Surg. 1992;127:392.
3. Messina JL, et al. Selective lymphadenectomy in patients with Merkel cell (cutaneous neuroendocrine) carcinoma. Ann Surg Oncol. 1997;4:389–95.
4. Kitai T, Inomoto T, Miwa M, Shikayama T. Fluorescence navigation with indocyanine green

for detecting sentinel lymph nodes in breast cancer. Breast Cancer. 2005;12:211–5.

5. Kusano M, Kokudo N, Toi M, Kaibori M. ICG fluorescence imaging and navigation surgery. Berlin: Springer; 2016.

6. Balch CM, et al. Prognostic factors analysis of 17,600 melanoma patients: validation of the American Joint Committee on Cancer melanoma staging system. J Clin Oncol. 2001;19:3622–34.

7. Geller AC, et al. Melanoma incidence and mortality among US whites, 1969–1999. JAMA. 2002;288:1719–20.

8. Gershenwald JE, et al. Melanoma staging: Evidence-based changes in the American Joint Committee on Cancer eighth edition cancer staging manual. CA Cancer J Clin. 2017;67:472–92.

9. Morton DL, et al. Final trial report of sentinel-node biopsy versus nodal observation in melanoma. N Engl J Med. 2014;370:599–609.

10. Coit D. Sentinel lymph node biopsy for melanoma: a plea to let the data speak. Ann Surg Oncol. 2014;21:3359–61.

11. Gershenwald JE, et al. Multi-institutional melanoma lymphatic mapping experience: the prognostic value of sentinel lymph node status in 612 stage I or II melanoma patients. J Clin Oncol. 1999;17:976.

12. Troyan SL, et al. The flare™ intraoperative near-infrared fluorescence imaging system: a first-in-human clinical trial in breast cancer sentinel lymph node mapping. Ann Surg Oncol. 2009;16:2943–52.

13. Fujiwara M, Mizukami T, Suzuki A, Fukamizu H. Sentinel lymph node detection in skin cancer patients using real-time fluorescence navigation with indocyanine green: preliminary experience. J Plast Reconstr Aesthet Surg. 2009;62:e373–8.

14. Themelis G, Yoo JS, Ntziachristos V. Multispectral imaging using multiple-bandpass filters. Opt Lett. 2008;33:1023.

15. Keereweer S, et al. Optical image-guided surgery—where do we stand? Mol Imaging Biol. 2011;13:199–207.

16. Lo MCI, et al. A feasibility study of indocyanine green fluorescence mapping for sentinel lymph node detection in cutaneous melanoma. J Plast Reconstr Aesthet Surg. 2019;72:137–71.

17. Knackstedt RW, Couto RA, Gastman B. Indocyanine green fluorescence imaging with lymphoscintigraphy for sentinel node biopsy in head and neck melanoma. J Surg Res. 2018;228:77–83.

18. Vahabzadeh-Hagh AM, Blackwell KE, Abemayor E, St John MA. Sentinel lymph node biopsy in cutaneous melanoma of the head and neck using the indocyanine green SPY Elite system. Am J Otolaryngol. 2018;39:485–8.

19. McGregor A, Pavri SN, Tsay C, Kim S, Narayan D. Use of indocyanine green for sentinel lymph node biopsy: case series and methods comparison. Plast Reconstr Surg Glob Open. 2017;5:e1566.

20. KleinJan GH, et al. Introducing navigation during melanoma-related sentinel lymph node procedures in the head-and-neck region. EJNMMI Res. 2017;7:65.

21. Göppner D, et al. Indocyanine green-assisted sentinel lymph node biopsy in melanoma using the 'FOVIS' system. J Dtsch Dermatol Ges. 2017;15:169–78.

22. Mondal SB, et al. Binocular Goggle Augmented Imaging and Navigation System provides real-time fluorescence image guidance for tumor resection and sentinel lymph node mapping. Sci Rep. 2015;5:12117.

23. Stoffels I, Leyh J, Pöppel T, Schadendorf D, Klode J. Evaluation of a radioactive and fluorescent hybrid tracer for sentinel lymph node biopsy in head and neck malignancies: prospective randomized clinical trial to compare ICG-(99m)Tc-nanocolloid hybrid tracer versus (99m)Tc-nanocolloid. Eur J Nucl Med Mol Imaging. 2015;42:1631–8.

24. Stoffels I, Dissemond J, Pöppel T, Schadendorf D, Klode J. Intraoperative fluorescence imaging for sentinel lymph node detection: prospective clinical trial to compare the usefulness of Indocyanine green vs technetium Tc 99m for identification of sentinel lymph nodes. JAMA Surg. 2015;150:617–23.

25. van den Berg NS, et al. Multimodal surgical guidance during sentinel node biopsy for melanoma: combined gamma tracing and fluorescence imaging of the sentinel node through use of the hybrid tracer indocyanine green-(99m)Tc-nanocolloid. Radiology. 2015;275:521–9.

26. Cloyd JM, Wapnir IL, Read BM, Swetter S, Greco RS. Indocyanine green and fluorescence lymphangiography for sentinel lymph node identification in cutaneous melanoma. J Surg Oncol. 2014;110:888–92.

27. Korn JM, Tellez-Diaz A, Bartz-Kurycki M, Gastman B. Indocyanine green SPY elite-assisted sentinel lymph node biopsy in cutaneous melanoma. Plast Reconstr Surg. 2014;133:914–22.

28. Jain V, Phillips BT, Conkling N, Pameijer C. Sentinel lymph node detection using laser-assisted indocyanine green dye lymphangiography in patients with melanoma. Int J Surg Oncol. 2013;2013:904214.

29. Murawa D, Polom K, Murawa P. One-year postoperative morbidity associated with near-infrared-guided indocyanine green (ICG) or ICG in conjugation with human serum albumin (ICG:HSA) sentinel lymph node biopsy. Surg Innov. 2014;21:240–3.

30. Gilmore DM, et al. Effective low-dose escalation of indocyanine green for near-infrared fluorescent sentinel lymph node mapping in melanoma. Ann Surg Oncol. 2013;20:2357–63.

31. Namikawa K, Tsutsumida A, Tanaka R, Kato J, Yamazaki N. Limitation of indocyanine green fluorescence in identifying sentinel lymph node prior to skin incision in cutaneous melanoma. Int J Clin Oncol. 2014;19:198–203.

32. van der Vorst JR, et al. Dose optimization for near-infrared fluorescence sentinel lymph node mapping in patients with melanoma. Br J Dermatol. 2013;168:93–8.

33. Brouwer OR, et al. Comparing the hybrid fluorescent-radioactive tracer indocyanine green-99mTc-nanocolloid with 99mTc-nanocolloid for sentinel node identification: a validation study using lymphoscintigraphy and SPECT/CT. J Nucl Med. 2012;53:1034–40.

34. Fujisawa Y, Nakamura Y, Kawachi Y, Otsuka F. Indocyanine green fluorescence-navigated sentinel node biopsy showed higher sensitivity than the radioisotope or blue dye method, which may help to reduce false-negative cases in skin cancer. J Surg Oncol. 2012;106:41–5.

35. Brouwer OR, et al. Feasibility of sentinel node biopsy in head and neck melanoma using a hybrid radioactive and fluorescent tracer. Ann Surg Oncol. 2012;19:1988–94.

36. Stoffels I, et al. Indocyanine green fluorescence-guided sentinel lymph node biopsy in dermato-oncology. J Dtsch Dermatol Ges. 2012;10:51–7.

37. Uhara H, et al. Applicability of radiocolloids, blue dyes and fluorescent indocyanine green to sentinel node biopsy in melanoma. J Dermatol. 2012;39:336–8.

38. Polom K, Murawa D, Rho YS, Spychala A, Murawa P. Skin melanoma sentinel lymph node biopsy using real-time fluorescence navigation with indocyanine green and indocyanine green with human serum albumin. Br J Dermatol. 2012;166:682–3.

39. Fujisawa Y, Nakamura Y, Kawachi Y, Otsuka F. A custom-made, low-cost intraoperative fluorescence navigation system with indocyanine green for sentinel lymph node biopsy in skin cancer. Dermatology. 2011;222:261–8.

40. Hayashi T, et al. Sentinel lymph node biopsy using real-time fluorescence navigation with indocyanine green in cutaneous head and neck/lip mucosa melanomas. Head Neck. 2012;34:758–61.

41. Niebling MG, et al. A systematic review and meta-analyses of sentinel lymph node identification in breast cancer and melanoma, a plea for tracer mapping. Eur J Surg Oncol. 2016;42:466–73.

42. Papathemelis T, et al. Sentinel lymph node biopsy in breast cancer patients by means of indocyanine green using the Karl Storz VITOM® fluorescence camera. Biomed Res Int. 2018;2018:1–8.

43. lidplussdesign. IC-flow™ imaging system—diagnostic green Germany. Diagnostic Green Germany. Available at: http://de.diagnosticgreen.com/ic-flow-imaging-system/. Accessed: 14 Mar 2019.

44. Sondak VK, Khushalani NI. Adjuvant and neoadjuvant therapy in high-risk stage III cutaneous melanoma. Int J Radiat Oncol Biol Phys. 2017;98:16–7.

45. Pleijhuis RG, et al. Obtaining adequate surgical margins in breast-conserving therapy for patients with early-stage breast cancer: current modalities and future directions. Ann Surg Oncol. 2009;16:2717–30.

46. Ntziachristos V. Fluorescence molecular imaging. Annu Rev Biomed Eng. 2006;8:1–33.

47. Murawa D, Hirche C, Dresel S, Hünerbein M. Sentinel lymph node biopsy in breast cancer guided by indocyanine green fluorescence. Br J Surg. 2009;96:1289–94.

48. Kang T, et al. Does blue dye contribute to success of sentinel node mapping for breast cancer? Ann Surg Oncol. 2010;17:280–5.

49. Bagaria SP, Faries MB, Morton DL. Sentinel node biopsy in melanoma: technical considerations of the procedure as performed at the John Wayne Cancer Institute. J Surg Oncol. 2010;101:669–76.

50. Derossis AM, et al. A trend analysis of the relative value of blue dye and isotope localization in 2,000 consecutive cases of sentinel node biopsy for breast cancer 1 1No competing interests declared. J Am Coll Surg. 2001;193:473–8.

51. King TA, et al. A prospective analysis of the effect of blue-dye volume on sentinel lymph node mapping success and incidence of allergic reaction in patients with breast cancer. Ann Surg Oncol. 2004;11:535–41.

52. Rughani MG, et al. Sentinel lymph node biopsy in melanoma: The Oxford ten year clinical experience. J Plast Reconstr Aesthet Surg. 2011;64:1284–90.

Index

© Springer Nature Switzerland AG 2020

E. M. Aleassa, K. M. El-Hayek (eds.), *Video Atlas of Intraoperative Applications of Near Infrared Fluorescence Imaging*, https://doi.org/10.1007/978-3-030-38092-2

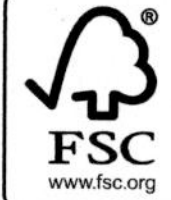